Systemic Lupus Erythematosus

Guest Editor

ELLEN M. GINZLER, MD, MPH

RHEUMATIC DISEASE CLINICS OF NORTH AMERICA

www.rheumatic.theclinics.com

February 2010 • Volume 36 • Number 1

SAUNDERS an imprint of ELSEVIER, Inc.

W.B. SAUNDERS COMPANY

A Division of Elsevier Inc.

1600 John F. Kennedy Blvd., Suite 1800 • Philadelphia, PA 19103-2899

http://www.theclinics.com

RHEUMATIC DISEASE CLINICS OF NORTH AMERICA Volume 36, Number 1

February 2010 ISSN 0889-857X, ISBN 13: 978-1-4377-1869-0

Editor: Rachel Glover
Developmental Editor: Theresa Collier

Rheumatic Disease Clinics of North America (ISSN 0889-857X) is published quarterly by Elsevier Inc., 360 Park Avenue South, New York, NY 10010-1710. Months of issue are February, May, August, and November. Business and editorial offices: 1600 John F. Kennedy Boulevard, Suite 1800, Philadelphia, PA 19103-2899. Periodicals postage paid at New York, NY and additional mailing offices. Subscription prices are USD 264.00 per year for US individuals, USD 455.00 per year for US institutions, USD 132.00 per year for US students and residents, USD 311.00 per year for Canadian individuals, USD 563.00 per year for Canadian institutions, USD 369.00 per year for international individuals, USD 563.00 per year for international institutions, and USD 185.00 per year for Canadian and foreign students/residents. To receive student/resident rate, orders must be accompanied by name of affiliated institution, date of term, and the *signature* of program/residency coordinator on institution letterhead. Orders will be billed at individual rate until proof of status received. Foreign air speed delivery is included in all *Clinics* subscription prices. All prices are subject to change without notice. **POSTMASTER:** Send address changes to *Rheumatic Disease Clinics of North America*, Elsevier Health Sciences Division, Subscription Customer Service, 3251 Riverport Lane, Maryland Heights, MO 63043. **Customer Service: 1-800-654-2452 (US and Canada). From outside of the US and Canada: 314-447-8871. Fax: 314-447-8029. For print support, e-mail: JournalsCustomerService-usa@elsevier.com. For online support, e-mail: JournalsOnline Support-usa@elsevier.com.**

Reprints. For copies of 100 or more of articles in this publication, please contact the Commercial Reprints Department, Elsevier Inc., 360 Park Avenue South, New York, New York, 10010-1710; Tel.: (+1) 212-633-3813, Fax: (+1) 212-462-1935, and E-mail: reprints@elsevier.com.

Rheumatic Disease Clinics of North America is covered in *MEDLINE/PubMed (Index Medicus), Current Contents/Clinical Medicine, Science Citation Index, ISI/BIOMED,* and *EMBASE/Excerpta Medica.*

Printed and bound by CPI Group (UK) Ltd, Croydon, CR0 4YY

Transferred to Digital Print 2011

Contributors

GUEST EDITOR

ELLEN M. GINZLER, MD, MPH
Distinguished Teaching Professor of Medicine; Chief, Division of Rheumatology, State
University of New York Downstate Medical Center, Brooklyn, New York

AUTHORS

JOSEPH M. AHEARN, MD
Lupus Center of Excellence, University of Pittsburgh School of Health Sciences,
Department of Medicine, University of Pittsburgh School of Medicine, Pittsburgh,
Pennsylvania

SADIA AHMED, MD
Fellow in Rheumatology, Division of Allergy, Immunology, and Rheumatology, Department
of Medicine, University of Rochester Medical Center, Rochester, New York

JENNIFER H. ANOLIK, MD, PhD
Associate Professor of Medicine, Division of Allergy, Immunology, and Rheumatology,
Department of Medicine, University of Rochester Medical Center, Rochester, New York

CYNTHIA ARANOW, MD
Associate Investigator, Feinstein Institute for Medical Research, Manhasset, New York

IAN N. BRUCE, MD, FRCP
Professor of Rheumatology, ARC Epidemiology Unit, Manchester Academic Health
Sciences Centre, The University of Manchester and The Kellgren Centre for
Rheumatology, Manchester Royal Infirmary, Manchester, United Kingdom

HERMINE I. BRUNNER, MD
Associate Professor, Division of Rheumatology, Department of Pediatrics, Cincinnati
Children's Hospital Medical Center, Cincinnati, Ohio

ROBERT CLANCY, PhD
Associate Professor of Medicine, NYU Langone School of Medicine; Tisch Hospital,
New York, New York

MARY K. CROW, MD
Benjamin M. Rosen Chair in Immunology and Inflammation Research, Mary Kirkland
Center for Lupus Research, Rheumatology Division, Hospital for Special Surgery;
Professor of Medicine, Weill Cornell Medical College, New York, New York

BETTY DIAMOND, MD
Investigator, Feinstein Institute for Medical Research, Manhasset, New York

MARY ANNE DOOLEY, MD, MPH
Associate Professor of Medicine, Department of Medicine, Division of Rheumatology and Immunology, University of North Carolina at Chapel Hill, Chapel Hill, North Carolina

ELLEN M. GINZLER, MD, MPH
Distinguished Teaching Professor of Medicine; Chief, Division of Rheumatology, State University of New York Downstate Medical Center, Brooklyn, New York

AMY H. KAO, MD, MPH
Lupus Center of Excellence, University of Pittsburgh School of Health Sciences, Department of Medicine, University of Pittsburgh School of Medicine, Pittsburgh, Pennsylvania

RACHEL S. KLEIN, BA
Philadelphia VA Medical Center, Department of Dermatology, University of Pennsylvania School of Medicine, Philadelphia, Pennsylvania

ANEESA NIRAVEL KRISHNAMURTHY, DO
Division of Rheumatology, State University of New York Downstate Medical Center, Brooklyn, New York

CHAU-CHING LIU, MD, PhD
Lupus Center of Excellence, University of Pittsburgh School of Health Sciences, Department of Medicine, University of Pittsburgh School of Medicine, Pittsburgh, Pennsylvania

MEGGAN MACKAY, MS, MD
Assistant Investigator, Feinstein Institute for Medical Research, Manhasset, New York

MICHAEL P. MADAIO, MD
Chairman of Medicine, Department of Medicine, Nephrology and Kidney Transplantation Section, Medical College of Georgia, Augusta, Georgia

ANUP MANOHARAN, MBBS
Department of Medicine, Nephrology and Kidney Transplantation Section, Medical College of Georgia, Augusta, Georgia

SUSAN MANZI, MD, MPH
Lupus Center of Excellence, University of Pittsburgh School of Health Sciences, Department of Medicine, University of Pittsburgh School of Medicine; Graduate School of Public Health, University of Pittsburgh, Pittsburgh, Pennsylvania

JENNIFER MERSEREAU, MD
Assistant Professor of Medicine, Department of Obstetrics and Gynecology, Division of Reproductive Endocrinology and Infertility, University of North Carolina at Chapel Hill, Chapel Hill, North Carolina

RINA MINA, MD
Fellow, Division of Rheumatology, Department of Pediatrics, Cincinnati Children's Hospital Medical Center, Cincinnati, Ohio

PAMELA A. MORGANROTH, MS
Philadelphia VA Medical Center, Department of Dermatology, University of Pennsylvania School of Medicine, Philadelphia, Pennsylvania

JEANNINE S. NAVRATIL, MS
Lupus Center of Excellence, University of Pittsburgh School of Health Sciences, Department of Medicine, University of Pittsburgh School of Medicine, Pittsburgh, Pennsylvania

BEN PARKER, MBChB, MRCP
Clinical Research Fellow, ARC Epidemiology Unit, Manchester Academic Health Sciences Centre, The University of Manchester, Manchester, United Kingdom

ARCHANA VASUDEVAN, MD
Clinical Assistant Professor, Division of Rheumatology, State University of New York Downstate Medical Center, Brooklyn, New York

VICTORIA P. WERTH, MD
Professor of Dermatology, Philadelphia VA Medical Center; Department of Dermatology, University of Pennsylvania School of Medicine; Perelman Center for Advanced Medicine, Philadelphia, Pennsylvania

JINOOS YAZDANY, MD, MPH
Department of Medicine, Division of Rheumatology, Rosalind Russell Medical Research Center for Arthritis, University of California, San Francisco, California

EDWARD YELIN, PhD
Department of Medicine, Division of Rheumatology, Rosalind Russell Medical Research Center for Arthritis, University of California, San Francisco, California

Contents

Changing Worldwide Epidemiology of Systemic Lupus Erythematosus

Archana Vasudevan and Aneesa Niravel Krishnamurthy

Developed countries have better systemic lupus erythematosus survival rates than developing countries, or countries with lower economic performance. This is in part because of a higher human development index, defined by standard of living (a marker for gross domestic product), literacy rates, and life expectancy, with contribution from ethnic variations within individual countries, and unique environmental factors.

Health-Related Quality of Life and Employment Among Persons with Systemic Lupus Erythematosus

Jinoos Yazdany and Edward Yelin

This article assesses the effect of systemic lupus erythematosus (SLE) on the shealth-related quality of life (HRQOL) and employment of persons with this condition. Far more than impaired health status can affect an individual's quality of life. The term "health-related quality of life" is used to connote the decrement in an individual's quality of life specifically attributable to a decrease in health status. The article presents evidence on employment because this plays a crucial role in determining the quality of life of most Americans of normal working age. However, evidence is also presented with respect to other domains of activity, because most people work to live but not many live to work.

Cutaneous Lupus and the Cutaneous Lupus Erythematosus Disease Area and Severity Index Instrument

Rachel S. Klein, Pamela A. Morganroth, and Victoria P. Werth

This article provides an overview of cutaneous lupus erythematosus, including classification schemes, disease subtypes, and therapy. It also describes the Cutaneous Lupus Erythematosus Disease Area and Severity Index, a novel clinical outcome instrument that quantifies cutaneous activity and damage in cutaneous lupus erythematosus.

Pediatric Lupus—Are There Differences in Presentation, Genetics, Response to Therapy, and Damage Accrual Compared with Adult Lupus?

Rina Mina and Hermine I. Brunner

Some complement deficiencies predispose to systemic lupus erythematosus (SLE) early in life. Currently, there are no known unique physiologic or genetic pathways that can explain the variability in disease phenotypes. Children present with more acute illness and have more frequent renal, hematologic, and central nervous system involvement compared to adults with SLE. Almost all children require corticosteroids during the course of their disease; many are treated with immunosuppressive drugs. Mortality rates remain higher with pediatric SLE. Children and adolescents accrue more damage, especially in the renal, ocular and musculoskeletal organ systems. Conversely, cardiovascular mortality is more prevalent in adults with SLE.

SLE. Thus, autoantibodies contribute to autoimmunity by multiple mechanisms including immune complex mediated type III hypersensitivity reactions, type II antibody-dependent cytotoxicity, and by instructing innate immune cells to produce pathogenic cytokines including interferon α, tumor necrosis factor, and interleukin 1. Recent data have highlighted the critical role of toll-like receptors as a link between the innate and adaptive immune system in SLE immunopathogenesis. Given the large body of evidence implicating abnormalities in the B-cell compartment in SLE, there has been a therapeutic focus on developing interventions that target the B-cell compartment. Several different approaches to targeting B cells have been used, including B-cell depletion with monoclonal antibodies against B-cell–specific molecules, induction of negative signaling in B cells, and blocking B-cell survival and activation factors. Overall, therapies targeting B cells are beginning to show promise in the treatment of SLE and continue to elucidate the diverse roles of B cells in this complex disease.

Biomarkers in Lupus Nephritis

Anup Manoharan and Michael P. Madaio

Biomarkers have the potential to be useful tools for noninvasively evaluating and managing patients with lupus nephritis. Many candidate biomarkers have been identified, but they require validation in larger cohorts. It is likely that combinations or biomarker profiles, rather than individual markers, will emerge to help better predict the severity of inflammation, the extent of fibrosis, degree of drug responsiveness, and other variables. This approach has the potential to reduce the use of the renal biopsy, improve therapeutic efficacy, and limit toxicity. We predict algorithms based on genotype and biomarkers combined with clinical presentation will emerge to help guide physicians in management. Assays that show the most potential include serum erythrocyte bound complement C4d, interleukin 17, interleukin 23, interferon score/chemokine score ratio, and anti-C1q antibodies. Such urinary biomarkers as fractional excretion of endothelial-1, monocyte chemoattractant protein–1, vascular cell adhesion molecule–1, and TWEAK (tumor necrosis factor–like weak inducer of apoptosis) may also be useful but require validations.

Endothelial Function and its Implications for Cardiovascular and Renal Disease in Systemic Lupus Erythematosus

Robert Clancy and Ellen M. Ginzler

Vascular manifestations associated with systemic lupus erythematosus (SLE) span a broad range, including vasculopathy. An understudied pathway of this morbidity is a repair component. Recent studies have elevated the anti-injury biomarkers, adiponectin and membrane endothelial protein C receptor (EPCR), for consideration with roles to antagonize premature atherosclerosis and SLE nephritis, respectively. For example, adiponectin was found to serve as an independent predictor of carotid plaque, and its elevations were persistent over more than one visit. Unexpectedly, this biomarker was present despite clinical quiescence. In vasculopathy as a comorbidity to SLE nephritis, the persistent expression of membrane

EPCR at peritubular capillaries may represent a response to the local cues of a deficit of active protein C. Under conditions of unresolved morbidity, higher levels of adiponectin and membrane EPCR may represent a physiologic attempt to limit further endothelial damage, and the observed increase in plaque and progression of SLE nephritis represent an overwhelming of this reparative process by disease-provoking stimuli.

Systemic lupus erythematosus is arguably the most clinically and serologically diverse autoimmune disease. This article highlights the biomarkers helpful in diagnosing this disease. The authors' own research is presented.

The long history of elevated interferon (IFN)-α in association with disease activity in patients who have systemic lupus erythematosus (SLE) has assumed high significance in the past decade, with accumulating data strongly supporting broad activation of the type I IFN pathway in cells of patients who have lupus, and association of IFN pathway activation with significant clinical manifestations of SLE and increased disease activity based on validated measures. In addition, a convincing association of IFN pathway activation with the presence of autoantibodies specific for RNA-binding proteins has contributed to delineation of an important role for Toll-like receptor activation by RNA-containing immune complexes in amplifying innate immune system activation and IFN pathway activation. Although the primary triggers of SLE and the IFN pathway remain undefined, rapid progress in lupus genetics is helping define lupus-associated genetic variants with a functional relationship to IFN production or response in patients. Together, the explosion of data and understanding related to the IFN pathway in SLE have readied the lupus community for translation of those insights to improved patient care. Patience will be needed to allow collection of clinical data and biologic specimens across multiple clinical centers required to support testing of IFN activity, IFN-inducible gene expression and chemokine gene products as candidate biomarkers. Meanwhile, promising clinical trials are moving forward to test the safety and efficacy of monoclonal antibody inhibitors of IFN-α. Other therapeutic approaches to target the IFN pathway may follow close behind.

The recent appreciation that a subset of anti-DNA antibodies cross-reacts with the N-methyl-d-aspartate receptor encourages a renewed examination of antibrain reactivity in systemic lupus erythematosus (SLE) autoantibodies. Moreover, investigations of their autospecificity present a paradigm for studies of antibrain reactivity and show that (1) serum antibodies access brain tissue only after a compromise of blood-brain barrier integrity, (2) the same antibodies have differential effects on brain function depending on the region of brain exposed to the antibodies, and (3) insults to the blood-brain barrier are regional rather than diffuse. These studies suggest that an anatomic classification scheme for neuropsychiatric SLE may facilitate research on etiopathogenesis and the design of clinical trials.

RELATED INTEREST
Neurologic Clinics
February 2010 (Volume 28, Issue 1)
Neurology and Systemic Disease
Alireza Minagar, MD, *Guest Editor*

THE CLINICS ARE NOW AVAILABLE ONLINE!

Access your subscription at:
www.theclinics.com

Preface

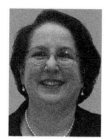

Ellen M. Ginzler, MD, MPH
Guest Editor

During the past 5 years since the last issue of *Rheumatic Disease Clinics of North America* was devoted to systemic lupus erythematosus (SLE), new paradigms for treatment have emerged, and advances in immunologic mechanisms and pathophysiology of clinical manifestations have provided a framework for further developments in care and response to therapy. The following 12 articles are directed toward improving the understanding of cutting-edge improvements in lupus biology and providing suggestions for new regimens designed to increase efficacy and minimize adverse events.

Vasudevan and Krishnamurthy discuss the changing worldwide epidemiology and outcomes of SLE, correlating them with a unique association with the human development index and standards of living in various regions of the world. Yazdany and Yelin continue a discussion of health-related quality of life and employment among lupus patients. Articles covering specific features of SLE and their relationship to therapy include those by Klein, Morganroth, and Werth regarding cutaneous manifestations and the newly validated CLASI instrument; differences between pediatric and adult lupus by Mina and Brunner; and the metabolic syndrome in SLE by Parker and Bruce. Recommendations for gonadal protection in association with immunosuppressive therapy are made by Mersereau and Dooley, whereas Ahmed and Anolik discuss investigational therapies for lupus as they relate to B-cell biology. Detection of flares of lupus nephritis and response to therapy should be aided by Manoharan and Madaio's discussion of biomarkers, leading to the article by Clancy and Ginzler regarding endothelial function and its implications for cardiovascular and renal disease in SLE. Finally, three articles review exciting discoveries in the immunology of lupus: cell-bound complement biomarkers by Liu and coworkers; Crow's interferon-α as a therapeutic target; and the significance of glutamate receptor biology in neuropsychiatric biology by Aranow, Diamond, and Mackay.

Ellen M. Ginzler, MD, MPH
Division of Rheumatology
State University of New York Downstate Medical Center
450 Clarkson Avenue
Brooklyn, NY 11203, USA

E-mail address:
ellen.ginzler@downstate.edu

Rheum Dis Clin N Am 36 (2010) xiii
doi:10.1016/j.rdc.2009.12.013
0889-857X/10/$ – see front matter © 2010 Elsevier Inc. All rights reserved.

Changing Worldwide Epidemiology of Systemic Lupus Erythematosus

Archana Vasudevan, MD*, Aneesa Niravel Krishnamurthy, DO

KEYWORDS

- Systemic lupus erythematosus • Human development index
- Gross domestic product • Ethnicity • Sociodemographics
- Epidemiology

Systemic lupus erythematosus (SLE) has been reported from most countries around the world. Epidemiologic studies have detailed worldwide SLE incidence and prevalence, along with the effects of gender, race, and age on presentation and mortality.[1,2] It is known that developed countries, which have a high gross domestic product (GDP), have significantly better survival rates than developing countries, defined as those having lower economic performances.[3] However, this does not explain differences in SLE outcomes among countries of varying GDPs, which are in part due to factors such as access to health care, physician availability, educational level, and treatment compliance. The human development index (HDI) provides a more three-dimensional view of life, by addressing the previously mentioned factors. The HDI accounts not just for standard of living (an indirect marker of GDP), but also literacy rates (a measure of educational levels), and life expectancy (an index of a population's quality of health and access to health care).[4]

There is no clear definition of a developed country. For the sake of this article, however, the authors include Western Europe, the United States of America, Canada, Japan, South Korea, Singapore, Kuwait, and the United Arab Emirates, all of which share a universally high GDP and very high HDI.[3]

Within the developing countries, China, India, South Africa, Brazil, Mexico, and a few Southeast Asian countries are separately categorized as newly industrialized countries, as they have outpaced their counterparts in the developing world in terms of economic growth and social development. The newly industrialized countries have medium- to high-level HDIs, with rapidly growing GDPs.[5] Finally, excluding South

---

Division of Rheumatology, SUNY Downstate Medical Center, 450 Clarkson Avenue, Box 42, Brooklyn, NY 11203, USA
* Corresponding author.
E-mail address: archanarvas@gmail.com (A. Vasudevan).

Rheum Dis Clin N Am 36 (2010) 1–13
doi:10.1016/j.rdc.2009.12.005
0889-857X/10/$ – see front matter © 2010 Elsevier Inc. All rights reserved.

Africa and Tunisia, many of the countries of sub-Saharan Africa have among the lowest GDPs and HDIs in the world, and are thus considered least developed among the developing countries.[6]

Outcomes in SLE survival depend on a complex interplay of many factors. In this article, the authors have categorized countries by HDI and GDP, to correlate the effects of both social and economic prosperity with SLE outcomes.

SLE IN THE DEVELOPED WORLD
Western Europe

Since the 1990s, several lupus registries have been established, most in the developed world. Within the German Collaborative Arthritis Database, 5% of the patients have SLE.[7] Five-year SLE survival rates from Germany are reported as high as 96.6%, with a 10-year survival rate between 83% and 90%.[8] In a small cohort of lupus nephritis patients in Germany, those diagnosed in the 1990s, compared with patients diagnosed in the 1980s, had significantly lower proteinuria, lower rates of renal failure, and less chronicity on kidney biopsy histopathology, due to earlier diagnosis and treatment.[9] In 1999 Camilleri reported his experience with 62 SLE patients from Malta, the country with the lowest GDP of the high HDI European countries (**Table 1**). The duration of follow-up, however, was not reported, and about 10% of the patients died.[10] In a pan-European cohort of 187 SLE patients with disease duration of greater than 10 years, renal and central nervous system (CNS) involvement increased to 47% and 65%, respectively, while cutaneous, musculoskeletal, and hematologic manifestation rates remained stable.[43,44]

The EuroLupus project consisting of 1000 patients from Western and European countries is perhaps the best-known European lupus registry. Within this cohort, active lupus nephritis was seen in 27.9% of patients. The 10-year survival rate was 92%, with deaths caused by active SLE in 26.5% of patients, infections in 25%, and thromboses (cerebral, coronary, and pulmonary) in 26.5%.[18] The cause of death in SLE patients is increasingly attributed to cardiovascular events rather than active disease, probably due to increased survival.[8]

Japan

Japan's national SLE registry of over 50,000 patients has survival rates mirroring that of other developed countries. SLE survival in Japan has improved from 72% in the 1950s and 1960s to 94% by the 1980s. Also noted was the decrease in death from active SLE over time, while deaths caused by fatal infections and pulmonary hypertension (PAH) increased.[45]

South Korea

As seen in German studies, even though the 5-year survival rates were at 93%, the overall SMR (standardized mortality ratio) was 3.02. The most common causes of death were PAH and interstitial lung disease.[19–21] Another cohort from South Korea reported infection (gram-negative bacilli), active SLE, and PAH as the main causes of mortality in patients.[46]

ETHNIC DIVERSITY AND SLE OUTCOMES IN DEVELOPED COUNTRIES
Singapore

Singapore has a diverse population consisting mainly of Chinese (70% to 80%), followed by Malays and Indians. In a retrospective review of 67 SLE patients from

1992 to 1995, active SLE and infection (gram-negative bacilli and tuberculosis) each accounted for over 40% of deaths.[22]

United States of America and Canada

Unlike Europe, which has a predominantly white cohort, the United States and Canada have increasingly diverse patient populations. People identified as belonging to minority ethnic populations within developed countries have higher prevalence of SLE, more severe disease manifestations, and younger age at onset of disease. These populations also tend to belong to a lower socioeconomic stratum and have a lower survival rate than the white population.[1,9]

Systemic Lupus Erythematosus International Collaborating Clinics (SLICC) is an SLE registry that includes patients from the United States and Canada, along with other developed countries such as South Korea and the United Kingdom. Bernatsky and colleagues[47] reported in 2006 that SLE patients had a higher SMR of 2.4. When this was further broken down by race for patients from the United States, African Americans had a higher SMR (2.6) than whites (SMR of 1.4).

The Lupus in Minorities: Nature versus nurture (LUMINA) cohort was started in 1994 to study the epidemiology of SLE in three different ethnic groups: Hispanics, African Americans, and whites, enrolling patients from the United States, and Puerto Rico. Lupus nephritis also was found to be at least two times more prevalent among African Americans and Hispanics than whites.[14–17] Among Hispanics, Texan Hispanics, who are of American Indian/Mestizo descent, had more serositis (60% vs 8.6%), renal involvement (41% vs 13.6%), and overall disease activity, than Puerto Rican Hispanics, who are of mixed white/African/American Indian descent.[48,49] Nonwhite patients also were found to be more likely to be living below the poverty line, less educated, and more noncompliant with clinic visits.[50]

SLE prevalence has been reported to be much more prevalent in those of African ancestry within the developed countries.[51] Even though Afro-Caribbeans and Asians had similar high rates of lupus nephritis (>55%) in a Canadian cohort, Afro-Caribbeans had higher damage scores and damage accumulation than Asians. Afro-Caribbeans also had lower household income and educational level than the other ethnic groups.[52]

In Hawaii, the prevalence of SLE was found to be higher in all three major Asian groups: Chinese, Filipinos, and Japanese, when compared with whites. In addition, the Asian group had a threefold higher mortality rate than whites.[53] Kaslow found that the age- and sex-adjusted mortality rates were three times higher for African Americans and two times higher for the Asian population, compared with the Caucasian population.[54]

Middle East

Kuwait and the United Arab Emirates enjoy a high GDP, very high HDI, and a high number of physicians per 10,000 population (**Table 1**). These countries have a majority expatriate population from other Arab and South Asian countries. Al-Jarallah and colleagues reported a 99% 5-year survival rate for their SLE patients from Kuwait.[24,25] AlSaleh and colleagues[23] reported a similarly high 5-year survival rate for patients from Dubai, in the United Arab Emirates.

SLE IN NEWLY INDUSTRIALIZED COUNTRIES
China

Of the newly industrialized countries, China has the fastest growing GDP and the third largest economy in the world, but a medium level HDI, and low GDP per capita. The

Table 1
Comparison of GDP per capita, HDI and the 5-year SLE survival by country

	GDP per Capita 1990 in US Dollars[12]	GDP per Capita in 2008 in US Dollars[12]	Government Health Care Expenditure as Percent of Total Expenses[13]	HDI[4]	Number of Physicians per 10,000 Population[13]	SLE 5-year Survival	SLE 10-year Survival	Percentage of Patients in the Cohort with Lupus Nephritis
Developed countries								
United States[11,14-16]	32,132.00	43,156.00	19.3%	VH (0.956)	26	97%	93%	28%–38%
Japan[17]	28,875.00	34,855.00	17.9%	VH (0.960)	21	94%	92%	NA
Germany[8]	28,585.00	36,248.00	17.9%	VH (0.947)	34	96.6%	89.9%	42%
EuroLupus cohort[18]	21,966.71	31,595.71	14.2%	VH (0.923)	30	NA	92%	28%
South Korea[19]	8,761.00	19,716.00	6.0%	VH (0.937)	33	93%	NA	37%
Sweden[20]	29,853.00	42,192.00	13.80%	VH (0.963)	33	93%	83%	NA
Greece[21]	14,044.00	22,561.00	11.60%	VH (0.942)	50	96.2%	87.4%	20%
Singapore[22]	15,686.00	30,394.00	6.7%	VH (0.944)	15	70%	60%	64%
United Arab Emirates[23]	29,514.00	34,207.00	8.7%	VH (0.903)	17	94%	NA	51%
Kuwait[24]	20,189.00	32,121.00	4.9%	VH (0.916)	7	99%	NA	37%
Iceland[25]	38,786.00	54,642.00	18%	VH (0.969)	38	84%	78%	20%
Malta[10]	9566.00	15,450.00	14.7%	VH (0.902)	39	NA	NA	30%

Newly industrialized countries							
China[26,27]	470.00	2342.00	9.9%	M (0.772)	14	93%	NA	45%–70%
Brazil[28]	4398.00	5736.00	7.2%	H (0.813)	12	NA	NA	NA
India[29,30]	385.00	850.00	3.4%	M (0.612)	6	70%	50%	57%
Mexico[31]	5884.00	7657.00	11.8%	H (0.854)	20	95%	NA	NA
South Africa[32]	4062.00	5183.00	9.1%	M (0.683)	8	57%–72%	NA	44%
Thailand[33]	1720.00	3236.00	11.3%	M (0.783)	4	84%	75%	NA
Malaysia[34,35]	3117.00	6283.00	7.0%	H (0.829)	7	82%	70%	74%
Phillipines[1]	967.00	1281.00	6.1%	M (0.751)	12	75%	NA	47%
Russia[36]	5921.00	6919.00	10.8%	H (0.817)	43	NA	NA	NA
Developing countries							
Saudi Arabia[37]	12,296.00	12,369.00	8.7%	H (0.843)	14	98%	97%	47.5%
Iran[38]	1967.00	3456.00	11.5%	M (0.782)	9	95.6%	NA	48%
Pakistan[39]	524.00	793.00	1.3%	M (0.572)	8	80%	77%	38%
Tunisia[40]	3415.00	5289.00	6.7%	M (0.769)	13	86%	NA	43%
Sri Lanka[41]	652.00	1315.00	8.3%	M (0.759)	6	93.4% (3-year survival)	NA	69%
Zimbabwe[42]	52.00	29.00	8.9%	M (0.513)	2	71% (1-year survival)	NA	71%

The HDI numbers within parentheses are index values: Very high (≥ 0.900). High (≥ 0.800 to 0.900). Medium (≥ 0.500 to 0.800). Least (<0.500).
Abbreviations: H, highly developed; M, medium development; VH, very highly developed.

main studies on survival in SLE patients in China are from Hong Kong, which is an autonomous region of China,[55] and has its own separate HDI ranking of very high.[4] These cohorts from the 1990s have 5-year survival rates comparable to Western cohorts; with greater than 90% survival, even with a higher prevalence of lupus nephritis, ranging from 45% to 70%. Mortality was mainly due to active disease or infection, once again, with each cohort reporting one to two deaths from PAH.[26,27]

India

Comparing two cohorts, the 5- and 10-year survival rates were 88% and 82% in southern India and 70% and 50% in northern India, respectively. Clinically, both regions had relatively high rates of renal involvement, with northern Indians having rates of about 70%, and southern Indians, about 50%. The exact causes of most deaths were not known, as they occurred outside of the hospital setting.[29–31] Active SLE, renal failure, and infection (bacterial infections and tuberculosis) are reported causes of mortality.[56]

South Africa

South Africa is the only country from Africa that is considered newly industrialized. In a review of case records from a lupus clinic in South Africa, over half of the 226 mainly black SLE patients were either dead or lost to follow-up at 55 months. The 5-year survival rates ranged from 57% to 72%, depending on whether those lost to follow-up were classified as dead or alive. Those patients with lupus nephritis (44% of their cohort) had a 5-year survival rate of 60%. Infection was the most common known cause of death (32.7%), mostly attributed to pneumonia, sepsis, or tuberculosis. Very few deaths were caused by cardiovascular morbidity.[32,33]

Southeast Asia—Philippines and Thailand

Analysis of over 1000 patients in a lupus database from a university hospital in Manila, Philippines, revealed renal involvement in 47% of the patients.[57] The reported survival rates from a 1988 study in the Philippines were 75% at 5 years and 60% at 1 year, similar to rates in other now newly industrialized countries around the same time period.[1] In Thailand, the survival rate for 569 patients with lupus nephritis followed from 1984 to 1991 was 76.9% . The most common cause of death was infection (52%), followed by renal failure. Tuberculosis remains a common infection as seen in other endemic countries.[58]

ETHNIC DIVERSITY AND SLE OUTCOMES IN NEWLY INDUSTRIALIZED COUNTRIES
Brazil and Mexico

Latin America is very ethnically diverse, as seen in the Grupo Latinoamericano de Estudio del Lupus (GLADEL), an SLE cohort that includes patients from Brazil and Mexico, among other Latin American countries. Of the 1214 patients in GLADEL, 44% are mixed European/American Indians (Mestizo); 42% are white, and 13% are African–Latin Americans (ALAs). Renal disease was more frequent in the Mestizo and ALA groups (>55%), than in whites (44%). Despite having a higher frequency of renal involvement, ALA patients had lower damage scores than both Mestizos and whites. Overall, with a 4-year survival rate of 95%, no difference in mortality was seen between ethnicities. Lack of medical coverage and lower education levels and socioeconomic status were associated with higher damage levels and mortality rates. Active disease and infection were the most common causes of death.[59] In another review at a single urban hospital in Brazil over a 14 year period, 13.9% of SLE inpatients died, of which the most common cause of death (58%) was infection, with 13% due to tuberculosis and fungus.[28]

Malaysia

The estimated prevalence of SLE in Malaysia is 43 cases per 100,000 population, with the immigrant Chinese having the highest rates at 57 cases per 100,000 population, the Indians with the lowest at 14 cases per 100,000 population, and the ethnic Malays in the middle at 33 cases per 100,000 population. Although there was no significant difference in renal involvement (approximately 65% to 75% affected) between the groups, Indians had the worst survival rates. The overall 5- and 10-year survival rates were 82% and 70%, respectively.[35] Infections followed by active SLE remain the main causes of mortality in Malaysia.[34]

SLE IN DEVELOPING COUNTRIES
Middle East

Saudi Arabia recently was promoted from a medium to high HDI. Iran still has a medium HDI.[4] As seen in the developed Middle Eastern countries and most Western European and North American countries, Iran and Saudi Arabia have high SLE survival rates of greater than 95%. Although hematological abnormalities appear to be the most common manifestation of SLE, renal involvement parallels that seen in ethnic minorities reported from the US LUMINA study and the United Kingdom.[37,38]

Eastern Europe

Studies from Russia (former Soviet Union) have shown an increased prevalence of SLE in native Siberian, Tadzhik, and Uzbek populations compared with populations from Dushanbe or Moscow.[36,60] A similar pattern has been reported in the aboriginal populations of Australia, with a higher prevalence of SLE, and more severe disease manifestations.[61]

South Asia

Lower 5- and 10-year survival rates of 80% and 77%, respectively, were reported in SLE patients from Pakistan. In this study, however, 49 of the 198 patients met only 3 of 11 criteria for SLE and were still included in the final analysis. Moreover, even though 21% of the patients were lost to follow-up, they were considered alive when calculating the survival rates. Another study reported a greater than 90% 3-year survival for 111 patients in Sri Lanka; however only 80% of these patients fulfilled criteria for SLE. Both the Pakistan (45%) and Sri Lankan studies (69%) had high rates of renal involvement.[39,41]

Caribbean Islands

High prevalence, severity, and poor outcome have been reported uniformly in all cohorts for patients of Afro-Caribbean ethnicity.[52,62] The prevalence of SLE in Jamaica is nearly as high as that of rheumatoid arthritis. Most countries in the Caribbean have medium to high HDIs, but the survival rates for patients with SLE are consistently poor, even in patients without nephritis. Reports from the island Curacao confirms this, with 5-year survival rates ranging between 55% and 60% [63,64]

Africa

Most countries in Africa have the lowest GDP, HDI, and number of physicians per 10,000 population, in the world (see **Table 1**). From published reports, SLE appears to be rare in Africa and is in contrast to the high prevalence of SLE in those of African ancestry within the developed countries, although this may be due to reporting bias.[51] Zimbabwe has a very high SLE mortality, with a reported 29% dead by 1 year, while Tunisia, one of the more prosperous countries in Africa, has a 5-year survival rate of 86%. The African continent has prevalent lupus nephritis, ranging from 43% to 70%, and the main causes of SLE death are infection and active disease.[40,65] There is very little published data on SLE in the least developed countries of Africa.

DISCUSSION

With the introduction of immunosuppressive agents, steroids, newer antihypertensives, dialysis, and renal transplant, SLE mortality rates have improved most significantly in the developed world,[66] characterized by high economic productivity (GDP), standards of living, education, and life expectancy (HDI).

Countries with higher economic productivity and HDIs spent more of their GDP on health care, with associated improvement in SLE survival ($P = .021$ per the authors' calculations). Germany has a lupus nephritis rate of 42%, relatively high for the rest of Europe, yet it still boasts a 5-year survival rate of over 95%. This is because of its very high HDI, and the fact that Germany spends close to 18% of its GDP on health expenditure. Zimbabwe, in contrast, has one of the highest reported rates of renal involvement, spends only 8.9% of its small GDP on health care, has only 2 physicians per 10,000 population, and has a very low 1-year survival rate of 71% (see **Table 1**).

Five-year SLE survival increases with GDP per capita ($P = .024$ per the authors' calculations), but the strongest correlation is with HDI ($P = .006$) (**Fig. 1**). This can be seen within the newly industrialized countries, where Malaysia, Mexico, and Brazil have high HDIs, and thus a trend toward improved survival, when compared with the medium HDI countries in the same group. An obvious exception is China, which has

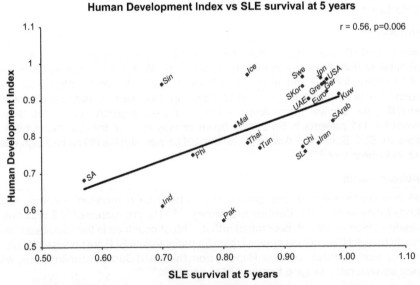

Fig. 1. HDI versus SLE survival at 5 years. *Abbreviations:* Chi, China; Eur, EuroLupus cohort; Ger, Germany; Gre, Greece; Ice, Iceland; Ind, India; Jpn, Japan; Kor, South Korea; Kuw, Kuwait; Mal, Malaysia; Pak, Pakistan; Phi, Philippines; SArab, Saudi Arabia; Sin, Singapore; SL, Sri Lanka (3-year survival data); Swe, Sweden; Thai, Thailand; Tun, Tunisia; UAE, United Arab Emirates; USA, United States of America.

a medium HDI, although most of the Chinese epidemiologic studies were reported from Hong Kong, which has both a high GDP and very high HDI ranking.

As a whole, developed countries with high GDP and HDI enjoy overall better health. It is becoming increasingly evident, however, that within the diaspora of ethnically diverse countries, there are discrepancies in health outcomes. As seen in the United States and Canada, the nonwhite SLE populations suffer from higher disease activity and damage. The microcosm of ethnic minorities with their lower socioeconomic strata, education level, and higher mortality suggests a lower HDI for these communities even within the developed countries.

Socioeconomic differences are apparent within developing countries also. India is a newly industrialized country with a growing GDP and medium HDI. Despite the overall improvement in the country's economy and standard of living, there are glaring regional differences. India's four southern states are characterized by higher production and literacy and lower birth rates than seen in the northern states.[67] This may explain the disparate 5-year survival rates of southern India versus northern India.

Socioeconomics also affect follow-up rates and survival outcomes. This was especially evident in South Africa, where the loss to follow-up swayed survival rates by 15% or more, and in India, where half the reported deaths were of unknown cause, occurring outside of the hospital setting.

With the changing economies and the improved standard of living, causes of mortality have adapted also. In developed countries and parts of the Middle East, mortality has trended from active disease and infection, toward cardiovascular disease. Within the developing world, which contains areas endemic for tuberculosis, mycobacterial infections cause significant morbidity.

The unique infectious agents and environment of lower HDI countries may have implications for SLE. Higher frequency of infections such as mumps and rubella during the development of the immune system (within the first year of life) has been associated with increased risk of having ANAs.[68] The diagnosis of SLE may be confounded in developing countries, where human immunodeficiency virus (HIV) and tuberculosis are endemic, affecting reported prevalence rates and outcomes.[1] Ultraviolet radiation and hormones may modulate the expression of human endogenous retroviruses, thus altering the epigenetics of lupus, and may explain the differences in disease expression between various ethnic groups.[69]

Large lupus registries such as the EuroLupus project and SLICC have revealed much about the epidemiology of SLE in the developed world. Despite the establishment of cohorts like GLADEL, there is little data from the newly industrialized and developing world, mostly due to a lack of resources. Within countries with high GDP and HDI, new epidemiologic data has increased awareness of higher cardiovascular morbidity in SLE patients. Studies from other countries may shed more light on the locally prevalent causes of morbidity and mortality such as PAH and tuberculosis. This would be beneficial in improving mortality in the developing world. As more countries join the developed world, understanding of SLE will grow along with the economies and standards of living.

REFERENCES

1. Tikly M, Navarra SV. Lupus in the developing world—is it any different? Best Pract Res Clin Res Rheumatol 2008;22(4):643–55.
2. Pons-Estel GJ, Alarcon GS, Scofield L, et al. Understanding the epidemiology and progression of systemic lupus erythematosus. Semin Arthritis Rheum 2009.

3. Developed countries. Available at: http://en.wikipedia.org/wiki/Developed_countries. Accessed November 22, 2009.

4. Human development index. Available at: http://en.wikipedia.org/wiki/List_of_countries_by_Human_Development_Index. Accessed November 22, 2009.

5. Newly industrialized country. Available at: http://en.wikipedia.org/wiki/Newly_industrialized_country. Accessed November 22, 2009.

6. Least developed country. Wikipedia website. Available at: http://en.wikipedia.org/wiki/Least_Developed_Country. Accessed November 22, 2009.

7. Zink A, Listing J, Klindworth C, et al. The national database of the German Collaborative Arthritis Centres: I. Structure, aims, and patients. Ann Rheum Dis 2001;60(3):199–206.

8. Manger K, Manger B, Repp R, et al. Definition of risk factors for death, end stage renal disease, and thromboembolic events in a monocentric cohort of 338 patients with systemic lupus erythematosus. Ann Rheum Dis 2002;61(12):1065–70.

9. Fiehn C, Hajjar Y, Mueller K, et al. Improved clinical outcome of lupus nephritis during the past decade: importance of early diagnosis and treatment. Ann Rheum Dis 2003;62(5):435–9.

10. Camilleri F, Mallia C. Male SLE patients in Malta. Adv Exp Med Biol 1999;455: 173–9.

11. Pistiner M, Wallace DJ, Nessim S, et al. Lupus erythematosus in 1980s: a survey of 570 patients. Semin Arthritis Rheum 1991;21(1):55–64.

12. United States Department of Agriculture. Economic research service. Available at: http://www.ers.usda.gov/Data/macroeconomics/Data/HistoricalRealPerCapitaIncomeValues.xls. Accessed November 22, 2009.

13. Kaiser Family Foundation. Available at: http://www.globalhealthfacts.org/. Accessed November 22, 2009.

14. Bastian HM, Roseman JM, McGwin G, et al. Systemic lupus erythematosus in three ethnic groups. XII. Risk factors for lupus nephritis after diagnosis. Lupus 2002;11(3):152–60.

15. Kumar K, Chambers S, Gordon C. Challenges of ethnicity in SLE. Best Pract Res Clin Rheumatol 2009;23(4):549–61.

16. Cooper GS, Parks CG, Treadwell EL, et al. Differences by race, sex, and age in the clinical and immunologic features of recently diagnosed systemic lupus erythematosus patients in the southeastern United States. Lupus 2002;11(3): 161–7.

17. Hashimoto H, Shiokawa Y. Changing patterns in the clinical features and prognosis of systemic lupus erythematosus—A Japanese experience. J Rheumatol 1982;9(3):386–9.

18. Cervera R, Khamashta MA, Hughes GRV. The EuroLupus project: epidemiology of systemic lupus erythematosus in Europe. Lupus 2009;18(10):869–74.

19. Chun BC, Bae SC. Mortality and cancer incidence in Korean patients with systemic lupus erythematosus: results from the Hanyang Lupus cohort in Seoul, Korea. Lupus 2005;14(8):635–8.

20. Stahl-Hallengren C, Jonsen A, Nived O, et al. Incidence studies of SLE in Southern Sweden: increasing age, decreasing frequency of renal manifestations, and good prognosis. J Rheumatol 2000;27(3):685–91.

21. Alamanos Y, Voulgari PV, Siozos C, et al. Epidemiology of systemic lupus erythematosus in northwest Greece 1982–2001. J Rheumatol 2003;30(12):731–5.

22. Koh ET, Seow A, Leong KH, et al. SLE mortality in an Oriental population. Lupus 1997;6(1):27–31.

23. AlSaleh J, Jassim V, ElSayed M, et al. Clinical and immunological manifestations in 151 SLE patients living in Dubai. Lupus 2008;17(1):62–6.
24. Al-Jarallah K, Al-Awadi A, Siddiqui H, et al. Systemic lupus erythematosus in Kuwait—hospital-based study. Lupus 1998;7(7):434–8.
25. Gudmundsson S, Steinsson K. Systemic lupus erythematosus in Iceland 1975 through 1984. A nationwide epidemiological study in an unselected population. J Rheumatol 1990;17(9):1162–7.
26. Mok CC, Lee KW, Ho CT, et al. A prospective study of survival and prognostic indicators of systemic lupus erythematosus in a southern Chinese population. Rheumatology (Oxford) 2000;39(4):399–406.
27. Mok CC, Mak A, Chu WP, et al. Long-term survival of southern Chinese patients with systemic lupus erythematosus: a prospective study of all age-groups. Medicine (Baltimore) 2005;84(4):218–24.
28. Iriya SM, Capelozzi VL, Calich I, et al. Causes of death in patients with systemic lupus erythematosus in Sao Paulo, Brazil: a study of 113 autopsies. Arch Intern Med 2001;161(12):1557.
29. Chandrasekaran AN, Radhakrishna B. Rheumatoid arthritis and connective tissue disorders: India and Southeast Asia. Baillieres Clin Rheumatol 1995;9(1):45–57.
30. Malaviya AN, Chandrasekaran AN, Kumar A, et al. Systemic lupus erythematosus in India. Lupus 1997;6(9):690–700.
31. Zonana-Nacach A, Yanez P, Jimenez-Balderas FJ, et al. Disease activity, damage, and survival in Mexican patients with acute severe systemic lupus erythematosus. Lupus 2007;16(12):997–1000.
32. Wadee S, Tikly M, Hopley M. Causes and predictors of death in South Africans with systemic lupus erythematosus. Rheumatology (Oxford) 2007;46(9):1487–91.
33. Kasitanon N, Louthrenoo W, Sukitawut W. Causes of death and prognostic factors in Thai patients with systemic lupus erythematosus. Asian Pac J Allergy Immunol 2002;20(2):85–91.
34. Yeap SS, Chow SK, Manivasagar M, et al. Mortality patterns in Malaysian systemic lupus erythematosus patients. Med J Malaysia 2001;56(3):308–12.
35. Wang F, Wang CL, Tan CT, et al. Systemic lupus erythematosus in Malaysia: a study of 539 patients and comparison of prevalence and disease expression in different racial and gender groups. Lupus 1997;6(3):248–53.
36. Bezrodnyhk AA, Karelin AP. Systemic lupus erythematosus and systemic scleroderma in patients from the aboriginal people and the newcomers of Yakutia under the extreme conditions of the far north. Ala Med 1994;36(2):102–6.
37. Al Arfaj AS, Khalil N. Clinical and immunological manifestations in 624 SLE patients in Saudi Arabia. Lupus 2009;18(5):465–73.
38. Nazarinia MA, Ghaffarpasand F, Shamsdin A, et al. Systemic lupus erythematosus in the Fars Province of Iran. Lupus 2008;17(3):221–7.
39. Rabbani MA, Habib HB, Islam M, et al. Ahmad. Survival analysis and prognostic indicators of systemic lupus erythematosus in Pakistani patients. Lupus 2009;18(9):848–55.
40. Houman MH, Smiti-Khan M, Ghorbell IB, et al. Systemic lupus erythematosus in Tunisia: demographic and clinical analysis of 100 patients. Lupus 2004;13(3):204–11.
41. Galapatthy P, Wazeel AN, Nanayakkara S, et al. Clinical features of systemic lupus erythematosus in Sri Lankan patients: results from a lupus clinic. Ceylon Med J 2000;45(4):162–5.
42. Taylor HG, Stein CM. Systemic lupus erythematosus in Zimbabwe. Ann Rheum Dis 1986;45(8):645–8.

43. Swaak AJ, van den Brink HG, Smeenk RJ, et al. Systemic lupus erythematosus: clinical features in patients with a disease duration of over 10 years, first evaluation. Rheumatology (Oxford) 1999;38(10):953–8.
44. Swaak AJ, van den Brink HG, Smeenk RJ, et al. Systemic lupus erythematosus. Disease outcome in patients with a disease duration of at least 10 years: second evaluation. Lupus 2001;10(1):51–8.
45. Kataoka H, Koike T. Lupus mortality in Japan. Autoimmun Rev 2004;3(6): 421–2.
46. Kim WU, Min JK, Lee SH, et al. Causes of death in Korean patients with systemic lupus erythematosus: a single center retrospective study. Clin Exp Rheumatol 1999;17(5):539–45.
47. Bernatsky S, Boivin JF, Joseph L, et al. Mortality in systemic lupus erythematosus. Arthritis Rheum 2006;54(8):2550–7.
48. Vila LM, Alarcon GS, McGwin G, et al. Early clinical manifestations, disease activity, and damage of systemic lupus erythematosus among two distinct US Hispanic subpopulations. Rheumatology (Oxford) 2004;43(3):358–63.
49. Uribe AG, McGwin G, Reveille JD, et al. What have we learned from a 10-year experience with the LUMINA (Lupus in Minorities; Nature vs nurture) cohort? Where are we heading? Autoimmun Rev 2004;3(4):321–9.
50. Uribe AG, Ho KT, Agee B, et al. Relationship between adherence to study and clinic visits in systemic lupus erythematosus patients: data from the LUMINA cohort. Lupus 2004;13(8):561–8.
51. Bae SC, Fraser P, Liang MH. The epidemiology of systemic lupus erythematosus in populations of African ancestry: a critical review of the prevalence gradient hypothesis. Arthritis Rheum 1998;41(12):2091–9.
52. Peschken CA, Katz SJ, Silverman E, et al. The 1000 Canadian faces of lupus: determinants of disease outcome in a large multiethnic cohort. J Rheumatol 2009;36(6):1200–8.
53. Maskarinec G, Katz AR. Prevalence of systemic lupus erythematosus in Hawaii: is there a difference between ethnic groups? Hawaii Med J 1995;54(2):406–9.
54. Kaslow RA. High rate of death caused by systemic lupus erythematosus among US residents of Asian descent. Arthritis Rheum 1982;25(4):414–8.
55. Mok CC, Lau CS. Lupus in Hong Kong Chinese. Lupus 2003;12(9):717–22.
56. Jindal B, Joshi K, Radotra BD, et al. Fatal complications of systemic lupus erythematosus—an autopsy study from north India. Indian J Pathol Microbiol 2000; 43(3):311–7.
57. Villamin CA, Navarra SV. Clinical Manifestations and clinical syndromes of Filipino patients with systemic lupus erythematosus. Mod Rheumatol 2008;18(2):161–4.
58. Shayakul C, Ongajyooth L, Chirawong P, et al. Lupus nephritis in Thailand: clinico-pathologic findings and outcome in 569 patients. Am J Kidney Dis 1995;26(2):300–7.
59. Pons-Estel BA, Catoggio LJ, Cardiel MH, et al. The GLADEL multinational Latin American prospective inception cohort of 1214 patients with systemic lupus erythematosus: ethnic and disease heterogeneity among Hispanics. Medicine (Baltimore) 2004;83(1):1–17.
60. Rasulov UR. Systemic lupus erythematosus in the native inhabitants of Tadzhikistan. Ter Arkh. 1990;62(4):90–4.
61. Danchenko N, Satia JA, Anthony MS. Epidemiology of systemic lupus erythematousus: a comparison of worldwide disease burden. Lupus 2006;15(5):308–18.
62. Patel M, Clarke AM, Bruce IN, et al. The prevalence and incidence of biopsy-proven lupus nephritis in the UK: evidence of an ethnic gradient. Arthritis Rheum 2006;54(9):2963–9.

63. Nossent JC. Course and prognostic value of systemic lupus erythematosus disease activity index in black Caribbean patients. Semin Arthritis Rheum 1993;23(1):16–21.
64. Nossent JC. Systemic lupus erythematosus on the Caribbean island of Curacao: an epidemiological investigation. Ann Rheum Dis 1992;51(11):1197–201.
65. Stein M, Davis P. Rheumatic disorders in Zimbabwe: a prospective analysis of patients attending a rheumatic diseases clinic. Ann Rheum Dis 1990;49(6):400–2.
66. Borchers AT, Keen CL, Shoenfeld Y, et al. Surviving the butterfly and the wolf: mortality trends in systemic lupus erythematosus. Autoimmun Rev 2004;3(6):423–53.
67. Haub C, Sharma OP. India's population reality: reconciling change and tradition. A publication of the Population Reference Bureau. Population 2006;61:3–19.
68. Edwards CJ, Syddall H, Goswami R, et al. Infections in infancy and the presence of antinuclear antibodies in adult life. Lupus 2006;15(4):213–7.
69. Blank M, Shoenfeld Y, Perl A. Cross-talk of the environment with the host genome and the immune system through endogenous retroviruses in systemic lupus erythematosus. Lupus 2009;18(13):1136–43.

Health-Related Quality of Life and Employment Among Persons with Systemic Lupus Erythematosus

Jinoos Yazdany, MD, MPH*, Edward Yelin, PhD

KEYWORDS

- Health-related quality of life • Employment
- Systemic lupus erythematosus

This article assesses the effect of systemic lupus erythematosus (SLE) on the health-related quality of life (HRQOL) and employment of persons with this condition. Far more than impaired health status can affect an individual's quality of life. The term "health-related quality of life" is used to connote the decrement in an individual's quality of life specifically attributable to a decrease in health status. The article presents evidence on employment because this plays a crucial role in determining the quality of life of most Americans of normal working age. However, evidence is also presented with respect to other domains of activity, because most people work to live but not many live to work.

Conceptualizing the effect of SLE on HRQOL is far more difficult than for rheumatoid arthritis (RA), let alone osteoarthritis (OA) or other nonsystemic musculoskeletal conditions. In RA, as opposed to OA, one has to take into account the effect of profound fatigue beyond the obvious effect of symmetric joint involvement and joint destruction. Symptoms like fatigue that are invisible to the observer may lead others to discount the effects of the condition. The disconnect between what others perceive and what the person with RA perceives may be a source of psychological disturbance. Also, the uncertainty associated with an uneven course of illness can also take a toll on the individual, not least because it makes planning for the future difficult. In SLE,

Grant Support: Multidisciplinary Clinical Research Center P60 AR053308, Arthritis Foundation, American College of Rheumatology Research and Education Foundation, and 5R01AR56476-7.

Department of Medicine, Division of Rheumatology, Rosalind Russell Medical Research Center for Arthritis, University of California, UCSF Box 0920, San Francisco, CA 94143-0920, USA

* Corresponding author.

E-mail address: jinoos.yazdany@ucsf.edu (J. Yazdany).

some of the same issues arise, but may be amplified because of the range of manifestations that may occur, adding complexity to invisibility of some symptoms and uncertainty of course.

Thus, measuring the effect of SLE on HRQOL may be a daunting challenge. It is nevertheless a propitious time to take stock. There is good evidence that improved treatment of SLE has resulted in decreased mortality associated with the condition, turning a frequently fatal condition into one in which concern about quantity of life has segued into a concern about its quality.

Reflecting decreased mortality, the literature on the effect of SLE on quality of life and employment has grown substantially in recent years. For example, a comprehensive literature review on employment and SLE[1] searched for articles on this topic from 1950 onward, but the earliest found was from 1994 and only another 8 were published before the end of the 1990s. Since 2000, 18 more have appeared, with 11 of these published after 2005.

However, the most important reason to take stock of the effect of SLE on quality of life and employment is that, for the first time in memory, new treatments may be imminent, particularly as the biologic era in rheumatology expands to encompass SLE. By estimating the effect of SLE on quality on life now, it will be possible to evaluate the effect of these new treatments as they diffuse into practice in the years to come.

A framework for discussing HRQOL in general is provided so that, from a review of some of the literature on HRQOL on SLE, the reader can see how groups of studies address the different elements in the framework. Often, literature reviews encompass studies across the elements without clarifying how these studies relate to the elements. The framework outlined incorporates integrative activities such as employment as the end result of a process that begins with the onset of SLE (or at an even earlier stage, the risk factors for onset), placing the studies of employment in the same framework as the remainder of the HRQOL literature.

Special attention is paid to the effect of SLE on employment among all of the integrative activities because SLE is typically diagnosed early in the career of those with the condition, perhaps limiting their ability to establish careers and, even if this is not the case, preventing them from gaining the kind of traction in work that normally occurs in the absence of a severe chronic disease.

HEALTH-RELATED QUALITY OF LIFE

Throughout the course of their disease, individuals with SLE face considerable physical, psychological, and social challenges. As long-term survival in SLE has become commonplace, measures that move beyond mortality or medical morbidity to capture the patient's perspective have become a critical aspect of appraising outcomes. Instruments that measure HRQOL attempt to characterize this subjective experience of illness. Rheumatologists have pioneered the measurement of HRQOL, dispelling notions that HRQOL is somehow not as important or valid as other traditionally used clinical end points. In fact, a growing body of literature demonstrates that HRQOL is a useful and valid end point for incorporation into clinical research and practice, and should be used alongside physician assessments and laboratory studies.

In SLE, considerable research has accumulated regarding HRQOL. This section defines the theoretical concepts underlying HRQOL and then, using a well-defined model, discusses what is known regarding HRQOL in SLE. The section ends with a brief discussion of the tools available to measure HRQOL in SLE, and recommends a general approach to selecting a measure for use in clinical practice or research studies.

Defining HRQOL

Although there is no universally accepted definition of HRQOL, the last several decades of scientific research suggest that it should be viewed as a multidimensional construct. This approach ensures that health status and quality of life are examined distinctly, with quality of life representing a more global view of the patients' social and psychological environment that may influence the response to illness.

In 1995, Wilson and Cleary[2] put forth what is now a classic model that emphasizes the multidimensional inputs to HRQOL (**Fig. 1**). Although more than a decade old, the model is still useful in thinking about the relationships among the conceptual areas represented. The model begins with biologic and physiologic variables, which, in the case of SLE, might reflect factors such as an individual patient's genetic predisposition to disease, autoantibody production, and organ manifestations. Second, the model contains symptom status, which relates the patient's perception of his or her symptoms. In SLE, this would include the physical, cognitive, and emotional symptoms experienced by the patient. Third, functional status is assessed, which incorporates physical, psychological, and social functioning. These preceding domains are related to the fourth concept, general health perceptions, which entail a subjective synthesis of the preceding factors in the model. Finally, the last domain is overall quality of life, a global concept that may incorporate notions such as life satisfaction and overall ratings of quality of life. The model's structure implies causal relationships between these content areas, with the dominant direction of causation proceeding from left to right. (The Wilson and Cleary[2] model of HRQOL is remarkably similar to the Nagi[3,4] model of work disability,[3,4] more recently amended by Verbrugge and Jette,[5] in which pathology, eg, SLE, begets impairment, eg, neuropsychiatric symptoms, which in turn beget functional limitations, eg, executive function, before affecting employment. The Nagi[3,4] model is used in employment or work disability research. For space reasons, and because HRQOL would certainly include employment, this article focuses on the Wilson and Cleary[2] HRQOL model.)

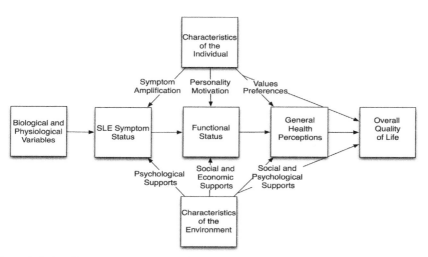

Fig. 1. Relationships among measures of patient outcome in an HRQOL conceptual model. (*Adapted from* Wilson I, Cleary P. Linking clinical variables with health-related quality of life. A conceptual model of patient outcomes. JAMA 1995;273(1):60; with permission.)

The next section breaks down the components of the Wilson and Cleary[2] model, highlighting examples of research in SLE that have examined the relationships between the relevant domains.

BIOLOGIC AND PHYSIOLOGIC VARIABLES AND SYMPTOM STATUS

The relationship between biologic and physiologic variables and symptoms (the patient's subjective physical, emotional, or cognitive state) is perhaps the most familiar concept to physicians and others involved in the clinical care of SLE. However, even this relationship proves surprisingly complex. Providers who care for patients with SLE intuitively realize this; in some patients, perceived symptoms correlate well with physician and laboratory assessments of disease activity. However, patients frequently experience symptoms in the absence of detectable disease activity, or have no symptoms in the face of obvious disease activity.

Although a patient's subjective report of symptoms correlates globally with formal disease activity measurements made by a physician, the correlation is only modest. This discrepancy is perhaps best illustrated by examining the growing literature on the validity of self-report measures of disease activity, such as the Systemic Lupus Activity Questionnaire (SLAQ).[6] For many items on the SLAQ, patient reports of symptoms correlate only weakly with physician assessments. For example, for skin disease the correlation coefficient comparing patient-reported symptoms with physician assessments was 0.34, for arthralgia/arthritis 0.50, and for myalgia/myositis 0.27.[6] In a validation study for the SLE Symptom Checklist (SSC), physician assessments of disease activity (as measured by the SLE Disease Activity Index [SLEDAI] or the physician global assessment) correlated only weakly to patient symptoms.[7] Similarly, several studies have documented significant differences between patient and physician assessments of disease activity.[8–10] For example, in the LUMINA cohort, 58% of patients had a significant disagreement regarding their disease activity compared with their physicians' assessments.[10]

Given that known biologic and physiologic parameters seem to only modestly affect individual perceptions of symptoms in SLE, what other factors have a role? As depicted in **Fig. 1**, a variety of things are postulated to influence the perception of symptoms. In SLE, a few studies have attempted to further investigate these influences. Adams and colleagues[11] found a relationship among psychological factors (stress, depression, anxiety, and anger) and SLE symptoms in a small study of 41 patients, particularly among a group whom they termed "stress responders." Similarly, in a study that followed 23 patients with SLE prospectively every 2 weeks for up to 40 weeks, Ward and colleagues[12] demonstrated that changes in depression and anxiety scores were correlated with simultaneous changes in patients' global assessments of their SLE activity. Other studies have also found that assessment of disease status by patients is influenced by their psychological well-being.[8,9]

Beyond understanding the multidimensional inputs into HRQOL, these findings have broader implications for patient care and medical care. Addressing the symptoms that patients experience requires a comprehensive approach that reaches beyond overt biologic and physiologic parameters. Similarly, in trying to understand the effects of costs associated with SLE, and why these differ significantly among patient groups, factors beyond assessments of disease activity must be considered.

Functional Status

The next central area depicted in the Wilson and Cleary[2] model is functional status. Functional status can be considered broadly as a patient's ability to perform a variety of activities, and encompasses not only physical function but also social role and psychological function. In **Fig. 1**, symptoms are one important influence on functional status, but a variety of other inputs are often present. Again, for clinicians, this may be intuitive; 2 patients with similar SLE symptoms may have vastly different functioning. Social support, levels of helplessness, illness-related behaviors, environment, and access to medical care are just some of factors that may influence functional outcomes.

Decrements in functional status in SLE have been well documented. All domains of function seem to be influenced by the disease, although some seem more affected than others. Reductions in physical function in SLE are substantial compared with individuals with other chronic medical conditions (hypertension, diabetes, depression, myocardial infarction) and the general population,[13–16] although they seem less severe than in RA. In the LUMINA cohort, Alarcon and colleagues[17] demonstrated that a variety of factors influence physical functioning in SLE beyond disease activity: lower socioeconomic status assessed at baseline predicted poorer physical functioning, as did higher degrees of helplessness, abnormal illness-related behaviors, and lower social support. Similarly, other studies have demonstrated that poor social support was associated with lower functional status.[14,18]

Social functioning, which is defined by normative behaviors in social situations, is also severely affected by SLE compared with the general population and to those with other chronic medical conditions; impairments in SLE are similar to those in individuals with depression.[13,14,16] In addition to higher disease activity, lower socioeconomic status, higher levels of helplessness, abnormal illness-related behaviors, and poorer social support all predict lower social functioning.[17]

Using a novel measure set, valued life activities (VLAs; a wide range of life activities deemed to be important by the individual), that moves beyond the basic functional status items examined in the studies mentioned earlier, Katz and colleagues[19] demonstrated significant impairments in SLE. Discretionary VLAs, such as leisure activities, social activities, and hobbies were more severely affected by SLE than obligatory VLAs, such as basic self-care, driving a car, or using transit. Although disease-related factors played a role, additional factors such as low educational attainment or cognitive impairment also influenced VLA impairment.

Reductions in psychological functioning in SLE are also substantial. Understanding the factors contributing to poor psychological function in SLE is complex, given that the disease itself has neuropsychiatric manifestations with direct effects on mood (eg, cerebrovascular accidents, cortical inflammation, and seizures). Studies evaluating the relationship between disease activity and psychological functioning are mixed, and comparisons are difficult because findings seem to depend on the disease activity measure that was assessed. For example, several studies using the SLEDAI found no significant relationship with the psychological functioning domain of SF-36,[15,20,21] although a study using the Mexican version of the SLEDAI did find a relationship.[22] Most, but not all, studies that have used the British Isles Lupus Activity Score (BILAG) or the Systemic Lupus Activity Measure (SLAM) seem to demonstrate some relationship between disease activity and psychological functioning.[23,24] In the LUMINA cohort, even after disease activity is accounted for, lower socioeconomic status, higher degrees of helplessness, abnormal illness-related behaviors, and poorer social support seem to have a role in psychological functioning.[17]

The Wilson and Cleary[2] model has directionality, implying that biologic and physiologic parameters are among the factors that lead to symptoms, and symptoms are among the factors that lead to decrements in functional status. Although the predominant causal relationships therefore run from left to right in the model, there may be instances in which reverse relationships also exist (eg, depression leading to altered biologic or physiologic variables). Painting a more accurate picture regarding the multidimensional inputs into functional status will require further research; however, the growing literature cited earlier supports the view that a broad-based, multidisciplinary approach is required to characterize and understand functional impairments in SLE.

General Health Perceptions and Overall Quality of Life

As patients subjectively respond to the previous factors discussed in the model (symptoms, functional status, individual characteristics, and the environment), the more global concept of general health perceptions emerges. One of the fascinating aspects of subjective assessments of general health relates to their powerful predictive value. Numerous studies have demonstrated that self-rated health is a predictor of mortality, even when specific health status indicators and other relevant covariates that are known to predict mortality are taken into account.[25]

In SLE, studies have demonstrated that a significant proportion of patients rate their general health as poor. For example, in a study using 3 large observational cohorts, individuals with SLE were more likely to rate their health as poor (47%) compared with individuals with RA (37%) or COPD (40%).[26] Whether or not these ratings are associated with mortality in SLE, as they are in a variety of other chronic health conditions, requires further investigation, although preliminary data from one small study in Brazil found that self-rated health was among the predictors of mortality in a group of 63 patients.[27]

The studies discussed earlier illustrate the validity of the Wilson and Cleary[2] model, and suggest that it provides a useful framework for thinking broadly about the concept of HRQOL in SLE.

Measuring HRQOL in SLE

The previous section illustrates the multidimensional inputs into the concept of HRQOL. With this framework in mind, how should HRQOL in patients be assessed? Several measures have been developed during the last several decades that attempt to measure HRQOL in SLE. However, commonly used instruments cover a variety of different domains (**Table 1**). Although there are several types of measures that conform to the general rubric of HRQOL, this article focuses on 2 main categories: generic HRQOL measures and SLE-specific measures. Other measures, such as utility-based measures (which incorporate preferences and are commonly used for economic evaluations), individualized measures (which allow patients to weigh the importance of items in their own life), and dimension-specific measures (which focus on a single area of HRQOL such as fatigue or depression) are not discussed here.[31]

Generic Instruments

A variety of generic measures are available and several have been validated in SLE (**Tables 1** and **2**). Generic HRQOL measures generally include a variety of domains. For example, the most commonly used generic HRQOL instrument in SLE, the Medical Outcomes Study Short Form 36 (SF-36), incorporates physical functioning, role limitations because of physical problems, bodily pain, general health, social functioning, mental health, role limitations because of emotional problems, and vitality.

Generic instruments have significant advantages but also notable disadvantages. A benefit is that they allow comparison of the HRQOL in one condition to other related conditions or to population norms, something that has been useful in documenting that SLE has similar or worse HRQOL decrements compared with other severe chronic conditions.[13] In addition, many generic instruments have undergone validation testing and may be available in different languages. The major drawback to generic instruments in SLE is that they may not capture symptoms or issues that are specific to the disease, and, therefore, may have reduced sensitivity to detect meaningful changes over time. For example, there is some literature to suggest that the SF-36 is insufficiently sensitive to change in longitudinal studies,[29,35] and may lack domains that are particularly relevant to a population with SLE, such as fatigue or sleep.[36] In contrast, results from recent clinical trials show that the instrument may respond to change over the short-term,[37,38] findings that emphasize the need to carefully examine the psychometric properties of an instrument before using it in different demographic groups, regions, or settings.

Generic instruments have been used for some time in observational studies of SLE, but the addition of these measures routinely to clinical trials is a new development. Many recent studies, including trials investigating treatment with dehydroepiandrosterone,[39] mycophenolate mofetil versus oral cyclophosphamide,[40] abetimus sodium,[41] and belimumab[38] have included HRQOL measures (and all used the SF-36 in addition to other measures). These trials demonstrated that generic HRQOL measures may demonstrate responses to treatment that are not necessarily captured with traditional disease activity and damage assessments. As the use of these instruments increases, further information about their psychometric properties and how to interpret improvements or decrements in scores related to specific therapies will likely be forthcoming. Therefore, several groups have recommended the use of HRQOL measures as routine end points in SLE studies in the future.[42,43]

SLE-specific Instruments

To date, 4 SLE-specific HRQOL instruments are available, although additional measures are in development (see **Table 1**). As opposed to generic instruments, these measures were designed to measure HRQOL among individuals with SLE, and therefore focus on the specific challenges and issues important to patients with the disease. Some were developed with structured input from patients regarding how the disease has affected their lives. For example, McElhone and colleagues[30] performed 30 face-to-face recorded interviews with patients as the first step in developing items for the LupusQoL. Instruments such as this are likely to capture the concepts relevant to individuals with SLE more accurately. However, because notions of HRQOL can vary significantly among persons from different demographic groups or from different countries, further validation work is needed before application in settings where the instruments have not been tested.

As illustrated in **Table 2**, preliminary validation work has been done for some of these instruments in defined populations, although further work is needed. Such measures will likely have a place in SLE studies in the future, although as mentioned earlier, their use precludes comparing HRQOL across conditions or in the general population.

Choosing an HRQOL Measure in SLE

The previous 2 sections outline a conceptual overview of HRQOL in SLE and briefly discuss available instruments and their characteristics. This section summarizes the relevant issues in selecting an HRQOL instrument for use in clinical practice or research.

Table 1
Examples of HRQOL measures used in SLE

Measures	No. of Items	Domains	Scores Derived	Item Responses	Score Range	Administration	Time to Complete
SLE-specific measures							
Lupus Quality of Life (L-QoL)[28]	25	Overall effect of SLE and its treatment on patient	Count of symptoms	Yes/no	0–25	Self-completed	<5 min
SLE Symptom Checklist (SSC)[7]	38	Checklist of disease and treatment related physical symptoms	Count of symptoms	Yes/no, followed by 4-point response for yes responses	0–38	Self-completed	<10 min
SLE Quality of Life (SLEQoL)[29]	40	6 (physical functioning, activities, symptoms, treatment, mood, self-image)	Summary score	7-point response	40–280	Self-completed	Not reported
Lupus Quality of Life (LupusQoL)[30]	34	8 (physical health, emotional health, body image, pain, fatigue, planning, intimate relationships, and burden to others)	Subscale scores for the 8 domains	5-point response	Scores are standardized to range 0–100	Self-completed	<10 min

Generic instruments

Instrument	Items	Domains	Scores	Response scale	Scoring/range	Administration	Time
Medical Outcomes Study Short Form (SF-36)[50]	36	8 (physical function, physical role function, vitality, bodily pain, mental health, emotional role function, social function, general health perceptions)	Subscale scores for the 8 domains. 2 summary scores (Physical and Mental Component Scores)	Mixture of 3, 5 and 6-point response scales	Scores are standardized to range 0–100	Self-completed to interviewer-administered	10–15 min
Quality of Life Scale (QOLs)[51]	16	5 (material and physical well-being, relationships, social/community/civic activities, personal development and fulfillment, recreation)	Total score	7-point scale	16–112	Self-administered or interview-administered	5 min
European Quality of Life Scale (EuroQoL)[32]	5	5 (mobility, self-care, usual activities, pain/discomfort, anxiety/depression) and VAS for overall general health	3 scores: a profile (5-digit descriptor indicating extent of problems in each domain), a population preference-weighted index, and VAS	3-level response and a VAS	Profile score: 5-digit descriptor (lists scores ranging from 1 to 3 for all 5 dimensions, eg, 33,333). Index score: –0.11 to 1	Self-completed	2 min

(continued on next page)

Table 1
(*continued*)

Measures	No. of Items	Domains	Scores Derived	Item Responses	Score Range	Administration	Time to Complete
Sickness Impact Profile (SIP)[33]	136	2 domains, 12 categories (sleep and rest, eating, work, home management, recreation and pastimes, ambulation, mobility, body care and movement, social interaction, alertness behavior, emotional behavior, communication)	12 category scores, 2 domain scores and a total score	Respondents check items that describe them on a given day; items weighted to reflect the relative severity of each statement	0–100	Self-completed or interviewer-administered	20–30 min
WHOQoL-Bref[34]	26	4 (physical health, psychological health, social relationships, environment) and overall quality of life and health	4 domain scores, raw scores can then be transformed to 0–100 scale	5-level response	0–100	Self-completed or interview-administered	10 min

	Construct Validity	Internal Consistency	Test-retest Reliability	Floor and Ceiling Effects	Responsiveness
Table 2					
Psychometric properties of commonly used HRQOL instruments in SLE					
Measures					
SLE-specific measures					
L-QoL[28]	✔'	✔	✔		
SSC[29,52]	✔	✔	✔		✔
SLEQoL[7,52]	✔	✔	✔	✔	✔
LupusQoL[30,53,54]	✔	✔	✔	✔	
Generic instruments					
SF-36[29,35,41,55]	✔	✔	✔	✔	✔
QOLs[56]	✔	✔	✔		
EuroQol[57,58]	✔	–	✔	✔	✔
SIP[59]	✔	✔	✔		
WHOQoL-Bref[60]	✔				

Checkmarks indicate that at least 1 published study has examined that psychometric property in patients specifically with SLE.

Abbreviations: L-QoL, Lupus Quality of Life; LupusQoL, Lupus Quality of Life; SF-36, Medical Outcomes Study Short Form 36; SIP, Sickness Impact Profile; SLEQoL, SLE Quality of Life; SSC, SLE Symptom Checklist.

There are 4 questions to consider when selecting an instrument:

1. Are the domains covered by the instrument relevant to the question or use at hand? As illustrated in **Table 1**, available HRQOL instruments in SLE cover a variety of different domains. Given the complexity and multiple inputs to HRQOL (see **Fig. 1**), available measures are unlikely to capture all relevant concepts. Increasingly, SLE researchers are using several instruments concomitantly (generic instruments and disease-specific instruments) in clinical trials and population-based studies.

2. Have sufficient validation studies been performed to assure that the instrument is psychometrically sound (valid, reliable, and responsive)? As illustrated in **Table 2**, HRQOL instruments currently used in SLE have undergone varying degrees of testing. Even if such testing has been performed, it is important to remember that validation of HRQOL instruments is always a work in progress. A single validation study in a particular demographic group or region does not always seamlessly apply to other populations. Generally, the more validation studies available demonstrating similar psychometric properties, the more likely that the instrument will behave similarly in future applications.

3. Are there floor and ceiling effects that are relevant? A ceiling effect is when individuals with the best score may still have substantial HRQOL impairment that is not captured by the instrument. Alternatively, a floor effect is when patients with the worst score may deteriorate further (see **Table 2**). In some cases, this lack of variability can seriously compromise the usefulness of the measurement.

4. What resources are available to assess HRQOL? All HRQOL instruments are subjective; that is, in attempting to capture the patient's perspective, they must be reported by the patient. Several methods are available to achieve this objective. Commonly used methods include in-person interviews, telephone interviews, and self-completed questionnaires. Therefore, choosing an instrument entails careful assessment of resources (in-person interviews are most expensive, self-completed

questionnaires less expensive, and telephone interview methods somewhere in between) and yield (methods based on in-person and telephone interviews generally have higher response rates, whereas self-completed questionnaires have lower response rates). Attention to whether the instrument has been validated using the chosen administration route is also important (see **Table 1**).

Employment

Although, as indicated at the beginning of this article, work may not be central to the lives of all persons of working age, it is often the portal to activities that are central. For example, it may provide the resources to travel or to partake in hobbies. It is also crucial to the accumulation of assets that can provide for an adequate standard of living in retirement. In the HRQOL scheme developed by Wilson and Cleary,[2] employment would be captured by the functional status domain. Because of the integrative set of skills necessary to sustain employment, it would be categorized in the subdomain of social role participation.

The literature on work loss associated with chronic disease in general emanates disproportionately from medical researchers rather than labor market analysts. The latter tend to be more precise in defining employment in a manner consistent with national unemployment statistics, with the consequence that not all the studies use the same terms to estimate the employment rate and to provide consistent inclusion and exclusion criteria.[1] However, the level of precision may not matter in SLE because the effect of this condition on employment is so great.

Fig. 2, from the review article by Baker and Pope,[1] summarizes the employment results from 23 studies. In all of the studies, the average age of the persons with SLE was between 34 and 47 years, usually the age range at which employment rates peak because almost all people have completed their education. The late 40s is the age at which most of us have achieved seniority in jobs but have not yet been

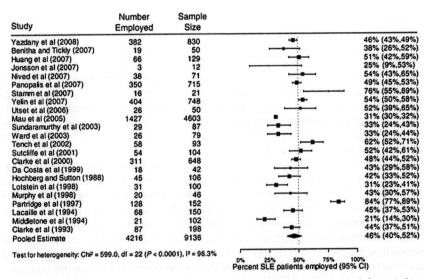

Study	Number Employed	Sample Size		
Yazdany et al (2008)	382	830		46% (43%,49%)
Benitha and Tickly (2007)	19	50		38% (26%,52%)
Huang et al (2007)	66	129		51% (42%,59%)
Jonsson et al (2007)	3	12		25% (9%,53%)
Nived et al (2007)	38	71		54% (43%,65%)
Panopalis et al (2007)	350	715		49% (45%,53%)
Stamm et al (2007)	16	21		76% (55%,89%)
Yelin et al (2007)	404	748		54% (50%,58%)
Utset et al (2006)	26	50		52% (39%,65%)
Mau et al (2005)	1427	4603		31% (30%,32%)
Sundaramurthy et al (2003)	29	87		33% (24%,43%)
Ward et al (2003)	26	79		33% (24%,44%)
Tench et al (2002)	58	93		62% (52%,71%)
Sutcliffe et al (2001)	54	104		52% (42%,61%)
Clarke et al (2000)	311	648		48% (44%,52%)
Da Costa et al (1999)	18	42		43% (29%,58%)
Hochberg and Sutton (1988)	45	106		42% (33%,52%)
Lotstein et al (1998)	31	100		31% (23%,41%)
Murphy et al (1998)	20	46		43% (30%,57%)
Partridge et al (1997)	128	152		84% (77%,89%)
Lacaille et al (1994)	68	150		45% (37%,53%)
Middletone et al (1994)	21	102		21% (14%,30%)
Clarke et al (1993)	87	198		44% (37%,51%)
Pooled Estimate	4216	9136		46% (40%,52%)

Test for heterogeneity: Chi² = 599.0, df = 22 (P < 0.0001), I² = 96.3%

0%   25%   50%   75%   100%
Percent SLE patients employed (95% CI)

Fig. 2. Meta-analysis of percentage of SLE patients employed. (*Adapted from* Baker K, Pope J. Employment and work disability in systemic lupus erythematosus: a systematic review. Rheumatology (Oxford) 2009;48(3):283; with permission.)

subjected to age-related job displacement. It is therefore telling that, on average, only 46% of persons with SLE reported being employed. The largest study[44] was from Germany, and reported one of the lowest employment rates. The next 4 largest studies used similar methods and reported employment rates of between 46% and 54%,[45–48] consistent with the overall results. The overall results, disproportionately affected by the other large studies, indicate that slightly less than half of working age adults with SLE are employed.

How does that compare with employment rates among people without SLE? In the United States as a whole, in 2007, fewer than 80% of persons aged 45 to 54 years were employed. In SLE, of course, most of those affected are women. In 2007, approximately 74% of women of these ages were employed. Thus, the employment rate of persons with SLE is 38% lower than the rate among women aged 45 to 54 years, and 43% lower than all people of these ages.

Overall employment rates mask the volatility of employment among persons with SLE. In 2 studies, the authors have estimated the frequency with which transitions between being employed and not employed occur. (We have avoided using the term "unemployed" to connote not working because "unemployed" in the United States means that one is not working but is actively looking for work. Most of those not employed are not actively looking for work.) In the first study,[48] we used retrospective data among those with SLE to estimate transitions in employment status between diagnosis of SLE and the study year, an average of slightly more than 12 years later. At diagnosis, 74% of the persons with SLE had been employed, but as of the study year, only 55% were employed. Accordingly, there was a substantial decline in the percentage employed. **Fig. 3**, reprinted from that study, shows the percentage employed by the number of years since diagnosis among those employed at that time. By 5 years after diagnosis, 15% had stopped working; by 10, 15, and 20 years, slightly more than a third, slightly more than a half, and slightly less than two-thirds had stopped working.

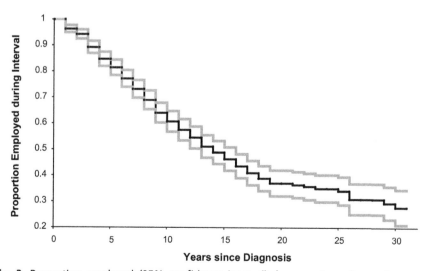

Fig. 3. Proportion employed (95% confidence interval), by year since diagnosis, among persons with SLE aged less than 65 years who were employed at diagnosis. (*Adapted from* Yelin E, Trupin L, Katz P, et al. Work dynamics among persons with systemic lupus erythematosus. Arthritis Rheum 2007;57(1):60; with permission.)

Overall, among those employed at diagnosis, 41% had stopped working by the study year, an average of about 13 years after diagnosis. However, among the 26% not employed at diagnosis, 40% started working. Thus, despite the overall decline in the percentage working, there was substantial movement into and out of employment.

In the second study,[49] we tracked transitions in employment prospectively from the baseline year of a longitudinal cohort and compared the frequency of such transitions to those of a matched sample nationally. Rates of work loss did not differ between persons with SLE and the matched sample until age 55 years. Presumably this is because, in the United States labor market, transitions out of work are the norm. However, rates of work entry were lower among persons with SLE less than 55 years old, suggesting that when they lose jobs they are less likely to reenter the labor market than their peers. Nor are they able to accommodate decreased ability to work by reduction in hours. Among all persons with SLE ever employed, annual work hours declined by about a third between the year of diagnosis and the study year, but such hours only declined by 1% among those continuously employed.[48]

Thus, because work entry once work loss occurs is less common than among their peers, and because reduction in work hours is uncommon, helping persons with SLE retain employment is crucial to their welfare.

In their review of the literature concerning work disability among persons with SLE, Baker and Pope[1] note that disease characteristics (higher levels of activity, longer duration, and select manifestations, particularly neurocognitive deficits); poorer physical function; demographics (age and race); lower socioeconomic status; and the nature of work (physically demanding work and jobs with high psychological demands and low levels of autonomy) all predispose to higher rates of work loss. To put these results in the context of the Wilson and Cleary[2] model, all of the precursor domains, including biologic and physiologic variables, symptoms, characteristics of individuals and of the environment contribute to employment outcomes.

In our prospective study of employment dynamics[49] we observed that persons with SLE who had been out of work a longer time were significantly less likely to enter new jobs, again indicating that helping persons with this condition to maintain employment may be the most effective strategy.

SUMMARY

SLE has a profound effect on HRQOL across a variety of domains, including symptoms, functional status, and general health perceptions, and results in significant reductions in employment. Current evidence supports the validity of examining HRQOL in SLE as a multidimensional construct influenced by a variety of individual characteristics, social circumstances, and environmental factors. As further studies elucidate the factors that affect HRQOL, measurement tools that capture meaningful change in this important construct will likely be forthcoming and will play a valuable role in the evaluation of outcomes in SLE clinical care, observational studies, and clinical trials. As these studies emerge, it will be helpful to evaluate them in the context of the model of HRQOL outlined by Wilson and Cleary[2] so that the reader can situate the results of each study in the context of the pathway from biologic and pathophysiologic factors at one end of the spectrum, to integrative measures of overall quality of life at the other.

REFERENCES

1. Baker K, Pope J. Employment and work disability in systemic lupus erythematosus: a systematic review. Rheumatology (Oxford) 2009;48(3):281–4.

2. Wilson I, Cleary P. Linking clinical variables with health-related quality of life. A conceptual model of patient outcomes. JAMA 1995;273(1):59–65.

3. Nagi S. An epidemiology of disability in the United States. Milbank Mem Fund Q Health Soc 1976;54:439–68.

4. Yelin E, Nevitt M, Epstein W. Toward an epidemiology of work disability. Milbank Mem Fund Q Health Soc 1980;58(3):386–415.

5. Verbrugge L, Jette A. The disablement process. Soc Sci Med 1994;38(1):1–14.

6. Karlson EW, Daltroy LH, Rivest C, et al. Validation of a Systemic Lupus Activity Questionnaire (SLAQ) for population studies. Lupus 2003;12(4):280–6.

7. Grootscholten C, Ligtenberg G, Derksen RH, et al. Health-related quality of life in patients with systemic lupus erythematosus: development and validation of a lupus specific symptom checklist. Qual Life Res 2003;12(6):635–44.

8. Neville C, Clarke AE, Joseph L, et al. Learning from discordance in patient and physician global assessments of systemic lupus erythematosus disease activity. J Rheumatol 2000;27(3):675–9.

9. Yen JC, Abrahamowicz M, Dobkin PL, et al. Determinants of discordance between patients and physicians in their assessment of lupus disease activity. J Rheumatol 2003;30(9):1967–76.

10. Alarcon GS, McGwin G Jr, Brooks K, et al. Systemic lupus erythematosus in three ethnic groups. XI. Sources of discrepancy in perception of disease activity: a comparison of physician and patient visual analog scale scores. Arthritis Rheum 2002;47(4):408–13.

11. Adams SG Jr, Dammers PM, Saia TL, et al. Stress, depression, and anxiety predict average symptom severity and daily symptom fluctuation in systemic lupus erythematosus. J Behav Med 1994;17(5):459–77.

12. Ward MM, Marx AS, Barry NN. Psychological distress and changes in the activity of systemic lupus erythematosus. Rheumatology (Oxford) 2002;41(2):184–8.

13. Jolly M. How does quality of life of patients with systemic lupus erythematosus compare with that of other common chronic illnesses? J Rheumatol 2005;32(9): 1706–8.

14. Sutcliffe N, Clarke AE, Levinton C, et al. Associates of health status in patients with systemic lupus erythematosus. J Rheumatol 1999;26(11):2352–6.

15. Gilboe IM, Kvien TK, Husby G. Health status in systemic lupus erythematosus compared to rheumatoid arthritis and healthy controls. J Rheumatol 1999;26(8): 1694–700.

16. Zheng Y, Ye DQ, Pan HF, et al. Influence of social support on health-related quality of life in patients with systemic lupus erythematosus. Clin Rheumatol 2009;28(3):265–9.

17. Alarcon GS, McGwin G Jr, Uribe A, et al. Systemic lupus erythematosus in a multi-ethnic lupus cohort (LUMINA). XVII. Predictors of self-reported health-related quality of life early in the disease course. Arthritis Rheum 2004;51(3):465–74.

18. Karlson EW, Daltroy LH, Lew RA, et al. The relationship of socioeconomic status, race, and modifiable risk factors to outcomes in patients with systemic lupus erythematosus. Arthritis Rheum 1997;40(1):47–56.

19. Katz P, Morris A, Trupin L, et al. Disability in valued life activities among individuals with systemic lupus erythematosus. Arth Care Res 2008;59(4):465–73.

20. Gladman DD, Urowitz MB, Gough J, et al. Fibromyalgia is a major contributor to quality of life in lupus. J Rheumatol 1997;24(11):2145–8.

21. Vu TV, Escalante A. A comparison of the quality of life of patients with systemic lupus erythematosus with and without endstage renal disease. J Rheumatol 1999;26(12):2595–601.

22. Khanna S, Pal H, Pandey RM, et al. The relationship between disease activity and quality of life in systemic lupus erythematosus. Rheumatology (Oxford) 2004; 43(12):1536–40.
23. Dobkin PL, Da Costa D, Dritsa M, et al. Quality of life in systemic lupus erythematosus patients during more and less active disease states: differential contributors to mental and physical health. Arthritis Care Res 1999;12(6):401–10.
24. Saba J, Quinet RJ, Davis WE, et al. Inverse correlation of each functional status scale of the SF-36 with degree of disease activity in systemic lupus erythematosus (m-SLAM). Joint Bone Spine 2003;70(5):348–51.
25. Idler EL, Benyamini Y. Self-rated health and mortality: a review of twenty-seven community studies. J Health Soc Behav 1997;38(1):21–37.
26. Katz P, Morris A, Gregorich S, et al. Valued life activity disability played a significant role in self-rated health among adults with chronic health conditions. J Clin Epidemiol 2009;62(2):158–66.
27. Freire E, Bruscato A, Ciconelli R. Quality of life in systemic lupus erythematosus patients in northeastern Brazil: is health-related quality of life a predictor of survival for these patients? Acta Reumatol Port 2009;34(2A):207–11.
28. Doward LC, McKenna SP, Whalley D, et al. The development of the L-QoL: a quality-of-life instrument specific to systemic lupus erythematosus. Ann Rheum Dis 2009;68(2):196–200.
29. Leong KP, Kong KO, Thong BY, et al. Development and preliminary validation of a systemic lupus erythematosus-specific quality-of-life instrument (SLEQOL). Rheumatology (Oxford) 2005;44(10):1267–76.
30. McElhone K, Abbott J, Shelmerdine J, et al. Development and validation of a disease-specific health-related quality of life measure, the LupusQol, for adults with systemic lupus erythematosus. Arthritis Rheum 2007;57(6):972–9.
31. Garratt A, Schmidt L, Mackintosh A, et al. Quality of life measurement: bibliographic study of patient assessed health outcome measures. BMJ 2002; 324(7351):1417.
32. EuroQol–a new facility for the measurement of health-related quality of life. The EuroQol Group. Health Policy 1990;16(3):199–208.
33. Bergner M, Bobbitt RA, Carter WB, et al. The sickness impact profile: development and final revision of a health status measure. Med Care 1981;19(8): 787–805.
34. The World Health Organization Quality of Life Assessment (WHOQOL): development and general psychometric properties. Soc Sci Med 1998;46(12):1569–85.
35. Kuriya B, Gladman DD, Ibanez D, et al. Quality of life over time in patients with systemic lupus erythematosus. Arthritis Rheum 2008;59(2):181–5.
36. Moses N, Wiggers J, Nicholas C, et al. Prevalence and correlates of perceived unmet needs of people with systemic lupus erythematosus. Patient Educ Couns 2005;57(1):30–8.
37. Strand V, Aranow C, Cardiel MH, et al. Improvement in health-related quality of life in systemic lupus erythematosus patients enrolled in a randomized clinical trial comparing LJP 394 treatment with placebo. Lupus 2003;12(9):677–86.
38. Wallace DJ, Stohl W, Furie RA, et al. A phase II, randomized, double-blind, placebo-controlled, dose-ranging study of belimumab in patients with active systemic lupus erythematosus. Arthritis Rheum 2009;61(9):1168–78.
39. Nordmark G, Bengtsson C, Larsson A, et al. Effects of dehydroepiandrosterone supplement on health-related quality of life in glucocorticoid treated female patients with systemic lupus erythematosus. Autoimmunity 2005;38(7): 531–40.

40. Tse KC, Tang CS, Lio WI, et al. Quality of life comparison between corticosteroid-and-mycofenolate mofetil and corticosteroid- and-oral cyclophosphamide in the treatment of severe lupus nephritis. Lupus 2006;15(6):371–9.

41. Strand V, Crawford B. Improvement in health-related quality of life in patients with SLE following sustained reductions in anti-dsDNA antibodies. Expert Rev Pharmacoecon Outcomes Res 2005;5(3):317–26.

42. Bertsias G, Gordon C, Boumpas DT. Clinical trials in systemic lupus erythematosus (SLE): lessons from the past as we proceed to the future–the EULAR recommendations for the management of SLE and the use of end-points in clinical trials. Lupus 2008;17(5):437–42.

43. Gladman D, Urowitz M, Fortin P, et al. Systemic Lupus International Collaborating Clinics conference on assessment of lupus flare and quality of life measures in SLE. Systemic Lupus International Collaborating Clinics Group. J Rheumatol 1996;23(11):1953–5.

44. Mau W, Listing J, Huscher D, et al. Employment across chronic inflammatory rheumatic diseases and comparison with the general population. J Rheumatol 2005;32(4):571–4.

45. Yazdany J, Yelin E, Panopalis P, et al. Validation of systemic lupus erythematosus activity questionnaire in a large observational cohort. Arth Care Res 2008;59(1):136–43.

46. Panopalis P, Julian L, Yazdany J, et al. Impact of memory impairment on employment status in persons with systemic lupus erythematosus. Arthritis Rheum 2007;57(8):1453–60.

47. Clarke A, Penrod J, St Pierre Y, et al. Underestimating the value of women: assessing the indirect costs of women with systemic lupus erythematosus. J Rheumatol 2000;27:2597–604.

48. Yelin E, Trupin L, Katz P, et al. Work dynamics among persons with systemic lupus erythematosus. Arthritis Rheum 2007;57(1):56–63.

49. Yelin E, Tonner C, Trupin L, et al. Work loss and work entry among persons with systemic lupus erythematosus: comparisons with a national matched sample. Arthritis Rheum 2009;61(2):247–58.

50. Ware JE Jr, Sherbourne CD. The MOS 36-item short-form health survey (SF-36). I. Conceptual framework and item selection. Med Care 1992;30(6):473–83.

51. Burckhardt CS, Anderson KL. The Quality of Life Scale (QOLS): reliability, validity, and utilization. Health Qual Life Outcomes 2003;1:60.

52. Leong KP, Kong KO, Thong BY, et al. Psychometric properties of a new systemic lupus erythematosus-specific quality-of-life instrument (SLEQOL). Ann Acad Med Singap 2004;33(Suppl 5):S35–7.

53. Gonzalez-Rodriguez V, Peralta-Ramirez MI, Navarrete-Navarrete N, et al. [Adaptation and validation of the Spanish version of a disease-specific quality of life measure in patients with systemic lupus erythematosus: the lupus quality of life]. Med Clin (Barc) 2010;134(1):13–6 [in Spanish].

54. Jolly M, Pickard AS, Wilke C, et al. Lupus specific health outcome measure for US patients: the LupusQoL-US Version(C). Ann Rheum Dis 2010;69:29–33.

55. Stoll T, Gordon C, Seifert B, et al. Consistency and validity of patient administered assessment of quality of life by the MOS SF-36; its association with disease activity and damage in patients with systemic lupus erythematosus. J Rheumatol 1997;24(8):1608–14.

56. Burckhardt CS, Archenholtz B, Bjelle A. Measuring the quality of life of women with rheumatoid arthritis or systemic lupus erythematosus: a Swedish version of the Quality of Life Scale (QOLS). Scand J Rheumatol 1992;21(4):190–5.

57. Aggarwal R, Wilke CT, Pickard AS, et al. Psychometric properties of the EuroQol-5D and Short Form-6D in patients with systemic lupus erythematosus. J Rheumatol 2009;36(6):1209–16.

58. Wang C, Mayo NE, Fortin PR. The relationship between health related quality of life and disease activity and damage in systemic lupus erythematosus. J Rheumatol 2001;28(3):525–32.

59. Lash A. Quality of life in systemic lupus erythematosus. Appl Nurs Res 1998; 11(3):130–7.

60. Abu-Shakra M, Keren A, Livshitz I, et al. Sense of coherence and its impact on quality of life of patients with systemic lupus erythematosus. Lupus 2006;15(1): 32–7.

Cutaneous Lupus and the Cutaneous Lupus Erythematosus Disease Area and Severity Index Instrument

Rachel S. Klein, BA[a,b], Pamela A. Morganroth, MS[a,b], Victoria P. Werth, MD[a,b],*

KEYWORDS

- Cutaneous lupus erythematosus • Disease classification
- Rowell syndrome • CLASI • Clinical outcome instrument

This article provides an overview of cutaneous lupus erythematosus (CLE), including classification schemes, disease subtypes, and therapy. It also describes the Cutaneous Lupus Erythematosus Disease Area and Severity Index (CLASI), a novel clinical outcome instrument that quantifies cutaneous activity and damage in CLE.

OVERVIEW OF CUTANEOUS LUPUS ERYTHEMATOSUS
Disease Classification

CLE skin lesions have been divided into two categories based on histopathology: lupus erythematosus (LE)–specific (histopathology shows interface dermatitis, which is specific for LE) and LE-nonspecific (no interface dermatitis; histopathology is not specific for LE).[1,2] The diagnosis of CLE can be confirmed by the presence of LE-specific lesions, whereas LE-nonspecific lesions may be seen in several diseases and thus are not sufficient for establishing a diagnosis of CLE. LE-specific skin lesions

---

R.S. Klein and P.A. Morganroth contributed equally.

This material is based upon work supported by the National Institutes of Health, including NIH grant K24-AR 02207 (Werth) and NIH training grant T32-AR007465-25 (Klein). This work was also partially supported by a Merit Review Grant from the Department of Veterans Affairs, Veterans Health Administration, Office of Research and Development, Biomedical Laboratory Research and Development.

[a] Philadelphia VA Medical Center, Philadelphia, PA, USA

[b] Department of Dermatology, University of Pennsylvania School of Medicine, Suite 1-330A, 3400 Civic Center Boulevard, Philadelphia, PA 19104, USA

* Corresponding author. Department of Dermatology, University of Pennsylvania School of Medicine, Suite 1-330A, 3400 Civic Center Boulevard, Philadelphia, PA 19104.

E-mail address: werth@mail.med.upenn.edu (V.P. Werth).

Rheum Dis Clin N Am 36 (2010) 33–51

doi:10.1016/j.rdc.2009.12.001

rheumatic.theclinics.com

can be further subdivided based on clinical characteristics into acute CLE (ACLE), subacute CLE (SCLE), and chronic CLE (CCLE).[2] **Box 1**[2-4] summarizes the classification of skin lesions seen in lupus erythematosus patients.

The risk of systemic LE (SLE) is highest in ACLE and lowest in CCLE, with SCLE falling in between. In one study of 191 patients with LE-specific skin lesions, the prevalence of underlying SLE was 72% in all patients with ACLE lesions, 58% in all patients with SCLE lesions, 28% in all patients with discoid LE (DLE) lesions (the most common type of CCLE), and 6% in all patients with localized DLE lesions (limited to the head and neck).[6] Many patients from this study had lesions from more than one clinical category (ACLE, SCLE, or CCLE), and some had lesions from all three categories. In patients with DLE lesions but no ACLE or SCLE lesions, the underlying prevalence of SLE was 15%.

Chronic cutaneous lupus erythematosus and the lupus erythematosus tumidus controversy

CCLE is a photosensitive dermatosis characterized by chronic lesions that may last for many months and produce scarring and atrophy. SLE and lupus-associated antibodies are uncommon in DLE.[6,7] Classic DLE, which can be either localized (confined to head and neck) or generalized (above and below the neck), is the most frequent presentation of CCLE.[6] Systemic symptoms and laboratory abnormalities occur more frequently in patients with generalized DLE than in patients with localized DLE.[6,8] DLE lesions are typically erythematous indurated plaques with keratotic scale. Follicular plugging (dilated follicles plugged with keratin) is also characteristic. When lesions heal, they classically leave behind atrophic scars (scarring alopecia on the scalp) and dyspigmentation. Variants of DLE include hypertropic DLE (thick hyperkeratotic plaques, which may be confused with squamous cell carcinoma clinically and histologically),[9] mucosal DLE (oral, conjunctival, nasal, and genital lesions),[10] and lichenoid DLE (DLE and lichen planus overlap).[11]

Other types of CCLE lesions include lupus panniculitis (lupus profundus) and chilblain (acral) LE. Lupus panniculitis manifests clinically as deep, tender subcutaneous nodules that heal with lipoatrophy.[12] DLE lesions or ulceration may overlay the subcutaneous nodules. A biopsy is needed to exclude subcutaneous panniculitis-like T cell lymphoma from the clinical differential diagnosis.[13] As with DLE, the risk of SLE in lupus panniculitis patients is low: In one case series of 40 lupus panniculitis patients, 10% fulfilled the criteria for SLE.[14] Chilblain LE, a rare type of CCLE induced by cold temperatures, presents as erythematous papules localized to acral areas.[15] In a series of 15 patients with chilblain LE, 20% had underlying SLE.[16]

Most dermatologists also include LE tumidus (papulomucinous LE) in the CCLE category, but this is controversial. LE tumidus lesions are erythematous plaques with an urticaria-like morphology and no clinically visible epidermal changes.[17] Like the other subtypes of CCLE, LE tumidus is a photosensitive dermatosis characterized by chronic or recurrent lesions and a low prevalence of lupus-associated autoantibodies and SLE. One study of 40 LE tumidus patients demonstrated a 10% prevalence of positive antinuclear antibody testing and a 0% prevalence of SLE.[17] However, unlike other CCLE lesions, LE tumidus lesions heal without scarring and atrophy, and LE tumidus lesions are more photosensitive than other forms of CCLE.[18] Furthermore, LE tumidus lesions lack the interface dermatitis that characterizes other LE-specific skin lesions. In a study of 91 LE tumidus biopsy specimens from 80 patients, vacuolar degeneration of the dermoepidermal junction was either absent or was slight and focal.[19] The most frequent histopathologic findings were mucin deposition and a superficial lymphocytic perivascular and periadnexal infiltrate. Some suggest that LE tumidus should be classified as intermittent CLE to reflect the idea that LE tumidus is a distinct clinicopathologic entity with an intermittent, relapsing clinical course and a favorable prognosis.[20] Others argue furthermore that, because LE tumidus lacks the characteristic interface dermatitis of LE-specific lesions and the association with SLE that defines LE-nonspecific lesions, LE tumidus should not be classified among the LE spectrum of skin diseases at all.[21] LE tumidus patients share some clinical and histologic features with non-LE photosensitive skin diseases, such as polymorphous light eruption, lymphocytic infiltrate of Jessner, and reticular erythematous mucinosis,[19] and it may be reasonable to classify LE tumidus within this clinical continuum. As new data enter the literature, the ideal classification of LE tumidus will become more apparent.

Subacute cutaneous lupus erythematosus
The term *subacute* CLE was chosen to reflect the observation that SCLE lesions last longer than the transient malar rash of ACLE but do not produce the chronic, destructive scarring and atrophy seen in CCLE.[22] SCLE typically presents as photosensitive papulosquamous or annular-polycyclic plaques on the back, shoulders, extensor arms, and V-neck. The lesions lack the scale and follicular plugging that characterize DLE lesions. Vesiculobullous lesions can occur, especially around the annular plaques (vesiculobullous annular SCLE).[4] Very rarely, a toxic epidermal necrolysis–like bullous eruption can evolve from otherwise typical SCLE lesions.[23] Patients with SCLE often have the human histocompatibility antigen HLA-DR3 and high titers of antibodies to SSA and SSB.[24] Approximately 50% of SCLE patients fulfill the criteria for SLE,[6] but SLE patients with SCLE appear to have fewer organ systems involved than do SLE patients without SCLE. One study that compared inpatients with both SLE and SCLE to inpatients with only SLE found an increased prevalence of central nervous system disease, renal disease, arthritis, anemia, and pleuritis in the SLE-only group.[25] Another study, which compared outpatients with SCLE (some also had SLE) to outpatients with SLE alone, found an increased frequency of serositis (pleuritis or pericarditis) and hematologic abnormalities (hemolytic anemia, thrombocytopenia, or leukopenia) in the SLE-only group.[26]

Although drug-induced DLE is very rare, numerous drugs have been reported to induce SCLE. Drug-induced SCLE resembles idiopathic SCLE both clinically (papulosquamous or annular-polycyclic photodistributed lesions) and serologically (high prevalence of positive anti-SSA and positive anti-SSB).[27,28] The medication classes that have been implicated most frequently in drug-induced SCLE are antifungals, calcium channel blockers, diuretics, antihistamines, beta-blockers, and chemotherapeutics.[28] Previous reports have documented drug-induced SCLE occurring anywhere from weeks to years following initiation of the culprit drug, and the skin disease may persist for several months after stopping the offending medication.

Acute cutaneous lupus erythematosus
Of the LE-specific lesions, ACLE is most frequently associated with SLE.[6] The usual clinical presentation of ACLE is a transient (hours to days) erythematous photosensitive rash on the malar area (butterfly rash). Less commonly, ACLE patients may have a generalized photosensitive morbilliform rash.[29] ACLE rashes typically spare the nasolabial folds and knuckles, which helps distinguish ACLE from dermatomyositis.[3] Rarely, patients present with a widespread subepidermal bullous eruption resembling toxic epidermal necrolysis, which evolves from otherwise typical photodistributed ACLE lesions.[4]

Box 1
Skin lesions seen in LE, based on the Gilliam classification,[2] the modified Gilliam classification,[5] and the vesiculobullous classification[4]

I. LE-specific skin disease (characterized by interface dermatitis)

A. CCLE

   1. Classic discoid lupus erythematosus (DLE)

      i. Localized DLE

      ii. Generalized DLE

   2. Hypertrophic/verrucous DLE

   3. Lupus panniculitis/lupus profundus

   4. Mucosal DLE

      i. Oral DLE

      ii. Conjunctival DLE

      iii. Nasal DLE

      iv. Genital DLE

   5. LE tumidus/papulomucinous LE[a]

   6. Chilblain LE

   7. Lichenoid DLE (LE–lichen planus overlap)

B. (SCLE)

   1. Annular SCLE

   2. Papulosquamous/psoriasiform

   3. Vesiculobullous annular SCLE

   4. Toxic epidermal necrolysis–like SCLE

C. ACLE

   1. Localized ACLE (malar rash)

   2. Generalized ACLE (morbiliform)

   3. Toxic epidermal necrolysis–like ACLE

II. LE-nonspecific skin disease (no interface dermatitis)

A. Cutaneous vascular disease

   1. Small-vessel cutaneous leukocytoclastic vasculitis secondary to LE

      i. Dependent palpable purpura

      ii. Urticarial vasculitis

   2. Vasculopathy

      i. Degos disease–like lesions

      ii. Secondary atrophie blanche

   3. Periungual telangiectasia

   4. Livedo reticularis

   5. Thrombophlebitis

   6. Raynaud phenomenon

   7. Erythromelalgia

B. Nonscarring alopecia

   1. Lupus hair

   2. Telogen effluvium

   3. Alopecia areata

C. Sclerodactyly

D. Rheumatoid nodules

E. Calcinosis cutis

F. LE-nonspecific bullous lesions (bullous SLE)[b]

G. Urticaria

H. Papulonodular mucinosis

I. Cutis laxa/anetoderma

J. Acanthosis nigricans

K. Erythema multiforme

L. Leg ulcers

M. Lichen planus

[a] LE tumidus lesions do not show interface dermatitis on histopathology. Some propose that LE-tumidus should be classified as intermittent CLE or should not be classified among the LE-spectrum of skin disease.

[b] Includes dermatitis herpetiformis–like, epidermolysis bullosa acquisita–like, and bullous pemphigoid–like vesiculobullous LE

Debate over the existence of Rowell syndrome

Rowell syndrome is a clinical entity that has been a source of confusion in the dermatology literature. In 1963, Rowell and colleagues defined a new syndrome based on four patients who had erythema multiforme–like lesions occurring in association with LE as well as the following immunologic serum abnormalities: speckled pattern of antinuclear antibody, anti-SjT antibody, and rheumatoid factor.[30] Over the next 4 decades, several other investigators reported new cases of Rowell syndrome, but these cases did not meet the same immunologic serum criteria as Rowell's initial patients, possibly because testing for SjT antibody became obsolete. In 2000, Zeitouni[31] proposed new major and minor criteria for Rowell syndrome (diagnosis requires three major criteria and one minor criteria). The new major criteria were LE (systemic, discoid, or subacute), erythema multiforme–like lesions, and speckled antinuclear antibody; and the minor criteria were chilblains, anti-SSA or anti-SSB antibody, and positive rheumatoid factor.

Although dermatologists continue to publish reports of Rowell syndrome in the literature, some doubt that Rowell syndrome is a unique clinical syndrome. These investigators suggest that Rowell syndrome is merely erythema multiforme and LE coexisting in the same patient and that any common serologic abnormalities are likely coincidental.[32] The lack of conservation of Rowell's original serologic criteria in subsequent cases supports this contention. In addition, later reports of Rowell syndrome failed to fit the clinical and demographic profile described in Rowell's original case series.[32] Rowell's patients were females in the third to seventh decade of life who suffered from DLE years before the onset of erythema multiforme lesions and rarely had mucosal erythema multiforme lesions. Later cases deviated from all of these commonalities. Furthermore, a recent report describes two patients who presented with clinical features of combined LE and erythema multiforme but were found to have LE-specific histopathology when the erythema multiforme–like lesions were biopsied. The authors of that report suggest that prior reports of Rowell syndrome may actually represent LE masquerading as erythema multiforme.[33] Further studies will help clarify the significance of erythema multiforme–like lesions in patients with LE.

Lupus erythematosus–nonspecific skin lesions

The wide variety of lesions seen in patients with SLE which lack LE-specific histopathology have been previously divided into the following categories: cutaneous vascular disease, nonscarring alopecia, and miscellaneous other dermatoses.[3] Cutaneous vascular diseases seen in SLE patients include vasculitis, vasculopathy, livedo reticularis, erythromelalgia, periungual telangiectasia, thrombophlebitis, and Raynaud phenomenon.[2] In a recent study of 670 SLE patients, 11% had vasculitis.[34] Of those with vasculitis, 89% had cutaneous manifestations. The most common vasculitis in SLE patients is small-vessel leukocytoclastic vasculitis, which frequently presents with palpable purpura or erythematous punctuate lesions on the hands (which may rarely enlarge and ulcerate). The small-vessel vasculitis may be associated with urticarial lesions lasting longer than 24 hours (urticarial vasculitis). Livedo reticularis is a nonspecific finding with an increased prevalence in several vascular diseases associated with SLE, including vasculitis, vasculopathy, and antiphospholipid antibody syndrome.[35]

Nonscarring alopecia in SLE patients may have several causes, including lupus hairs (thinning at the frontal hairline; found during SLE flares),[36] alopecia areata (patches of hair loss; has an increased incidence in lupus patients),[37] and telogen effluvium (diffuse hair thinning). Other nonspecific skin lesions that may be observed in SLE patients include sclerodactyly, rheumatoid nodules, calcinosis cutis, urticaria, papulonodular mucinosis, cutis laxa, acanthosis nigricans, leg ulcers, lichen planus, and erythema multiforme.[2]

Subclassification of bullous systemic lupus erythematosus (lupus erythematosus–nonspecific bullous lesions)

Bullous SLE (BSLE) is an autoantibody-mediated subepidermal vesiculobullous skin disease that is LE-nonspecific (does not occur as an extension of the skin lesions showing the interface dermatitis characteristic of LE). BSLE typically presents as a nonscarring generalized bullous eruption, which can be responsive to dapsone treatment.[38,39] A diagnosis of BSLE requires (1) SLE, (2) vesiculobullous eruption, (3) histology showing subepidermal blister and neutrophilic upper dermal infiltrate, and (4) immunoglobulin and complement deposition at the basement membrane zone on direct immunofluorescence (immune reactants on or beneath the lamina densa ultrastructurally).[40,41] Immunoblotting and indirect immunofluorescence on sodium chloride–split skin show that some BSLE patients have serum antibodies to type VII collagen and that their serum may react with a dermal epitope, an epidermal epitope, or both.[40–42] The clinical, histopathological, and immunologic patterns seen in BSLE can resemble epidermolysis bullosa aquisita (EBA), dermatitis herpetiformis (DH), and bullous pemphigoid (BP), but BSLE patients have features that are not consistent with any single primary bullous disease.

A recent report argues that BSLE is a vague term that includes a heterogeneous group of vesiculobullous lesions and recommends using immunologic and histologic characteristics to divide BSLE into the following categories: DH-like vesiculobullous LE, EBA-like vesiculobullous LE, and BP-like vesiculobullous LE.[4] Patients with DH-like vesiculobullous LE have histology showing neutrophilic microabscesses in dermal papillae, granular deposition of IgA or IgG at the basement membrane zone on direct immunofluorescence, and no evidence of serum basement membrane zone antibodies on indirect immunofluorescence.[43–45] These findings are immunohistologically similar to those seen in idiopathic DH. In EBA-like vesiculobullous LE, there are serum antibodies to basement membrane zone type VII collagen (the EBA antigen), and serum binds a dermal epitope on sodium chloride–split skin (the same indirect immunofluorescence pattern seen in idiopathic EBA).[46,47] BP-like vesiculobullous LE is characterized by the linear deposition of IgG and C3 at the dermoepidermal junction found in idiopathic BP.[48] However, immunoelectron microscopy demonstrates that IgG deposits are largely below the basal lamina, and indirect immunofluorescence is negative for serum basement membrane zone antibodies. In contrast, idiopathic BP patients have IgG deposits that are localized to the lamina lucida area, and their serum frequently shows positive indirect immunofluorescence (binds to the epidermal portion of sodium chloride–split skin).[49] BP-like, EBA-like, and DH-like vesiculobullous LE should be distinguished from the rare cases of otherwise typical primary idiopathic BP, EBA, and DH that have been reported in patients with SLE.[4]

Cutaneous lesions and systemic lupus erythematosus criteria

The current American College of Rheumatology classification criteria for SLE include four cutaneous findings: malar rash, discoid rash, photosensitivity, and oral ulcers.[50] Using these criteria, some patients with disease limited to the skin can be classified as having SLE.[51] Other limitations of these criteria include (1) the association between the malar rash and photosensitivity, (2) the association between the discoid rash and oral ulcers, (3) the difficulty of definitively diagnosing the malar rash or discoid lupus without a biopsy, and (4) the lack of specificity of oral ulcers for LE.[52] Integrating dermatologic input into the next revision of the American College of Rheumatology criteria for SLE would help to rectify the current limitations.

Therapy

For all patients, management of CLE begins with prevention of disease exacerbation though avoidance of sunlight and vigilant use of sunscreen. First-line therapeutic agents for CLE include topical corticosteroids, topical calcineurin inhibitors,[53] and intralesional corticosteroids (for scalp lesions). Patients who are refractory to topical therapy or who have widespread or scarring skin disease are generally treated systemically with the antimalarials hydroxychloroquine (<6.5 mg/kg/d) or chloroquine (<3.5 mg/kg/d).[3] Hydroxychloroquine is usually used before chloroquine because of the lower eye toxicity associated with hydroxychloroquine use. Quinacrine (100 mg/d) may be added for nonresponders. Other systemic medications that can be useful in certain subsets of CLE patients include dapsone, retinoids, azathioprine, methotrexate, thalidomide, and, occasionally, systemic corticosteroids.

The ability to perform clinical trials evaluating CLE treatments has been hampered by the lack of validated outcome measures for cutaneous lupus. Thus, clinical practices are predominantly based on expert opinion, case reports, and case series. However, the recently developed and validated CLASI provides a useful tool to facilitate future systematic research.[54,55] Several recent studies using the CLASI have already provided valuable data to help improve clinical therapy.[56–60]

In a recent retrospective study of 36 patients with LE tumidus, 61% showed complete or almost complete resolution of skin lesions following treatment with hydroxychloroquine or chloroquine.[56] Compared with nonsmokers, smokers had a higher initial CLASI score and a lower CLASI score reduction with antimalarial use. Another retrospective study of 34 SLE and CLE patients with skin lesions unresponsive to hydroxychloroquine therapy demonstrated that combination therapy with hydroxychloroquine and quinacrine was effective in reducing CLASI activity scores in patients with DLE, ACLE, and chilblain lesions, but not in those with SCLE or lupus profundus.[57]

Several small studies have used the CLASI activity score to assess newer treatments for refractory CLE. In one prospective study of 10 SCLE patients who had failed at least one standard therapy, treatment with mycophenolate sodium was both effective and safe.[58] Another open prospective study showed promising results in 12 DLE patients refractory to at least one standard therapy who were treated with pulsed dye laser.[59] In addition, a preliminary study describing use of lenalidomide to treat 2 patients with severe, generalized DLE refractory to multiple treatments demonstrated partial improvement and no serious adverse events attributable to the study medication in 1 patient.[60] Future trials using validated measures of CLE are needed to further evaluate the treatments in these small studies and to assess other new treatments for CLE. Such studies will help clinicians to practice evidence-based medicine and will ultimately improve patient care.

THE CUTANEOUS LUPUS ERYTHEMATOSUS DISEASE AREA AND SEVERITY INDEX
Rationale

The development of novel therapeutic agents offers promise for managing patients with SLE. Since SLE is so heterogeneous, consideration of approval of drugs for single-organ indications may facilitate new drug development. To address this problem, the Food and Drug Administration has recommended focusing on organ-specific therapies, which may be easier to approve than medications that target multiple organ systems.[61]

To demonstrate efficacy in one organ system, it is important to have an organ-specific index of disease activity. Even though cutaneous findings are prevalent in patients with lupus,[5] no clinical tool was available until recently to measure cutaneous findings. At least 60 indices are available for measuring disease activity in SLE, including the SLE Disease Activity Index (SLEDAI) and the Systemic Lupus Activity Measure (SLAM). However, only 3 of these tools have some utility in measuring cutaneous activity, and even these have limitations.[62,63] Thus, CLASI was developed in 2005 as a means of specifically tracking cutaneous activity and damage in patients with CLE.[54,64]

The CLASI provides a quantitative measure of the skin-specific burden of disease, which enables standardized assessments of disease progression. Such a standardized approach facilitates the organization of clinical trials, analysis of results, and comparisons among studies. Similarly, in an outpatient setting, CLASI enables more objective monitoring of patients undergoing a change in therapy.

General Overview

The CLASI is a simple, single-page tool that separately quantifies disease activity and damage (**Fig. 1**). Each part of the body, from the scalp to the feet, is listed separately. The instrument also includes sections focusing on mucous membrane involvement and alopecia. For the activity score, points are given for the presence of erythema, scale, mucous membrane lesions, recent hair loss, and inflammatory alopecia. For the damage score, points are given for the presence of dyspigmentation, scarring, and scarring alopecia. For both activity and damage, higher scores are awarded for more severe manifestations. Thus, for example, faint erythema receives one point, whereas violaceous erythema receives three. Similarly, scarring receives one point, whereas severely atrophic scarring receives two. In addition, total dyspigmentation scores are doubled when most of the dyspigmentation has been present for more than 1 year. Scores for each area are assigned based on the most severe lesion within the area of interest. Affected body parts are weighted equally regardless of surface area and number of lesions present. Separate composite scores for activity and damage are calculated by simply summing the individual component scores.[54]

Development

General principles

The design of the CLASI was based on guidelines established by Finlay[65] for the development of an outcome instrument for atopic dermatitis. Each criterion is discussed in greater detail below. According to the guidelines, instruments should:

Be easy to administrate

Clearly separate scores assigned by the clinician from scores assigned by the patient

Ensure that the signs graded are unambiguous and amenable to change; and make clear that, if there is a high correlation between the presence of two different signs, only one is recorded

Base areas of involvement on assessments of the sites involved rather than on estimates of total surface area involvement

Make certain that validity testing should demonstrate good intra- and inter-rater reliability.[65]

Ease of administration

The CLASI can be used even in a busy clinical practice. The layout is easy to follow, and the scoring is self-explanatory. It can be completed without disrupting office routine and without the use of invasive tests. The average time needed to complete the CLASI is 5.25 minutes, ranging from 1 to 11 minutes.[54]

Separation of patient and physician scores

The CLASI includes only those scores determined by the clinician, all of which are based on clinical signs. Patient-derived scores are recorded on separate visual analog scales that measure subjective symptoms, including pain, itch, and fatigue.

Clinical signs: activity and damage

As discussed earlier, the clinical signs that comprise the activity score include erythema, scale, mucous membrane lesions, and inflammatory alopecia. The clinical signs that comprise the damage score include dyspigmentation, scarring, and scarring alopecia. The erythema score is considered a particularly reliable reflection of disease activity because it is easily identified in most skin types.[54,64] Physiologically, erythema mirrors disease activity well because it results directly from the hyperemia associated with inflammation.[64] The physician's visual estimation of erythema is considered an accurate measurement of activity because several studies have demonstrated a good correlation between subjective visual assessments of erythema and objective laser Doppler assessments of blood flow.[66,67]

Following a common trend in rheumatology, the CLASI clearly differentiates between activity and damage, providing two independent summary scores. This distinction is seen in other outcomes measures for SLE. For example, the SLEDAI and SLAM-R specifically measure activity, whereas the Systemic Lupus International Collaborative Clinics–American College of Rheumatology Damage Index specifically

Cutaneous LE Disease Area and Severity Index (CLASI)

Select the score in each anatomical location that describes the most severely affected cutaneous lupus-associated lesion

Anatomical Location	activity		damage		Anatomical Location
	Erythema	Scale/Hypertrophy	Dyspigmentation	Scarring/Atrophy/Panniculitis	
	0-absent 1-pink; faint erythema 2- red; 3-dark red; purple/violaceous/ crusted/hemorrhagic	0-absent; 1-scale 2-verrucous/ hypertrophic	0-absent, 1-dyspigmentaton	0 – absent 1 – scarring 2 – severely atrophic scarring or panniculitis	
Scalp				See below	Scalp
Ears					Ears
Nose (incl. malar area)					Nose (incl. malar area)
Rest of the face					Rest of the face
V-area neck (frontal)					V-area neck (frontal)
Post. Neck &/or shoulders					Post. Neck &/or shoulders
Chest					Chest
Abdomen					Abdomen
Back, buttocks					Back, buttocks
Arms					Arms
Hands					Hands
Legs					Legs
Feet					Feet

Fig. 1. The CLASI. (*From* Albrecht J, Taylor L, Berlin JA, et al. The CLASI (Cutaneous Lupus Erythematosus Disease Area and Severity) Index: an outcome instrument for cutaneous lupus erythematosus. J Invest Dermatol 2005;125(5):892; with permission.)

Mucous membrane

Mucous membrane lesions (examine if patient confirms involvement)	
0-absent; 1-lesion or ulceration	

Dyspigmentation

Report duration of dyspigmentation after active lesions have resolved (verbal report by patient – tick appropriate box)	
☐ Dyspigmentation usually lasts less than 12 months (dyspigmentation score above remains) ☐ Dyspigmentation usually lasts at least 12 months (dyspigmentation score is doubled)	

Alopecia

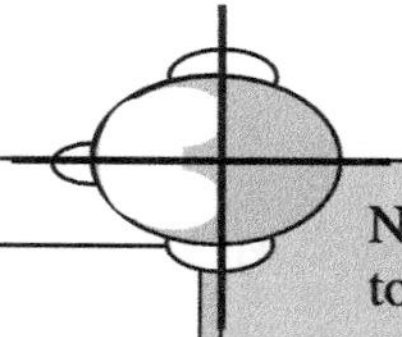

Recent Hair loss (within the last 30 days / as reported by patient)	
1-Yes 0-No	

NB: if scarring and non-scarring aspects seem to coexist in one lesion, please score both

Divide the scalp into four quadrants as shown. The dividing line between right and left is the midline. The dividing line between frontal and occipital is the line connecting the highest points of the ear lobe. A quadrant is considered affected if there is a lesion within the quadrant.

Alopecia (clinically not obviously scarred)	
0-absent 1-diffuse; non-inflammatory 2-focal or patchy in one quadrant; 3-focal or patchy in more than one quadrant	

Scarring of the scalp (judged clinically)	
0- absent 3- in one quadrant 4- two quadrants 5- three quadrants 6- affects the whole skull	

Total Activity Score

(For the activity score please add up the scores of the left side i.e. for Erythema, Scale/Hypertrophy, Mucous membrane involvement and Alopecia)

Total Damage Score

(For the damage score, please add up the scores of the right side, i.e. for Dyspigmentation, Scarring/Atrophy/Panniculitis and Scarring of the Scalp)

Fig. 1. *(continued)*

measures damage.[68] This separation is critical because activity and damage embody two different aspects of the disease. The activity score reflects ongoing inflammation, which has the potential to decrease with treatment. The damage score represents the aftermath of inflammation, which cannot itself be treated, only prevented. As such, the activity score is most appropriate for short-term drug studies, whereas the damage score is helpful in long-term preventative studies.[64]

There is little clinical utility in combining scores because of the potential for scores that are deceptively stable despite significant clinical changes. Clinical experience has shown that patients who respond to therapy can have a simultaneous decrease in the activity score and increase in the damage score, reflecting the alleviation of active inflammation amidst organ damage caused by previous inflammation.[55] Thus, it is most appropriate to treat each score as a separate indicator of disease burden.

Area of involvement

An important decision in the development of any outcome measurement for cutaneous diseases is how best to capture the extent of the disease. One method considered was lesion counting, as is commonly used in acne. This system was rejected for two reasons. First, the interrater reproducibility is poor.[69] Second, the lesions in CLE tend to range in size, and improvement can lead to a paradoxic increase in the number of lesions, as large confluent lesions fragment into smaller lesions.[64]

Another popular method is the estimation of surface area involvement, as has been used in the PASI (Psoriasis Area and Severity Index) and the SCORAD (Severity Scoring of Atopic Dermatitis).[70–72] This method was rejected for two reasons. First, studies have shown that area assessments are difficult to perform, resulting in poor interrater reproducibility and a high incidence of errors.[73,74] Second, this method fails to account for the particular concern that patients have about noticeable lesions, regardless of the total surface area involved.

Cutaneous lupus tends to affect photo-exposed areas, such as the face, V-neck area, scalp, and extensor surfaces of the arms—the areas most visible to others. Studies in psoriasis have shown that patients with visible lesions who feel stigmatized by their disease suffer from impaired quality of life.[75] Furthermore, it has also been shown that patients with visible skin lesions suffer from more psychiatric symptoms than patients with lesions in unexposed areas.[76] As such, these areas require special attention and aggressive treatment, even if the area of involved skin is small. To account for this, the CLASI separates exposed areas into a number of distinct categories, thereby effectively weighing those areas more heavily in the total score. The head, for example, is divided into the scalp, ears, nose, and rest of face. Each of these individually carries the same weight as much larger areas of the body, such as the back/buttocks and abdomen.

Inter- and intra-rater reliability

Inter- and intra-rater reliability is discussed in detail in the following section on validation.

Validation

Content validity

Content validity refers to the inclusion of essential features of the disease in the outcome instrument. This was accomplished by collaborating with a group of seven dermato-rheumatologists with expertise in CLE during the development of the CLASI. The instrument was further assessed by a group of dermatologists and rheumatologists at the American College of Rheumatology Response Criteria Committee on SLE at a meeting in Germany in 2004. Finally, during the initial testing of the CLASI, the raters were interviewed extensively, and their feedback was used to make several improvements to the instrument.[54]

Inter-rater reliability

Interrater reliability refers to the similarity between measurements made by two different observers on the same subject. For both activity and damage scores, the interrater reliability was high: Eleven physicians scored nine different patients and achieved intraclass Pearson's correlation coefficients of 0.86 (95% CI, 0.73–0.99) and 0.92 (95% CI, 0.85–1.00) for the activity and damage scales, respectively.[54]

Intra-rater reliability

Intra-rater reliability refers to agreement of multiple measurements made by one observer on a single subject. For this assessment, eight physicians scored four patients, one of whom was evaluated twice. The intra-rater reliability was also found to be quite high. For the activity score, the Spearman's correlation coefficient was 0.96 (95% CI, 0.89–1.00), with a mean difference between scores of two points. For the damage score, the Spearman's correlation coefficient was 0.99 (95% CI, 0.97–1.00), with a mean difference between scores of zero points.[54]

Clinical responsiveness

To assess clinical responsiveness, changes in the CLASI were monitored for 2 months (56 days) following initiation of a new therapy. These scores were correlated with changes in other clinical outcome instruments, including the physician's global skin assessment, the patient's global skin assessment, and the patient's assessment of pain and itch. Eight subjects with CLE (four DLE, two SCLE, and two DLE/SLE) were included. The results indicated a high correlation between changes in the CLASI activity score and in the physician's global skin assessment ($r_p = 0.97$, $P = .003$, $n = 7$), the patient's global skin assessment ($r_p = 0.85$, $P = .007$, $n = 8$), and the pain score ($r_p = 0.98$, $P = .004$, $n = 5$).[55] These early findings suggested that the CLASI is responsive to changes in disease activity.

Recent studies performed by other groups have further validated the clinical responsiveness of the CLASI. Kreuter and colleagues[56] showed that CLASI activity scores in patients with tumid LE decreased significantly after 3 months of therapy with an antimalarial medication. In another study, Kreuter and colleagues[58] illustrated that CLASI activity scores decrease significantly after 3 months of therapy with mycophenolate sodium, which correlated with improvements on ultrasound and colorimetry. A third study, by Erceg,[59] demonstrated that CLASI activity scores in patients with DLE decreased significantly after 6 to 18 weeks of pulsed dye laser therapy.

Extension to rheumatology

Because rheumatologists frequently encounter patients with CLE, further validation studies were performed to assess the CLASI when used by rheumatologists rather than dermatologists. Internal structure reliability (inter- and intra-rater reliability) and diagnostic skill were evaluated. Diagnostic skill was assessed to ensure that the CLASI is used for CLE to the exclusion of mimicker skin diseases. Fourteen subjects were enrolled, including 10 with CLE, 3 with CLE plus a mimicker disease, and 1 with a mimicker disease only. The subjects were evaluated by five rheumatologists and five dermatologists.[77]

The results indicated that the CLASI has high reliability when used by rheumatologists. The interrater reliability correlation coefficients were 0.83 (95% CI, 0.70–0.96) for activity and 0.86 (95% CI, 0.75–0.97) for damage. The intrarater reliability correlation

Table 1
Disease severity based on the CLASI activity score

	CLASI Activity Score Range	Sensitivity (%)	Specificity (%)
Mild	0–9	93	78
Moderate	10–20	—	—
Severe	21–70	80	95

coefficients were 0.91 (95% CI, 0.71–1.00) for activity and 0.99 (95% CI, 0.94–1.00) for damage. The diagnostic skill assessment, however, suggested that rheumatologists may not have the training to reliably distinguish between CLE and mimicker diseases. Several mimicker lesions were misdiagnosed as CLE, resulting in poor specificity compared with dermatologists (0.46 vs 0.74, respectively).[77] These results indicate that it may be prudent for rheumatologists to consult with dermatologists when recruiting patients for studies using the CLASI.

Practical Applications

With the design and validation of the CLASI complete, more recent work has focused on practical applications of the CLASI, particularly for use in clinical trials. The quantified scores enable an objective measure of disease burden, which can be used to standardize patient assessments.

Severity

Many clinical trials only enroll patients with moderate or severe disease. It is therefore important to have a standardized method of assessing disease severity to ensure that that the patient populations included in different trials are comparable. This was accomplished by categorizing 37 patients (45 visits) as "mild," "moderate," or "severe" based on the principal investigator's subjective assessment. Corresponding CLASI activity scores were also calculated and analyzed with crosstab row percents and receiver operating characteristic curves. The results indicated that mild, moderate, and severe disease corresponded with CLASI activity score ranges of 0 to 9 (sensitivity 93%, specificity 78%), 10 to 20, and 21 to 70 (sensitivity 80%, specificity 95%), respectively **(Table 1)**.[78]

Future directions

CLASI can be used in a number of potential applications. The CLASI activity score can be used for assessments of disease progression, including response to therapy, flare, stability, and remission. The CLASI damage score can evaluate residual changes in skin after the activity has resolved. Finally, changes in either score can be correlated with changes in quality of life to better understand the tangible ramifications of disease progression.

SUMMARY
Overview of Cutaneous Lupus Erythematosus

Cutaneous lupus lesions are classified as LE-specific or LE-nonspecific based on histology. LE-specific lesions are subclassified as acute, subacute, or chronic based on clinical information. Outstanding issues in the classification of cutaneous lupus include the categorization of LE tumidus and bullous systemic LE and the significance of Rowell syndrome. There are few controlled studies of CLE treatments, and therapy is largely based on expert opinion. Future trials using validated outcome measures to document skin disease activity are needed to help guide clinical practice.

The Cutaneous Lupus Erythematosus Disease Area and Severity Index

The CLASI is a clinical tool that quantifies activity and damage in CLE. It was designed to be easy to use, to be completed by physicians, and to include the most significant signs of disease burden (erythema, scale, dyspigmentation, and scarring). The CLASI measures disease extent based on the number of involved areas, giving more weight to those that are most visible. Total surface area of affected skin is not estimated. Validation studies have demonstrated good content validity, inter- and intrarater reliability, and clinical responsiveness. The CLASI is reliable when used by both dermatologists and rheumatologists. Some practical applications of the CLASI include standardized assessments of disease severity and responsiveness to new therapies.

REFERENCES

1. Gilliam JN, Sontheimer RD. Distinctive cutaneous subsets in the spectrum of lupus erythematosus. J Am Acad Dermatol 1981;4(4):471–5.
2. Sontheimer RD. The lexicon of cutaneous lupus erythematosus—a review and personal perspective on the nomenclature and classification of the cutaneous manifestations of lupus erythematosus. Lupus 1997;6(2):84–95.
3. Werth V. Current treatment of cutaneous lupus erythematosus. Dermatol Online J 2001;7(1):2.
4. Ting W, Stone MS, Racila D, et al. Toxic epidermal necrolysis-like acute cutaneous lupus erythematosus and the spectrum of the acute syndrome of apoptotic pan-epidermolysis (ASAP): a case report, concept review and proposal for new classification of lupus erythematosus vesiculobullous skin lesions. Lupus 2004; 13(12):941–50.
5. Werth VP. Clinical manifestations of cutaneous lupus erythematosus. Autoimmun Rev 2005;4(5):296–302.
6. Watanabe T, Tsuchida T. Classification of lupus erythematosus based upon cutaneous manifestations. Dermatological, systemic and laboratory findings in 191 patients. Dermatology 1995;190(4):277–83.
7. Callen JP, Fowler JF, Kulick KB. Serologic and clinical features of patients with discoid lupus erythematosus: relationship of antibodies to single-stranded deoxyribonucleic acid and of other antinuclear antibody subsets to clinical manifestations. J Am Acad Dermatol 1985;13(5 Pt 1):748–55.
8. Callen JP. Chronic cutaneous lupus erythematosus. Clinical, laboratory, therapeutic, and prognostic examination of 62 patients. Arch Dermatol 1982;118(6): 412–6.
9. Perniciaro C, Randle HW, Perry HO. Hypertrophic discoid lupus erythematosus resembling squamous cell carcinoma. Dermatol Surg 1995;21(3):255–7.
10. Burge SM, Frith PA, Juniper RP, et al. Mucosal involvement in systemic and chronic cutaneous lupus erythematosus. Br J Dermatol 1989;121(6):727–41.
11. Nagao K, Chen KR. A case of lupus erythematosus/lichen planus overlap syndrome. J Dermatol 2006;33(3):187–90.
12. Fraga J, Garcia-Diez A. Lupus erythematosus panniculitis. Dermatol Clin 2008; 26(4):453, 63, vi.
13. Massone C, Kodama K, Salmhofer W, et al. Lupus erythematosus panniculitis (lupus profundus): clinical, histopathological, and molecular analysis of nine cases. J Cutan Pathol 2005;32(6):396–404.

14. Martens PB, Moder KG, Ahmed I. Lupus panniculitis: clinical perspectives from a case series. J Rheumatol 1999;26(1):68–72.
15. Viguier M, Pinquier L, Cavelier-Balloy B, et al. Clinical and histopathologic features and immunologic variables in patients with severe chilblains. A study of the relationship to lupus erythematosus. Medicine (Baltimore) 2001;80(3):180–8.
16. Doutre MS, Beylot C, Beylot J, et al. Chilblain lupus erythematosus: report of 15 cases. Dermatology 1992;184(1):26–8.
17. Kuhn A, Richter-Hintz D, Oslislo C, et al. Lupus erythematosus tumidus—a neglected subset of cutaneous lupus erythematosus: report of 40 cases. Arch Dermatol 2000;136(8):1033–41.
18. Kuhn A, Sonntag M, Richter-Hintz D, et al. Phototesting in lupus erythematosus tumidus—review of 60 patients. Photochem Photobiol 2001;73(5):532–6.
19. Kuhn A, Sonntag M, Ruzicka T, et al. Histopathologic findings in lupus erythematosus tumidus: review of 80 patients. J Am Acad Dermatol 2003;48(6): 901–8.
20. Kuhn A, Bein D, Bonsmann G. The 100th anniversary of lupus erythematosus tumidus. Autoimmun Rev 2009;8(6):441–8.
21. Callen JP. Clinically relevant information about cutaneous lupus erythematosus. Arch Dermatol 2009;145(3):316–9.
22. Sontheimer RD, Thomas JR, Gilliam JN. Subacute cutaneous lupus erythematosus: a cutaneous marker for a distinct lupus erythematosus subset. Arch Dermatol 1979;115(12):1409–15.
23. Perera GK, Black MM, McGibbon DH. Bullous subacute cutaneous lupus erythematosus. Clin Exp Dermatol 2004;29(3):265–7.
24. Sontheimer RD, Maddison PJ, Reichlin M, et al. Serologic and HLA associations in subacute cutaneous lupus erythematosus, a clinical subset of lupus erythematosus. Ann Intern Med 1982;97(5):664–71.
25. Lopez-Longo FJ, Monteagudo I, Gonzalez CM, et al. Systemic lupus erythematosus: clinical expression and anti-Ro/SS—a response in patients with and without lesions of subacute cutaneous lupus erythematosus. Lupus 1997;6(1):32–9.
26. Black DR, Hornung CA, Schneider PD, et al. Frequency and severity of systemic disease in patients with subacute cutaneous lupus erythematosus. Arch Dermatol 2002;138(9):1175–8.
27. Vedove CD, Del Giglio M, Schena D, et al. Drug-induced lupus erythematosus. Arch Dermatol Res 2009;301(1):99–105.
28. Sontheimer RD, Henderson CL, Grau RH. Drug-induced subacute cutaneous lupus erythematosus: a paradigm for bedside-to-bench patient-oriented translational clinical investigation. Arch Dermatol Res 2009;301(1):65–70.
29. Cardinali C, Giomi B, Caproni M, et al. Maculopapular lupus rash in a young woman with systemic involvement. Lupus 2000;9(9):713–6.
30. Rowell NR, Beck JS, Anderson JR. Lupus erythematosus and erythema multiforme–like lesions. A syndrome with characteristic immunological abnormalities. Arch Dermatol 1963;88:176–80.
31. Zeitouni NC, Funaro D, Cloutier RA, et al. Redefining Rowell's syndrome. Br J Dermatol 2000;142(2):343–6.
32. Shteyngarts AR, Warner MR, Camisa C. Lupus erythematosus associated with erythema multiforme: Does Rowell's syndrome exist? J Am Acad Dermatol 1999;40(5 Pt 1):773–7.
33. Modi GM, Shen A, Mazloom A, et al. Lupus erythematosus masquerading as erythema multiforme: does Rowell syndrome really exist? Dermatol Online J 2009;15(2):5.

34. Ramos-Casals M, Nardi N, Lagrutta M, et al. Vasculitis in systemic lupus erythematosus: prevalence and clinical characteristics in 670 patients. Medicine (Baltimore) 2006;85(2):95–104.

35. Gibbs MB, English JC 3rd, Zirwas MJ. Livedo reticularis: an update. J Am Acad Dermatol 2005;52(6):1009–19.

36. Alarcon-Segovia D, Cetina JA. Lupus hair. Am J Med Sci 1974;267(4):241–2.

37. Werth VP, White WL, Sanchez MR, et al. Incidence of alopecia areata in lupus erythematosus. Arch Dermatol 1992;128(3):368–71.

38. Vassileva S. Bullous systemic lupus erythematosus. Clin Dermatol 2004;22(2): 129–38.

39. Ludgate MW, Greig DE. Bullous systemic lupus erythematosus responding to dapsone. Australas J Dermatol 2008;49(2):91–3.

40. Yell JA, Allen J, Wojnarowska F, et al. Bullous systemic lupus erythematosus: revised criteria for diagnosis. Br J Dermatol 1995;132(6):921–8.

41. Gammon WR, Briggaman RA, Bullous SLE. A phenotypically distinctive but immunologically heterogeneous bullous disorder. J Invest Dermatol 1993; 100(1):28S–34S.

42. Chan LS, Lapiere JC, Chen M, et al. Bullous systemic lupus erythematosus with autoantibodies recognizing multiple skin basement membrane components, bullous pemphigoid antigen 1, laminin-5, laminin-6, and type VII collagen. Arch Dermatol 1999;135(5):569–73.

43. Camisa C, Sharma HM. Vesiculobullous systemic lupus erythematosus. Report of two cases and a review of the literature. J Am Acad Dermatol 1983;9(6):924–33.

44. Harris-Stith R, Erickson QL, Elston DM, et al. Bullous eruption: a manifestation of lupus erythematosus. Cutis 2003;72(1):31–7.

45. Pedro SD, Dahl MV. Direct immunofluorescence of bullous systemic lupus erythematosus. Arch Dermatol 1973;107(1):118–20.

46. Gammon WR, Woodley DT, Dole KC, et al. Evidence that anti-basement membrane zone antibodies in bullous eruption of systemic lupus erythematosus recognize epidermolysis bullosa acquisita autoantigen. J Invest Dermatol 1985; 84(6):472–6.

47. Yoon J, Moon TK, Lee KH, et al. Fatal vascular involvement in systemic lupus erythematosus following epidermolysis bullosa acquisita. Acta Derm Venereol 1995;75(2):143–6.

48. Olansky AJ, Briggaman RA, Gammon WR, et al. Bullous systemic lupus erythematosus. J Am Acad Dermatol 1982;7(4):511–20.

49. Sato M, Shimizu H, Ishiko A, et al. Precise ultrastructural localization of in vivo deposited IgG antibodies in fresh perilesional skin of patients with bullous pemphigoid. Br J Dermatol 1998;138(6):965–71.

50. Hochberg MC. Updating the American College of Rheumatology revised criteria for the classification of systemic lupus erythematosus. Arthritis Rheum 1997; 40(9):1725.

51. Parodi A, Rebora A. ARA and EADV criteria for classification of systemic lupus erythematosus in patients with cutaneous lupus erythematosus. Dermatology 1997;194(3):217–20.

52. Albrecht J, Berlin JA, Braverman IM, et al. Dermatology position paper on the revision of the 1982 ACR criteria for systemic lupus erythematosus. Lupus 2004;13(11):839–49.

53. Tzellos TG, Kouvelas D. Topical tacrolimus and pimecrolimus in the treatment of cutaneous lupus erythematosus: an evidence-based evaluation. Eur J Clin Pharmacol 2008;64(4):337–41.

54. Albrecht J, Taylor L, Berlin JA, et al. The CLASI (Cutaneous Lupus Erythematosus Disease Area and Severity Index): an outcome instrument for cutaneous lupus erythematosus. J Invest Dermatol 2005;125(5):889–94.

55. Bonilla-Martinez ZL, Albrecht J, Troxel AB, et al. The Cutaneous Lupus Erythematosus Disease Area and Severity Index: a responsive instrument to measure activity and damage in patients with cutaneous lupus erythematosus. Arch Dermatol 2008;144(2):173–80.

56. Kreuter A, Gaifullina R, Tigges C, et al. Lupus erythematosus tumidus: response to antimalarial treatment in 36 patients with emphasis on smoking. Arch Dermatol 2009;145(3):244–8.

57. Cavazzana I, Sala R, Bazzani C, et al. Treatment of lupus skin involvement with quinacrine and hydroxychloroquine. Lupus 2009;18(8):735–9.

58. Kreuter A, Tomi NS, Weiner SM, et al. Mycophenolate sodium for subacute cutaneous lupus erythematosus resistant to standard therapy. Br J Dermatol 2007; 156(6):1321–7.

59. Erceg A, Bovenschen HJ, van de Kerkhof PC, et al. Efficacy and safety of pulsed dye laser treatment for cutaneous discoid lupus erythematosus. J Am Acad Dermatol 2009;60(4):626–32.

60. Shah A, Albrecht J, Bonilla-Martinez Z, et al. Lenalidomide for the treatment of resistant discoid lupus erythematosus. Arch Dermatol 2009;145(3):303–6.

61. U.S. Department of Health and Human Services, FDA, Center for Drug Evaluation and Research (CDER). Guidance for industry: systemic lupus erythematosus—developing drugs for treatment. Available at: http://www.fda.gov/downloads/Drugs/GuidanceComplianceRegulatoryInformation/Guidances/ucm072063. pdf. Accessed September 30, 2009.

62. Parodi A, Massone C, Cacciapuoti M, et al. Measuring the activity of the disease in patients with cutaneous lupus erythematosus. Br J Dermatol 2000;142(3): 457–60.

63. Merrill JT. Measuring disease activity in systemic lupus: progress and problems. J Rheumatol 2002;29(11):2256–7.

64. Albrecht J, Werth VP. Development of the CLASI as an outcome instrument for cutaneous lupus erythematosus. Dermatol Ther 2007;20(2):93–101.

65. Finlay AY. Measurement of disease activity and outcome in atopic dermatitis. Br J Dermatol 1996;135(4):509–15.

66. Quinn AG, McLelland J, Essex T, et al. Quantification of contact allergic inflammation: a comparison of existing methods with a scanning laser Doppler velocimeter. Acta Derm Venereol 1993;73(1):21–5.

67. Lahti A, Kopola H, Harila A, et al. Assessment of skin erythema by eye, laser Doppler flowmeter, spectroradiometer, two-channel erythema meter and Minolta chroma meter. Arch Dermatol Res 1993;285(5):278–82.

68. Lam GK, Petri M. Assessment of systemic lupus erythematosus. Clin Exp Rheumatol 2005;23(5 Suppl 39):S120–32.

69. Lucky AW, Barber BL, Girman CJ, et al. A multirater validation study to assess the reliability of acne lesion counting. J Am Acad Dermatol 1996;35(4):559–65.

70. Severity scoring of atopic dermatitis: the SCORAD index. Consensus Report of the European Task Force on Atopic Dermatitis. Dermatology 1993;186(1):23–31.

71. Garduno J, Bhosle MJ, Balkrishnan R, et al. Measures used in specifying psoriasis lesion(s), global disease and quality of life: a systematic review. J Dermatolog Treat 2007;18(4):223–42.

72. Ramsay B, Lawrence CM. Measurement of involved surface area in patients with psoriasis. Br J Dermatol 1991;124(6):565–70.

73. Tiling-Grosse S, Rees J. Assessment of area of involvement in skin disease: a study using schematic figure outlines. Br J Dermatol 1993;128(1):69–74.
74. Charman CR, Venn AJ, Williams HC. Measurement of body surface area involvement in atopic eczema: an impossible task? Br J Dermatol 1999;140(1):109–11.
75. Vardy D, Besser A, Amir M, et al. Experiences of stigmatization play a role in mediating the impact of disease severity on quality of life in psoriasis patients. Br J Dermatol 2002;147(4):736–42.
76. Hughes JE, Barraclough BM, Hamblin LG, et al. Psychiatric symptoms in dermatology patients. Br J Psychiatry 1983;143:51–4.
77. Krathen MS, Dunham J, Gaines E, et al. The Cutaneous Lupus Erythematosus Disease Activity and Severity Index: expansion for rheumatology and dermatology. Arthritis Rheum 2008;59(3):338–44.
78. Klein RS, Moghadam-Kia S, LoMonico J, et al. Using the CLASI to assess disease severity and responsiveness to therapy in cutaneous lupus erythematosus. Arthritis Rheum 2009;60(10):S339.

Pediatric Lupus—Are There Differences in Presentation, Genetics, Response to Therapy, and Damage Accrual Compared with Adult Lupus?

Rina Mina, MD, Hermine I. Brunner, MD*

KEYWORDS

- Pediatric SLE • Children • Lupus • Adults
- Lupus nephritis • Complement

An estimated 10% to 20% of patients experience the onset of systemic lupus erythematosus (SLE) before adulthood. More precise estimates are difficult due to a lack of a clear age limit for the diagnosis of pediatric SLE. The maximum age at diagnosis most commonly used to define pediatric SLE is 16 years but ages range from 14 to 20 years in various studies.[1–8] This review article explores the differences and similarities between pediatric SLE and adult (aSLE), using studies that provide a direct comparison between groups. Issues pertaining to neonatal SLE are not addressed.

GENDER RATIO AND DISEASE ONSET

Albeit uncommon, onset of pediatric SLE is described even in children younger than 2 years of age.[9] The female-to-male ratio of pediatric SLE changes from 4:3 with disease onset during the first decade of life to 4:1 during the second decade to 9:1 in aSLE and decreases to 5:1 in SLE commencing after age 50.[10–13]

Dr Brunner is supported by NIAMS P60 AR47784. Dr Mina is supported by the NIH Training Grant T32 AR074594.

Division of Rheumatology, Department of Pediatrics, Cincinnati Children's Hospital Medical Center, 3333 Burnet Avenue, MC 4010, Cincinnati, OH 45229, USA

* Corresponding author.

E-mail address: Hermine.Brunner@cchmc.org (H.I. Brunner).

Pediatric SLE often presents with more acute and severe disease features than aSLE, based on studies providing direct comparisons.[2,8,14] Almost all published research suggests a higher frequency of renal, neurologic, and hematologic involvement with pediatric SLE than with aSLE at the time of diagnosis.[2,5–8,15] In a Canadian inception cohort of 67 pediatric SLE patients, the average disease activity score, as measured by the SLE Disease Activity Index, was 16.8 at diagnosis but only 9.3 in the comparison group of 131 patients with aSLE (P = .0001).[1] The most pronounced differences in disease activity between aSLE and pediatric SLE pertain to the renal or neurologic organ systems.[16]

Despite widely variable estimates, fever and lymphadenopathy are more frequently described with pediatric SLE than aSLE in studies directly comparing both groups (**Table 1**). Conversely, adults with SLE more commonly present with arthritis than children with SLE.[2,4,17] When comparing prepubertal to postpubertal onset of pediatric SLE, the former group presents more often with hemolytic anemia and renal involvement whereas in the latter group cutaneous and musculoskeletal features are more common at disease onset.[9,18] As with aSLE, approximately one-third of the children and adolescents with SLE present with anemia, thrombocytopenia, or lymphopenia at the time of SLE onset.[19–21] On the contrary, leukopenia is more common in pediatric SLE than aSLE at onset (31% to 35% vs 18%),[19,20,22] and 49% of children with SLE as compared to 18% to 65% of aSLE patients test Coombs positive at the time of diagnosis.[19,21,23] Equally frequent in pediatric SLE and aSLE at the time of initial presentation (5% to 20%) are anti-Smith (anti-Sm), antiribonucleoprotein (anti-RNP), anti-Ro, and anti-La antibodies, as suggested by one study.[2]

DISEASE COURSE

Besides significantly more active disease at the time of disease onset, there is also more active disease over time with pediatric SLE when compared to aSLE.[1,8] In the Canadian study discussed previously, the average time-adjusted mean SLE Disease Activity Index score was 5.7 with pediatric SLE but only 4.6 with aSLE (P = .012).[1] Similarly, there was a trend toward more active disease during the course of the disease in adolescent-onset SLE patients (SLE onset between ages 13 and 18 years) recruited to the Lupus in Minorities (LUMINA) study than in those with aSLE.[8]

At least five contemporary cohorts provide a direct comparison of disease features and laboratory abnormalities with pediatric SLE and aSLE over time. Specific details are presented in **Tables 2** and **3**.[2,4,5,17,24] The variability in the estimates between studies may be a reflection of sample sizes or recruitment criteria but true divergence of SLE features due to race, ethnicity, and specific environmental or health milieus is likely also important. This review excludes some earlier studies that compared pediatric SLE to historic aSLE cohorts or research not designed to allow for the delineation of statistically significant differences between the groups.[7,25]

MUCOCUTANEOUS AND MUSCULOSKELETAL MANIFESTATIONS

When directly comparing pediatric SLE to aSLE, inflammatory rashes, including the typical malar erythema, are significantly more frequent in children than adults.[2,5,24] Exceptions are photosensitivity and discoid skin lesions that are more prominently found with aSLE. Isolated discoid lupus erythematosus (DLE) is uncommon in childhood, with fewer than 5% of all DLE cases reported in patients under the age 15.[2,26] Lesions of DLE in children are indistinguishable from those in adults but children with DLE suffer less often from photosensitivity, and there is a less pronounced female predominance. Conversely, children with DLE more often have a positive family

Table 1
Clinical and laboratory features in pediatric and adult systemic lupus erythematosus at disease onset[a]

Study	Carreno 1999[b]			Font 1998[c]		
Clinical Findings	pedSLE (n = 49)	aSLE (n = 130)	P Value	pedSLE (n = 34)	aSLE (n = 396)	P Value
Fever	20	15	NS	41	21	0.006
Lymphadenopathy	—	—	—	6	0.5	0.03
Malar rash	22	16	NS	44	35	NS
Discoid lupus	—	—	—	0	3	NS
Subcutaneous cutaneous lupus	—	—	—	0	3	NS
Livedo reticularis	—	—	—	3	0.5	NS
Oral ulcers	—	—	—	9	13	NS
Photosensitivity	—	—	—	23	20	NS
Arthritis	22	39	<0.05	65	62	NS
Arthalgias	26	23	NS	—	—	—
Myositis	—	—	—	3	4	NS
Nephropathy	—	—	—	20	9	0.04
Neurologic involvement	—	—	—	0	6	NS
Chorea	—	—	—	3	0	NS
Serositis	—	—	—	12	13	NS
Pleuritis	6	6	NS	—	—	—
Lung involvement	—	—	—	0	1	NS
Hemolytic anemia	—	—	—	9	3	NS
Thrombocytopenia	—	—	—	12	9	NS
Vasculitis	8	2	NS	—	—	—
Cutaneous vasculitis	—	—	—	—	—	—
Raynaud phenomenon	8	8	NS	12	16	NS
Thrombosis	—	—	—	0	1	NS
Sicca syndrome	—	—	—	0	0.5	NS

Abbreviations: NS, statistically not significant; pedSLE, pediataric systemic lupus erythematosus; —, No data in original article.
[a] Values expressed as percentages (%).
[b] Carreno L, Lopez-Longo FJ, Monteagudo I, et al. Immunological and clinical differences between juvenile and adult onset of systemic lupus erythematosus. Lupus 1999;8(4):287–92.
[c] Font J, Cervera R, Espinosa G, et al. Systemic lupus erythematosus (SLE) in childhood: analysis of clinical and immunological findings in 34 patients and comparison with SLE characteristics in adults. Ann Rheum Dis 1998;57(8):456–9.

history of DLE or SLE and, more importantly, 25% to 30% of the children with DLE progress to SLE as opposed to only 5% to 10% of adults.[26,27]

Painful nonerosive arthritis and arthralgias are common in aSLE and pediatric SLE. There may be a trend toward more overt arthritis with pediatric SLE, whereas arthralgias and myalgias seem more frequently encountered in aSLE.[2,4,5,24] Whether or not differences in the frequencies of subjective musculoskeletal features between groups are related to the underlying disease or are a reflection of more common joint symptoms in adulthood remains to be determined. Jaccoud arthropathy[28] and drug-induced myopathy, however, are more often described with aSLE.[29,30]

Table 2
Clinical features in pediatric and adult systemic lupus erythematosus over time[a]

Organ Systems	Hoffman 2009[b] pedSLE (n = 56)	aSLE (n = 194)	P Value	Ramirez-Gomez 2008[c] pedSLE (n = 230)	aSLE (n = 984)	P Value	Rood 1999[d] pedSLE (n = 31)	aSLE (n = 135)	P Value	Carreno 1999[e] pedSLE (n = 49)	aSLE (n = 130)	P Value	Font 1998[f] pedSLE (n = 34)	aSLE (n = 396)	P Value
Constitutional															
Fever	67.3	51	<0.05	63.5	55.2	0.02	—	—	—	—	—	—	62	43	NS
Fatigue	78.6	83.5	NS	—	—	—	87	—	—	—	—	—	—	—	—
Weight loss	—	—	—	—	—	—	71	—	—	—	—	—	—	—	—
Lymphadenopathy	—	—	—	—	—	—	36	—	—	—	—	—	6	1	NS
Mucocutaneous															
Malar rash	69.6	58.6	NS	70.4	59.1	0.002	71	40	<0.05	59.1	59.2	NS	79	51	0.002
Discoid lupus	18.9	28.4[g]	NS	12.6	11.6	NS	10	27	<0.05	26.5	13.8	<0.05	15	4	NS
Subcutaneous cutaneous lupus	9.6	2.2	<0.05	—	—	—	—	—	—	—	—	—	3	6	NS
Alopecia	41.1	45.1	NS	—	—	—	48	—	—	—	—	—	—	—	—
Generalized erythema	20	9.5	<0.05	—	—	—	—	—	—	—	—	—	—	—	—
Livedo reticularis	—	—	—	—	—	—	—	—	—	—	—	—	6	1	NS
Oral ulcers	28.6	23.5	NS	49.1	39.9	0.01	48	42	NS	40.8	37.6	NS	38	25	NS
Genital ulcers	3.6	4.3	NS	—	—	—	—	—	—	—	—	—	—	—	—
Photosensitivity	44.6	53.2	NS	53	56.8	NS	39	43	NS	40.8	50.7	NS	44	35	NS
Musculoskeletal															
Articular manifestations	—	—	—	—	—	—	—	—	—	85.7	96.1	<0.05	—	—	—
Arthritis	59.3	66.8	NS	83	82	NS	100	94	NS	—	—	—	88	81	NS
Arthralgia	75	98.7	<0.005	—	—	—	—	—	—	—	—	—	—	—	—

Myalgias	42.4	35.2	NS	11.7	18.9	0.01	—	—	—	—	—	—	—	—	—
Myositis	—	—	—	—	—	—	—	—	—	—	—	—	3	7	NS
Renal															
Proteinuria	63.6	4.2	<0.01	49.1	45.3	NS	61	43	NS	—	—	—	—	—	—
Urinary cell casts	57.1	32	<0.001	—	—	—	65	53	NS	—	—	—	—	—	—
Nephropathy	62.5	36	<0.001	—	—	—	—	—	—	67.3	48.4	<0.05	50	34	NS
Neuropsychiatric															
Chorea	—	—	—	2.2	0	0.000	—	—	—	—	—	—	9	0	<0.001
Seizures	14.5	6.9	NS	11.3	7.4	0.05	26	14	NS	—	—	—	—	—	—
Cerebro vascular accident	5.6	6.9	NS	5.2	2.2	0.01	—	—	—	—	—	—	—	—	—
Transient ischemic attack	—	—	—	0.9	0	0.03	—	—	—	—	—	—	—	—	—
Cranial nerve abnormalities	—	—	—	1.3	42	0.03	—	—	—	—	—	—	—	—	—
Pseudotumor cerebri	—	—	—	0.9	0	0	—	—	—	—	—	—	—	—	—
Headache	25.5	30.9	NS	—	—	NS	61	—	NS	—	—	—	—	—	—
Concentration disorder	20.4	17.8	NS	—	—	—	—	—	—	—	—	—	—	—	—
Psychosis	9.3	5.9	NS	4.8	3.9	NS	13	6	NS	—	—	—	—	—	—
Depression	12.7	15.8	NS	—	—	—	—	—	—	—	—	—	—	—	—
Enceph alopathy	20.4	5.3	<0.005	—	—	—	—	—	—	—	—	—	—	—	—
Neurologic disorder	—	—	—	—	—	—	—	—	—	36.7	20	<0.05	—	—	—
Cardiopulmonary															
Pericarditis	16.7	18.2	NS	17.0	17.3	NS	26	33	NS	16.3	13	NS	—	—	—

(continued on next page)

Table 2
(continued)

Study	Hoffman 2009[b]			Ramirez-Gomez 2008[c]			Rood 1999[d]			Carreno 1999[e]			Font 1998[f]		
Organ Systems	pedSLE (n = 56)	aSLE (n = 194)	P Value	pedSLE (n = 230)	aSLE (n = 984)	P Value	pedSLE (n = 31)	aSLE (n = 135)	P Value	pedSLE (n = 49)	aSLE (n = 130)	P Value	pedSLE (n = 34)	aSLE (n = 396)	P Value
Serositis	—	—	—	—	—	—	—	—	—	—	—	—	32	27	NS
Pleuritis	18.5	32.1	NS	17.4	23.2	NS	48	58	NS	28.5	33	NS	—	—	—
Pneumonitis	—	—	—	—	—	—	10	—	—	—	—	—	—	—	—
Lung involvement	—	—	—	—	—	—	—	—	—	—	—	—	6	4	NS
Miscellaneous															
Thrombosis	—	—	—	—	—	—	—	—	—	—	—	—	0	8	NS
Raynaud phenomenon	39.3	41.1	NS	—	—	—	26	—	—	36.7	34.6	NS	20	25	NS
Chillblains	9.4	1.1	<0.01	—	—	—	—	—	—	—	—	—	—	—	—
Cutaneous vasculitis	—	—	—	—	—	—	—	—	—	44.8	27.6	<0.05	—	—	—
Sicca syndrome	—	—	—	3.9	9.3	0.007	—	—	—	—	—	—	9	15	NS
Xerophthalmia	3.8	18.7	<0.01	1.7	6.6	0.004	—	—	—	—	—	—	—	—	—
Xerostomia	7.5	21.4	<0.05	—	—	—	—	—	—	—	—	—	—	—	—

Abbreviations: NS, statistically not significant; pedSLE, pediatric SLE; —, No data in original article.

[a] Values expressed as percentages (%).

[b] Hoffman IE, Lauwerys BR, De Keyser F, et al. Juvenile-onset systemic lupus erythematosus: different clinical and serological pattern than adult-onset systemic lupus erythematosus. Ann Rheum Dis 2009;68(3):412–5.

[c] Ramirez Gomez LA, Uribe Uribe O, Osio Uribe O, et al. Childhood systemic lupus erythematosus in Latin America. The GLADEL experience in 230 children. Lupus 2008;17(6):596–604.

[d] Rood MJ, ten Cate R, van Suijlekom-Smit LW, et al. Childhood-onset Systemic Lupus Erythematosus: clinical presentation and prognosis in 31 patients. Scand J Rheumatol 1999;28(4):222–6.

[e] Carreno L, Lopez-Longo FJ, Monteagudo I, et al. Immunological and clinical differences between juvenile and adult onset of systemic lupus erythematosus. Lupus 1999;8(4):287–92.

[f] Font J, Cervera R, Espinosa G, et al. Systemic lupus erythematosus (SLE) in childhood: analysis of clinical and immunological findings in 34 patients and comparison with SLE characteristics in adults. Ann Rheum Dis 1998;57(8):456–9.

[g] Localized and disseminated discoid lesions.

With a reported prevalence of approximately 40%, osteopenia (z scores <-1 or -1.5) is common in pediatric SLE, and osteoporotic fractures occur in 6% to 10% of the children.[31,32] This compares to reports of osteopenia at 40% and osteoporosis at 5% in premenopausal women with aSLE; much higher estimates are provided for aSLE cohorts that include postmenopausal patients.[33,34]

Traditional risk factors for osteoporosis that contribute to impaired bone health in aSLE are unlikely important in pediatric SLE.[35] Possibly due to inflammation, corticosteroid use, reduced physical activity, inadequate sun exposure, and low calcium and vitamin D intake, children and adolescents with SLE are often unable to reach their peak bone mass.[103,130,199] For reasons not fully understood, there is a higher prevalence of vitamin D deficiency in children and adults with SLE as compared to the general population.[36]

LUPUS NEPHRITIS

Lupus nephritis (LN) is often a presenting feature of pediatric SLE.[2] In comparative studies of pediatric SLE and aSLE, the prevalence of LN in adults with SLE is at 34% to 48%.[19,24,37] Despite large variations between racial groups, most studies report LN to be present in 50% to 67% of the children, at a higher frequency than with aSLE.[17,19,24,37] Consequently, proteinuria and urinary cell casts during the disease course are more common with pediatric SLE than aSLE.[4] A study by Brunner and colleagues[1] supports a similar distribution of LN histologic classes in pediatric SLE as compared to aSLE, with diffuse proliferative LN (class IV) occurring in 40% to 60%, focal proliferative LN (class III) in 10% to 20%, and membranous LN (class V) in 3% to 28% of pediatric SLE patients with renal disease.[38] Overlap between proliferative and membranous changes are reported in 12% of the cases on initial kidney biopsy.[38] Hypertension occurs in 40% of pediatric SLE patients with LN,[3,8,39,40] and African American children, in particular boys, may have a significantly higher risk of hypertension than white children.

NEUROPSYCHIATRIC SYSTEMIC LUPUS ERYTHEMATOSUS

Lack of specific laboratory tests and imaging modalities make the diagnostic process of neuropsychiatric involvement with SLE (NPSLE) difficult in children and adults with SLE. The types of NPSLE syndromes are similar in pediatric SLE and aSLE.[41,42]

NPSLE is at least as common in children as it is in adults.[43–46] Within the first year post diagnosis, 70% of the children, as compared to only 28% of adults, develop features compatible with NPSLE.[47,48] Depression is the most common mood disorder in children and adults without apparent differences in prevalence between groups.[4,41,42] The Grupo Latinoamericano de Estudio del Lupus (GLADEL) cohort reported a significantly higher prevalence of pseudotumor cerebri, transient ischemic attack, and seizures in their pediatric SLE cohort when directly compared with aSLE.[8] Despite a general lack of comorbid conditions, cerebrovascular disease is reported in up to 25% of children with NPSLE and may be more common than in aSLE.[4,24] Approximately 20% of children with NPSLE develop psychosis, which usually presents with visual hallucinations.[45,49] Psychosis, chorea, or any type of encephalopathy occurs preferentially with pediatric SLE.[2,8,44,50] Cerebral vein thrombosis is reported in 15% to 25% of the children with SLE, often presenting with severe headache in lupus anticoagulant (LAC)-positive patients.[51] Conversely, cranial nerve abnormalities are more frequently encountered in aSLE than pediatric SLE.[8]

Neurocognitive dysfunction is reported in as many as 30% to 60% of all children with SLE.[43–45,52] This wide range of numeric estimates reported in the literature is likely

Table 3
Laboratory findings in pediatric and adult systemic lupus erythematosus over time[a]

Study	Hoffman 2009[b]			Ramirez-Gomez 2008[c]			Rood 1999[d]			Carreno 1999[e]			Font 1998[f]		
Laboratory Test	pedSLE (n = 56)	aSLE (n = 194)	P Value	pedSLE (n = 230)	aSLE (n = 984)	P Value	pedSLE (n = 31)	aSLE (n = 135)	P Value	pedSLE (n = 49)	aSLE (n = 130)	P Value	pedSLE (n = 34)	aSLE (n = 396)	P Value
Antibodies															
Antinuclear AB	—	—	—	96.9	98.2	NS	100	99	NS	100	99.2	NS	—	—	—
Anti-dsDNA AB	60.7	24.9	<0.001	67	71.3	NS	93	66	<0.05	89.7	78.4	NS	—	—	—
Anti-Sm AB	17.9	12.4	NS	51.3	47.6	NS	30	32	NS	20.4	14.6	NS	—	—	—
Anti-Ro AB	23.2	33.5	NS	—	—	—	—	—	—	36.7	38.4	NS	—	—	—
Anti-La AB	7.1	17.0	NS	—	—	—	—	—	—	12.2	13	NS	—	—	—
Anti-RNP AB	14.3	17.5	NS	—	—	—	—	—	—	38.7	41.5	NS	—	—	—
Antiribosomal P AB	25	11.3	<0.001	—	—	—	—	—	—	—	—	—	—	—	—
Antihistone AB	39.3	25.8	<0.05	—	—	—	—	—	—	24.4	31.5	NS	—	—	—
Rheumatoid factor	—	—	—	—	—	—	54	—	—	—	—	—	—	—	—
aPL AB															
IgM aCL AB	—	—	—	47.5	36.8	0.05	—	—	—	—	—	—	—	—	—
IgG aCL AB	—	—	—	51.8	50.2	NS	—	—	—	—	—	—	—	—	—
LAC	—	—	—	34.4	29.6	NS	23	—	—	—	—	—	—	—	—
Hematology															

Anemia	—	—	—	—	—	—	84	56	<0.05	—	—	—	—	—	—
Hemolytic anemia	38.5	13	<0.001	16.1	10.8	0.02	—	—	—	20.4	10	NS	15	6	NS
Leukocytopenia	63.6	56.8	NS	46.1	41.5	NS	74	50	<0.05	55.1	56.9	NS	—	—	—
Lymphopenia	67.9	64.1	NS	60.4	59	NS	30	26	NS	30.6	21.4	NS	—	—	—
Thrombocytopenia	31.5	25	NS	25.2	17.8	0.01	48	36	NS	30.6	38.4	NS	26	23	NS

Abbreviations: AB, antibodies; NS, statistically not significant; pedSLE, pediatric SLE; —, No data in original article.

[a] Values expressed as percentages (%).

[b] Hoffman IE, Lauwerys BR, De Keyser F, et al. Juvenile-onset systemic lupus erythematosus: different clinical and serological pattern than adult-onset systemic lupus erythematosus. Ann Rheum Dis 2009;68(3):412–5.

[c] Ramirez Gomez LA, Uribe Uribe O, Osio Uribe O, et al. Childhood systemic lupus erythematosus in Latin America. The GLADEL experience in 230 children. Lupus 2008;17(6):596–604.

[d] Rood MJ, ten Cate R, van Suijlekom-Smit LW, et al. Childhood-onset Systemic Lupus Erythematosus: clinical presentation and prognosis in 31 patients. Scand J Rheumatol 1999;28(4):222–6.

[e] Carreno L, Lopez-Longo FJ, Monteagudo I, et al. Immunological and clinical differences between juvenile and adult onset of systemic lupus erythematosus. Lupus 1999;8(4):287–92.

[f] Font J, Cervera R, Espinosa G, et al. Systemic lupus erythematosus (SLE) in childhood: analysis of clinical and immunological findings in 34 patients and comparison with SLE characteristics in adults. Ann Rheum Dis 1998;57(8):456–9.

due to differences in design and case ascertainment between studies. Nonetheless, neurocognitive dysfunction seems similarly widespread among children and adults with SLE.[16] The 1999 American College of Rheumatology (ACR) case definitions of NPSLE have not been validated for use in children and adolescents, and the proposed 1-hour ACR battery of standardized tests to assess neuropsychiatric function is not suited for use in pediatrics.[53] More recently an alternative battery for children has been developed.[54]

CARDIOPULMONARY AND GASTROINTESTINAL INVOLVEMENT

Pericarditis is the most commonly diagnosed cardiac manifestation of SLE and presents in approximately 17% to 33 % of SLE patients, irrespective of age.[55] Symptomatic coronary artery disease and myocardial infarction are exceedingly rare in children and adolescents with SLE.[56] Conversely, clinically recognizable coronary artery disease is reported in 6% to 9% of adults with SLE, and ischemic heart disease remains a major factor for morbidity and mortality in aSLE.[57,58] Symptomatic and asymptomatic pulmonary manifestations are described in up to 60% of the children and adolescents with SLE,[59] which compares to estimates of 20% to 90% in aSLE.[60,61] In studies directly comparing children and adults with SLE, there is a trend toward more common occurrence of pleuritis with aSLE.[2,4,5,24] Among the most common pathologic features reported in pediatric SLE and aSLE are restrictive lung defects and impaired diffusion capacity.[62] Shrinking lung syndrome (eg, restrictive lung disease combined with diaphragmatic paralysis) is a rare complication of SLE with fewer than 150 cases in adults and fewer than 10 cases reported in pediatrics.[63,64] Pulmonary hemorrhage is still linked to high mortality rates in children and adults with SLE.[65]

The frequency of ascites in pediatric SLE is comparable to that in aSLE. Adults with SLE are commonly diagnosed with conventional age or medication-related abdominal pathology,[66,67] whereas in children symptoms are more often due to SLE itself.[68] In a review of 175 adults hospitalized for aSLE, 22% presented with acute abdominal pain, which was due to aSLE in 44% of the cases.[67] Conversely, some abdominal pain was reported in 19% of 201 French children with SLE.[68] In this review, in 87% of the cases the gastrointestinal pathology was attributed to pediatric SLE.[68]

Distinguishing surgical from nonsurgical cases of acute abdomen is challenging, especially in children with SLE. Acute onset of even mild abdominal pain and low-grade fever in an otherwise well-controlled patient on immunosuppressive medications may be due to bacterial peritonitis. Abnormalities on ultrasound are present in approximately half of the children with SLE with abdominal pathology, whereas abnormalities on CT are seen in 80% of the cases.[68]

HEMATOLOGIC MANIFESTATIONS

Chronic disease is the most common cause of anemia in pediatric SLE and aSLE. There is a higher incidence of anemia in the very young, affecting 77% of patients with infantile SLE (ie, SLE with onset before age 1 year), as compared to only 35% of children older than 1 year at onset of pediatric SLE.[9] Anemia in pediatric SLE is usually of a mild to moderate degree and normochromic normocytic but becomes microcytic and hypochromic over time.[43] Hemolytic anemia is more prevalent in pediatric SLE than aSLE, as suggested by several studies comparing pediatric SLE to aSLE.[2,4,24]

With a reported prevalence of between 42% and 74% during the course of the disease, leukopenia occurs with similar frequency in pediatric SLE and aSLE.[4,24]

Leukopenia may be less frequent in young children with SLE compared to pediatric SLE with onset at or after puberty.[9] Lymphopenia is as common with aSLE as it is with pediatric SLE over time. It changes with disease activity, is correlated with anti–double-stranded DNA (anti-dsDNA) antibody levels, and is associated with NPSLE and mucocutaneous involvement in pediatric SLE and aSLE.[69]

Neutropenia is similarly frequent in aSLE and pediatric SLE, occurring in approximately 12% to 15% of children and 4% to 20% of adults. Neutropenia has been associated with thrombocytopenia and NPSLE in pediatric SLE and aSLE.[19,70] Overall, the prevalence of thrombocytopenia seems somewhat higher in pediatric SLE than aSLE.[4,24] Thrombocytopenia occurs in approximately two-thirds of children with infantile SLE and in 25% to 30% of pediatric SLE patients with disease onset later in life.[9] Low platelet counts are associated with the presence of antiphospholipid (aPL) and antiplatelet autoantibodies.

Prior to developing pediatric SLE, children and adults with thrombocytopenia may have carried a diagnosis of idiopathic thrombocytopenic purpura (ITP).[71] In a study by Pamuk and colleagues,[72] six of 321 adults (2%) with ITP developed aSLE during a 4-year follow-up time. In this cohort, 27% of the adult patients with ITP tested positive for antinuclear antibodies (ANA). In contrast, in a single retrospective study of 365 Turkish children with ITP, ANA titers of 1:80 or higher were present in 9% of the children but none developed pediatric SLE during the mean follow-up of 3.6 years.[73] Given the low frequency of ANA positivity in the cohort, however, any potentially increased risk of ANA positive individuals to develop pediatric SLE might have been missed, and the observations from Turkey may not be typical for other parts of the world. In the authors' experience, careful follow-up is warranted for any child with ITP who is found to have ANA at high titers.

Hemolytic uremic syndrome or thrombotic thrombocytopenic purpura (TTP) are rarely features of the initial presentation of pediatric SLE.[74,75] ANA positivity and high grade proteinuria at the time of presentation are risk factors for children with TTP to subsequently develop pediatric SLE.[74] Based on a systematic review of the literature, at least 35% of children with TTP subsequently develop pediatric SLE, which compares to only 2% to 3% in adults with TTP.[74,76]

Although it has been described in all age groups, macrophage activation syndrome may be more common, or at least more recognized, in pediatric SLE than aSLE.[77,78] The morphologic features in the bone marrow of pediatric SLE and aSLE with macrophage activation syndrome are indistinguishable from those with other causes. Bone marrow dysplasia has been described in pediatric SLE and aSLE.[79]

ANTIPHOSPHOLIPID ANTIBODY AND SJÖGREN SYNDROMES

The prevalence of anticardiolipin (aCL) antibodies and LAC seems similar in groups of adults and children with SLE.[9] Thrombosis in patients who test positive for aPL antibodies is, however, more common in aSLE than pediatric SLE, likely reflective of underlying comorbidities and longer disease duration in adults.[80] In a cross-sectional Canadian cohort study, children with SLE who tested persistently positive for LAC had a 28-fold increased risk of experiencing a thrombotic event compared to those without LAC.[81] Approximately one-third of pediatric SLE patients with aPL syndrome experience recurrent thromboses within 13 months of the initial event, especially if anticoagulation is discontinued or when there are other predisposing thrombophilic factors.[81]

Although 6.5% of all aSLE patients have Sjögren syndrome, it is less common in children with SLE (see **Table 2**). Although a case series (n = 34) from Japan reports that 41% of the children with SLE have secondary Sjögren syndrome, the prevalence of sicca syndrome at 3.9% in pediatric SLE versus 9.3% in aSLE was considerably lower in the much larger GLADEL cohort.[24,82] Primary, as opposed to secondary, Sjögren syndrome is rare before adulthood. In a cohort study of 180 children with primary pediatric Sjögren syndrome, the mean age at diagnosis was 9.8 years.[83] Common clinical manifestations of pediatric Sjögren syndrome are bilateral parotid swelling, which is present in 70% of the cases. Extraglandular manifestations were reported in 5% of the children in one series of patients with pediatric Sjögren syndrome. ANA positivity is less frequently observed in children than in adults with Sjögren syndrome.[84]

ENDOCRINE ABNORMALITIES

Types of endocrine aberrations are comparable in adults and children with SLE.[85] An estimated 50% to 85% of pediatric SLE and aSLE have dyslipidemia.[86,87] Proatherogenic lipid profiles in children and adults with SLE exist even before commencing steroid therapy.[86–88] Low-density lipoprotein particles are smaller with active compared to inactive disease in pediatric SLE and aSLE, contributing to their atherogenicity.[89,90] Compared with healthy controls, adults and children with SLE have higher insulin levels which, if persistent, are associated with metabolic syndrome.[91,92] There may be higher rates of diabetes in aSLE compared with pediatric SLE.[1,7]

Autoimmune thyroid disorders are associated with SLE and present in approximately 15% to 20% of the patients without apparent differences in prevalence between adults and children.[93,94]

There is a trend toward higher levels of follicle stimulating hormone, luteinizing hormone, and prolactin in cSLE patients compared with healthy children.[95,96] Elevated prolactin levels occur in subsets of pediatric SLE and aSLE patients with active disease, especially those with NPSLE.[96,97]

Menarche in girls with pediatric SLE is, on average, delayed by 1 year. The delay in puberty progression increases with longer disease durations and the higher cumulative doses of corticosteroids used for treatment ($R^2 > 0.3$; $P<.009$).[98] Transient or permanent amenorrhea has been reported in 12% of 298 adolescents with pediatric SLE and is positively correlated with the presence of disease activity and damage. Ovarian failure is a well-known complication of intravenous cyclophosphamide therapy in aSLE. The risk of ovarian failure after cyclophosphamide is considerably lower in pediatric SLE than in aSLE.[99,100] Based on limited information from case series, the average risk of premature ovarian failure is 11% in female patients with pediatric SLE who are younger than 21 years of age.[98,101,102] In a cohort of 77 patients with pediatric SLE, of whom 47% were treated with cyclophosphamide, a reduced ovarian reserve, but not overt ovarian failure, was observed in 31% of the female patients who were treated with cyclophosphamide.[102] Different from aSLE, ovarian protection has not been studied in pediatric SLE but a randomized trial of a gonadotropin-releasing hormone agonist is ongoing to assess the benefits and risks of transient ovarian suppression.[102]

As with aSLE, semen abnormalities, low testicular volumes, and high gonadotropin levels all seem more frequent in male patients with pediatric SLE than their healthy peers, especially after cyclophosphamide therapy with initiation after the onset of puberty.[103,104] Sertoli cell dysfunction is more common in pediatric SLE male patients than in healthy adolescents. Semen abnormalities are more common with immunosuppressive use, especially with cyclophosphamide.[104]

IMMUNOLOGIC FEATURES

As with aSLE, circulating ANA are the hallmark of pediatric SLE and present in virtually all children.[105] An estimated 30% to 50% of children referred to pediatric rheumatologists who test ANA positive have a musculoskeletal pain syndrome and not pediatric SLE.[106] In a retrospective study of 110 children who tested positive for ANA, 10 children eventually developed pediatric SLE after follow-up of up to 4 years. The median ANA titer of the children who developed pediatric SLE was 1:1080,[107] whereas ANA titers of 1:320 or lower seemed not to confer a sizeable risk for the subsequent development of pediatric SLE.[107]

Most studies that directly compare pediatric SLE to aSLE suggest that elevated levels of anti-dsDNA antibodies are more common in pediatric SLE than in aSLE (61% to 93% vs 25% to 78%).[2,4,5,17,24] An estimated 92% of children with infantile SLE test positive for anti-dsDNA antibodies.[9] As with aSLE, changes in the levels of anti-dsDNA antibodies are used to monitor disease activity in pediatric SLE.[108] There are conflicting reports as to whether or not anti-dsDNA antibodies and complement levels are predictive of future pediatric SLE or aSLE flares.[109] Although traditionally viewed as specific to SLE, anti-dsDNA antibodies can be present with autoimmune hepatitis, Epstein-Barr virus infections, and rheumatoid arthritis and, rarely, in healthy people.[110]

Besides anti-dsDNA antibodies, antihistone and antiribosomal P antibodies are all more frequently encountered in pediatric SLE than aSLE.[4] Antiribosomal P antibodies are elevated in 25% to 42% of the patients with pediatric SLE[4] compared with only 6% to 11% of the patients with aSLE.[4,47,111] One study directly comparing pediatric SLE and aSLE for the presence of antihistone antibodies suggests a significantly higher prevalence in the former than the latter, 39% and 26%, respectively.[4]

The prevalence of anti-Sm, anti-RNP, anti-Ro/SSA, and anti-La/SSB antibodies seems not to differ between pediatric SLE and aSLE.[4] Anti-Sm antibodies are present in up to 51%, anti-RNP antibodies in approximately 37%, anti-Ro antibodies in 33%, and anti-La antibodies in 15% of pediatric SLE patients during the course of their disease, respectively.[2,4,5,16,17,24] The disease association of the antibody clustering in pediatric SLE may be different from that observed in aSLE.[112] Similar to what has been reported in aSLE, there are ethnic variations in the frequency of autoantibodies with pediatric SLE; anti-U1RNP and anti-Sm antibodies occur more frequently in nonwhite patients with pediatric SLE.[112,113] Despite a lack of comparative studies, the frequency of antinucleosome antibodies seems comparable in aSLE and pediatric SLE.[114,115] The rheumatoid factor is positive in 5% of the pediatric SLE patients at diagnosis and in 10% to 54% of them over time, exceeding the frequency at which rheumatoid facto is reported in juvenile idiopathic arthritis.[2,5,7,17] A comparative study of aSLE and pediatric SLE suggests a trend toward more common rheumatoid facto positivity among adults at diagnosis and during the course of the disease.[2]

GENETICS

There is limited knowledge about the relative risk of children of different races to develop SLE. As with aSLE, however, nonwhite children seem at a higher risk of being diagnosed with SLE. Genetic studies in pediatric SLE provide, for the most part, confirmation of genetic variants reported in aSLE and currently do not explain differences in disease presentation, activity, and outcomes between pediatric SLE and aSLE.[21,116]

Congenital complement deficiencies are present in approximately 1% of patients with SLE.[117] The closest association between SLE and complement deficiencies is seen with C1q deficiency, where there is a risk of more than 90% to develop a lupus-like illness early in life.[117,118] Deficiency of C1q is a rare condition with only approximately 50 cases reported in the literature. Other complement deficiencies include homozygous C4 deficiency with a 75% association rate with SLE[119] and C1s or C1r deficiency, which has a 50% association rate with SLE, again with onset early in life. Homozygous C2 deficiency is present in 1/10,000 to 1/30,000 whites, and 10% to 30% of them may develop SLE.[117]

The major histocompatibility complex class II and III alleles have long been implicated in conveying risk for developing SLE. HLA DRB1*15:03, DRB5*01:01, DQA1*01:02, and DQB1*06:02 are more common in American blacks with SLE, independent of age at disease onset.[120] HLA DRB1*03:01, DQA1*05:01, and DQB1*02:01 are more common in whites with SLE, again independent of age at disease onset.[121] Non–major histocompatibility complex loci that have been associated with pediatric SLE and aSLE are the 1858T single-nucleotide polymorphism (SNP) of PTPN22, a gene which encodes for the enzyme, lymphocyte phosphatase and inhibits T-cell activation.[116,122,123] A polymorphism (−28C/G polymorphism) of the RANTES (also CCL5) gene also has been associated with aSLE, and its importance was confirmed in a study of Chinese children with SLE.[124] A genome-wide scan in children and adults proposed that susceptibility to SLE is conveyed by the N673S polymorphism of the P-selectin gene, a cell adhesion molecule expressed on activated endothelial cells, and of the C203S polymorphism of the interleukin-1 receptor-associated kinase 1 gene, which is involved in the signaling cascade of the toll/interleukin-1 receptor family.[125] Another SNP, PD1.3G/A, located within the regulatory area of the programmed cell death 1 gene, is also a proposed susceptibility locus of aSLE and pediatric SLE from Mexico.[126]

THERAPY

Treatment approaches to pediatric SLE and aSLE vary across centers and are largely determined by organ involvement, disease activity and damage, access to medications, and institutional preferences.[18,127] Comparative studies of adults and children support that pediatric SLE is more often treated with high doses of corticosteroids and immunosuppressive medications than aSLE (**Table 4**). When comparing therapies of patients treated at two Canadian tertiary hospitals, children with SLE were more often prescribed oral corticosteroids than adults (97% of 67 pediatric SLE patients vs 70% of 131 aSLE patients).[1] In the same study, children with SLE were treated with intravenous methylprednisolone almost three times more often than adults.[1] This is similar to what has been reported from a cohorts of 90 pediatric SLE and 795 aSLE patients managed in the United States,[3] but no important differences in steroid use between aSLE and pediatric SLE were noted by others.[2,8]

More frequent use of any immunosuppressive medication with pediatric SLE compared with aSLE is reported by several investigators,[1–3,16] although the types of immunosuppressive drugs prescribed seem not to differ between children and adults, except for a more common use of methotrexate in aSLE than pediatric SLE (31% vs 9%).[1]

There is a trend toward a more frequent administration of intravenous cyclophosphamide in the adolescent-onset group compared with aSLE in the LUMINA study cohort.[8] How the increasing use of rituximab in recent years has affected overall medication profiles in pediatric SLE and aSLE is unknown at this point.

Patients with SLE of all ages older than 6 years are equally likely to be prescribed antimalarials.[1,3] Adults and children with SLE are comparable in their use of nonsteroidal anti-inflammatory medications,[2,3] except for cyclooxygenase 2 inhibitors, which seem less commonly prescribed to children and adolescents.[3]

Corticosteroids, intravenous immunoglobulins, dapsone, vincristine, and various immunosuppressive medications have all been used to treat SLE-associated thrombocytopenia

Table 4
Medication prescribed during follow-up in pediatric and adult systemic lupus erythematosus[a]

Study	Hersh 2009[b]			Brunner 2008[c]			Tucker 2008[d]			Font 1998[e]		
Medication	pedSLE (n = 90)	aSLE (n = 795)	P Value	pedSLE (n = 67)	aSLE (n = 131)	P Value	adoSLE (n = 31)	aSLE (n = 48)	P Value	pedSLE (n = 34)	aSLE (n = 396)	P Value
Traditional nonsteroidal anti-inflammatory drugs	81.8	88.1	NS	—	—	—	—	—	—	88	81	NS
Cyclooxygenase-2 inhibitors	23	49.9	<0.001	—	—	—	—	—	—	—	—	—
Antimalarials	87.6	83.8	NS	81	73	NS	—	—	—	85	82	NS
Oral corticosteroids	100	89.3	0.001	97	70	<0.0001	96.8	85.4	NS	94	84	NS
Pulse methylprednisolone	48.8	38.4	0.064	30	11	0.001	—	—	—	3	1	NS
Immunosuppressive medications	—	—	—	66	37	0.0001	—	—	—	—	—	—
Azathioprine	33.7	28.4	NS	64	75	NS	—	—	—	15	2	0.00004
Methotrexate[f]	26.9	30.9	NS	9	31	NS	—	—	—	—	—	—
Mycophenolate mofetil	28.1	13	<0.001	0	2	NS	—	—	—	—	—	—
Cyclosporine	18.6	9.9	0.014	2	0	NS	—	—	—	—	—	—
Intravenous cyclophosphamide	30.7	14.1	<0.001	25	21	0.009	16.1	4.2	NS	—	—	—
Oral cyclophosphamide	3.5	7.5	NS	—	—	—	—	—	—	9	4	NS

Abbreviations: adoSLE, the cohort pediatric SLE patients that had disease onset between the ages 13 and 18 years; NS, statistically not significant; pedSLE, pediatric SLE; —, No data in original article.

[a] Values expressed as percentages.
[b] Hersh AO, von Scheven E, Yazdany J, et al. Differences in long-term disease activity and treatment of adult patients with childhood- and adult-onset systemic lupus erythematosus. Arthritis Rheum 2009;15;61(1):13–20.
[c] Brunner HI, Gladman DD, Ibanez D, et al. Difference in disease features between childhood-onset and adult-onset systemic lupus erythematosus. Arthritis Rheum 2008;58(2):556–62.
[d] Tucker LB, Uribe AG, Fernandez M, et al. Adolescent onset of lupus results in more aggressive disease and worse outcomes: results of a nested matched case-control study within LUMINA, a multiethnic US cohort (LUMINA LVII). Lupus 2008;17(4):314–22.
[e] Font J, Cervera R, Espinosa G, et al. Systemic lupus erythematosus (SLE) in childhood: analysis of clinical and immunological findings in 34 patients and comparison with SLE characteristics in adults. Ann Rheum Dis 1998;57(8):456–9.
[f] Oral or injectable methotrexate.

in children and adults. Successful therapy of chronic treatment-resistant hemolytic anemia and thrombocytopenia in pediatric SLE with rituximab is reported from a single center; no serious infections were observed, despite prolonged B-cell depletion.[128]

Children and adolescents with NPSLE seem to have an excellent response to treatment, and the majority of them experience a resolution of symptoms. As with NPSLE in adults, high-dose glucocorticoids, often combined with immunosuppressive medications, including cyclophosphamide, are the mainstays of NPSLE treatment of children.[44,129] For NPSLE-associated cerebral vein thrombosis or arterial strokes anticoagulation is added to the anti-inflammatory drug regimen.[130] There are no longitudinal randomized studies addressing target parameters for anticoagulant therapy or antithrombotic prophylaxis in pediatric NPSLE. Academic delays of children and adolescents with NPSLE have not been quantified but are likely considerable. Educational interventions and psychologic support seem important for children with NPSLE, based on studies in aSLE.[131]

Treatment of LN in pediatric SLE is adapted from protocols used in adults. As with aSLE the best induction and maintenance therapy for pediatric SLE-associated LN remains to be determined.[132,133] In children with severe LN, cyclophosphamide use is associated with better renal survival compared with corticosteroids therapy alone.[134] Lehman and Onel[135] treated 16 patients with class III or IV LN with monthly intravenous pulse cyclophosphamide for 6 months, followed by three monthly infusions for a total of 36 months. A significant reduction of proteinuria, disease activity, and prednisone dosage at 1 year post initial diagnosis was observed as was improvement of LN on rebiopsy. No significant treatment complications were reported by this group during the 3-year study. The combination therapy of cyclophosphamide and methotrexate for refractory class IV therapy in children with SLE has been suggested but is rarely used in pediatric or adults clinical practice, given its potentially severe side effects.[136]

Different from aSLE, there are no randomized trials of mycophenolate mofetil for specifically pediatric SLE treatment. The efficacy and safety of mycophenolate mofetil in controlling LN in children has been reported: in a case series mycophenolate mofetil was effective in five of 13 patients (38%), partially effective in four (31%), and ineffective in four (31%). No severe side effects were observed.[137]

Some studies suggest that proliferative LN in children progresses in 9% to 15% of the cases to end-stage renal disease within 5 years,[38,138] which is comparable to what has been reported from some aSLE cohorts.[139] LN accounts for 3% of end-stage renal disease leading to kidney transplantations among children in North America,[140] whereas adults with SLE account for 1.9% of the adult kidney transplant population, based on the United States Renal Data System.

A review of the North American Pediatric Renal Transplant Cooperative Study database supports 1-year graft survival rates with pediatric SLE at 91% after living donor, and 78% after cadaveric transplants. This compares to estimates of graft survival in aSLE at 88% at 1 year, and 67% at 5 years. In aSLE and pediatric SLE, kidney graft survival is similar to that with other adult or pediatric diseases.[139,141,142]

PROGNOSIS AND SURVIVAL

Delay in aSLE diagnosis is associated with higher mortality and a reduced likelihood of achieving remission.[143] In adults with SLE, remission for 1-year is reported in as many as 6.5% of the patients.[144] Conversely, despite a lack of firm estimates, remission is exceedingly rare in pediatric SLE in North America.[3]

Historically, children and adolescents have higher mortality rates and are perceived to encounter more disease damage than adults with SLE.[1,8] The 5-year survival rates have improved in pediatric SLE from 30% to 40% in 1950s to more than 90% in the 1980s.[145–147] Similarly, survival has much improved with aSLE.[148] In aSLE and pediatric SLE, recent 5-year survival rates well over 90% are reported from developed countries.[149–152] Nevertheless, in the LUMINA study cohort, there is an almost twofold higher mortality with adolescent-onset SLE than with aSLE (19.4% vs 10.4%, $P = .37$).[24]

Major causes of death in pediatric SLE and aSLE include renal disease, severe disease flares, and infections.[146,147,153,154] Although NPSLE is a risk factor of poor outcome in pediatric SLE, cardiovascular disease remains an important cause of death in aSLE. There is an ongoing controversy as to whether or not age at SLE onset constitutes a risk factor for poor disease outcome (**Table 5**).[18,39,155] Male gender, black race, low socioeconomic status, thrombocytopenia, disease damage, and nonadherence to treatment have all been linked with worse survival.[149,156,157] Nonadherence to visits and medications is a universal challenge for SLE patients of all ages. In a single-center study, 39% of 55 adolescents and adults with SLE were nonadherent (adherence rates <80%) to prednisone and 51% to hydroxychloroquine, based on pharmacy refill data.[158] Significant risk factors of insufficient adherence included being single, low educational level, and presence of other comorbidities but not age at disease onset. Initial study suggests text messaging to be a promising venue to enhance adherence to pediatric SLE therapies.[159]

Despite improved survival rates in SLE patients of all ages, there remains substantial morbidity due to disease damage.[160,161] In aSLE, increasing age and longer duration of disease are correlated with disease damage. Approximately 50% to 70% of adults with SLE will have accrued some disease damage at 10 years post diagnosis.[149,162] In a study of 1015 pediatric SLE patients from 39 countries, 40% of the children acquired some disease damage during mean disease durations of 4 years. This percentage increased to 58% in those with disease durations of greater than 5 years,[163] with similar results reported by others.[16,18]

Statistically significant differences in the development of damage between aSLE and pediatric SLE were noted in the past. Comparison of Canadian inception cohorts found children with SLE to have mean Systemic Lupus International Collaborating Clinics/ ACR (SLICC/ACR) damage index scores of 1.7 and adults of 0.76.[1] Ocular and musculoskeletal damage were statistically more common in children but there was a trend toward higher rates of malignancy with aSLE (see **Table 5**).[1] In the LUMINA study cohort, there was a trend toward higher rates of any disease damage in the adolescent-onset group as compared with the aSLE group (mean SLICC/ACR damage index score at last available visit, 2.3 vs 1.6),[8] and renal damage was significantly less frequent in those with disease onset in adulthood ($P = .023$). In the LUMINA study cohort, patients with diagnosis during adolescence also had a trend toward more neuropsychiatric, ocular, and musculoskeletal damage but there were more diabetes and peripheral vascular damage in those with disease onset during adulthood.[8]

COST OF CARE

Cost of care is considerably higher in children than adults with SLE.[164,165] The estimated economic burden of pediatric SLE ranges from $146 to $650 million annually in the United States[164] In a study using administrative databases from two tertiary pediatric rheumatology centers in the United States, the annual cost of care of pediatric SLE

Table 5
Damage accrual in pediatric and adult systemic lupus erythematosus as measured by the Systemic Lupus International Collaborating Clinics/American College of Rheumatology damage index[a]

Study	Brunner 2008[b]			Tucker 2008[c]		
Damage Domain	pedSLE (n = 66)	aSLE (n = 131)	P Value	adoSLE (n = 31)	aSLE (n = 48)	P Value
SDI domains						
Ocular	42.2	13.0	<0.0001	9.7	4.3	NS
Neuropsychiatric	12.1	9.9	NS	29.0	19.6	NS
Renal	9.1	6.1	NS	45.2	17.4	0.023
Pulmonary	3.0	2.3	NS	3.2	6.5	NS
Cardiovascular	1.5	4.6	NS	6.5	4.3	NS
Peripheral vascular	3.0	1.5	NS	0	8.7	NS
Gastrointestinal	3.0	2.3	NS	3.2	10.9	NS
Musculoskeletal	24.2	9.9	0.007	19.4	15.2	NS
Integument	7.6	6.9	NS	9.7	15.2	NS
Gonadal	0	1.5	NS	12.9	10.9	NS
Diabetes	3.0	4.6	NS	3.2	8.7	NS
Malignancy	0	3.8	NS	3.2	0	NS
Mean (SD) of SDI score at study entry	—	—	—	0.7 (1.1)	0.5 (1.0)	NS
Mean (SD) in months of disease duration at study entry	1.13 (5.01)	2.83 (3.43)	0.014	1.7 (1.5)	1.6 (1.4)	NS
Mean (SD) of SDI score at the end of follow-up	1.76 (2.67)	0.76 (1.16)	0.008	2.3 (2.5)	1.6 (2.0)	NS
Mean (SD) in years of disease duration at the end of the study	3.2 (2)	3.5 (2.6)	NS	5.1 (3.0)	4.0 (2.8)	NS
Proportion[a] of patients with ANY damage as measured by the SDI	56.1	43.5	NS	64.5	66.7	NS

Abbreviations: adoSLE, the cohort pediatric SLE patients that had disease onset between the ages 13 and 18 years; NS, statistically not significant; pedSLE, pediatric SLE; SDI, SLICC/ACR damage index.
[a] Values are percentages of patients of the total group unless otherwise noted.
[b] Brunner HI, Gladman DD, Ibanez D, et al. Difference in disease features between childhood-onset and adult-onset systemic lupus erythematosus. Arthritis Rheum 2008;58(2):556–62.
[c] Tucker LB, Uribe AG, Fernandez M, et al. Adolescent onset of lupus results in more aggressive disease and worse outcomes: results of a nested matched case-control study within LUMINA, a multiethnic US cohort (LUMINA LVII). Lupus 2008;17(4):314–22.

was $14,944 (cost basis: 2000), excluding outpatient medication expenses. Cost was accrued mostly by hospitalizations (28%), laboratory testing (21%), and outpatient clinic visits (20%), whereas emergency department visits contributed to only 1% to the total cost of care. Renal replacement therapy, although required for only three of the 119 children, constituted 11% of the total cost. Previous studies examining the cost of health services in aSLE used a slightly different valuation system than that used for the study (discussed previously) in children. Nonetheless, using a conservative estimate, the direct cost of care for a child with SLE seems approximately three times higher than for an adult. Whether or not this difference in cost between adults and children is due to differences in health care delivery systems, adherence to therapies, or differences in disease severity remains to be determined.[166]

REFERENCES

1. Brunner HI, Gladman DD, Ibanez D, et al. Difference in disease features between childhood-onset and adult-onset systemic lupus erythematosus. Arthritis Rheum 2008;58(2):556–62.
2. Font J, Cervera R, Espinosa G, et al. Systemic lupus erythematosus (SLE) in childhood: analysis of clinical and immunological findings in 34 patients and comparison with SLE characteristics in adults. Ann Rheum Dis 1998;57(8): 456–9.
3. Hersh AO, von Scheven E, Yazdany J, et al. Differences in long-term disease activity and treatment of adult patients with childhood- and adult-onset systemic lupus erythematosus. Arthritis Rheum 2009;61(1):13–20.
4. Hoffman IE, Lauwerys BR, De Keyser F, et al. Juvenile-onset systemic lupus erythematosus: different clinical and serological pattern than adult-onset systemic lupus erythematosus. Ann Rheum Dis 2009;68(3):412–5.
5. Rood MJ, ten Cate R, van Suijlekom-Smit LW, et al. Childhood-onset Systemic Lupus Erythematosus: clinical presentation and prognosis in 31 patients. Scand J Rheumatol 1999;28(4):222–6.
6. Tucker LB. Making the diagnosis of systemic lupus erythematosus in children and adolescents. Lupus 2007;16(8):546–9.
7. Tucker LB, Menon S, Schaller JG, et al. Adult- and childhood-onset systemic lupus erythematosus: a comparison of onset, clinical features, serology, and outcome. Br J Rheumatol 1995;34(9):866–72.
8. Tucker LB, Uribe AG, Fernandez M, et al. Adolescent onset of lupus results in more aggressive disease and worse outcomes: results of a nested matched case-control study within LUMINA, a multiethnic US cohort (LUMINA LVII). Lupus 2008;17(4):314–22.
9. Pluchinotta FR, Schiavo B, Vittadello F, et al. Distinctive clinical features of pediatric systemic lupus erythematosus in three different age classes. Lupus 2007; 16(8):550–5.
10. Danchenko N, Satia JA, Anthony MS. Epidemiology of systemic lupus erythematosus: a comparison of worldwide disease burden. Lupus 2006;15(5):308–18.
11. Malleson PN, Fung MY, Rosenberg AM. The incidence of pediatric rheumatic diseases: results from the Canadian Pediatric Rheumatology Association Disease Registry. J Rheumatol 1996;23(11):1981–7.
12. Nossent HC. Systemic lupus erythematosus in the Arctic region of Norway. J Rheumatol 2001;28(3):539–46.
13. McCarty DJ, Manzi S, Medsger TA Jr, et al. Incidence of systemic lupus erythematosus. Race and gender differences. Arthritis Rheum 1995;38(9):1260–70.
14. Tucker LB, Uribe AG, Fernandez M. Clinical differences between juvenile and adult onset patients with systemic lupus erythematosus: results from a multiethnic longitudinal cohort. Arthritis Rheum 2006;54(6):S162.
15. Costallat LT, Coimbra AM. Systemic lupus erythematosus: clinical and laboratory aspects related to age at disease onset. Clin Exp Rheumatol 1994;12(6): 603–7.

16. Hiraki LT, Benseler SM, Tyrrell PN, et al. Clinical and laboratory characteristics and long-term outcome of pediatric systemic lupus erythematosus: a longitudinal study. J Pediatr 2008;152(4):550–6.

17. Carreno L, Lopez-Longo FJ, Monteagudo I, et al. Immunological and clinical differences between juvenile and adult onset of systemic lupus erythematosus. Lupus 1999;8(4):287–92.

18. Descloux E, Durieu I, Cochat P, et al. Paediatric systemic lupus erythematosus: prognostic impact of antiphospholipid antibodies. Rheumatology (Oxford) 2008; 47(2):183–7.

19. Bader-Meunier B, Armengaud JB, Haddad E, et al. Initial presentation of childhood-onset systemic lupus erythematosus: a French multicenter study. J Pediatr 2005;146(5):648–53.

20. Iqbal S, Sher MR, Good RA, et al. Diversity in presenting manifestations of systemic lupus erythematosus in children. J Pediatr 1999;135(4):500–5.

21. Hiraki L, Benseler S, Tyrrell P, et al. Ethnic differences in pediatric systemic lupus erythematosus. J Rheumatol 2009;36(11):2539–46.

22. Cooper GS, Parks CG, Treadwell EL, et al. Differences by race, sex and age in the clinical and immunologic features of recently diagnosed systemic lupus erythematosus patients in the southeastern United States. Lupus 2002;11(3): 161–7.

23. Gattorno M, Buoncompagni A, Molinari AC, et al. Antiphospholipid antibodies in paediatric systemic lupus erythematosus, juvenile chronic arthritis and overlap syndromes: SLE patients with both lupus anticoagulant and high-titre anticardiolipin antibodies are at risk for clinical manifestations related to the antiphospholipid syndrome. Br J Rheumatol 1995;34(9):873–81.

24. Ramirez Gomez LA, Uribe Uribe O, Osio Uribe O, et al. Childhood systemic lupus erythematosus in Latin America. The GLADEL experience in 230 children. Lupus 2008;17(6):596–604.

25. Meislin AG, Rothfield N. Systemic lupus erythematosus in childhood. Analysis of 42 cases, with comparative data on 200 adult cases followed concurrently. Pediatrics 1968;42(1):37–49.

26. Del Boz J, Martin T, Samaniego E, et al. Childhood discoid lupus in identical twins. Pediatr Dermatol 2008;25(6):648–9.

27. Sampaio MC, de Oliveira ZN, Machado MC, et al. Discoid lupus erythematosus in children–a retrospective study of 34 patients. Pediatr Dermatol 2008;25(2):163–7.

28. Santiago MB, Galvao V. Jaccoud arthropathy in systemic lupus erythematosus: analysis of clinical characteristics and review of the literature. Medicine (Baltimore) 2008;87(1):37–44.

29. Nord JE, Shah PK, Rinaldi RZ, et al. Hydroxychloroquine cardiotoxicity in systemic lupus erythematosus: a report of 2 cases and review of the literature. Semin Arthritis Rheum 2004;33(5):336–51.

30. Kanayama Y, Shiota K, Horiguchi T, et al. Correlation between steroid myopathy and serum lactic dehydrogenase in systemic lupus erythematosus. Arch Intern Med 1981;141(9):1176–9.

31. Alsufyani KA, Ortiz-Alvarez O, Cabral DA, et al. Bone mineral density in children and adolescents with systemic lupus erythematosus, juvenile dermatomyositis, and systemic vasculitis: relationship to disease duration, cumulative corticosteroid dose, calcium intake, and exercise. J Rheumatol 2005;32(4):729–33.

32. Trapani S, Civinini R, Ermini M, et al. Osteoporosis in juvenile systemic lupus erythematosus: a longitudinal study on the effect of steroids on bone mineral density. Rheumatol Int 1998;18(2):45–9.

33. Cervera R, Khamashta MA, Font J, et al. Morbidity and mortality in systemic lupus erythematosus during a 10-year period: a comparison of early and late manifestations in a cohort of 1,000 patients. Medicine (Baltimore) 2003;82(5):299–308.

34. Pineau CA, Urowitz MB, Fortin PJ, et al. Osteoporosis in systemic lupus erythematosus: factors associated with referral for bone mineral density studies, prevalence of osteoporosis and factors associated with reduced bone density. Lupus 2004;13(6):436–41.

35. Yeap SS, Fauzi AR, Kong NC, et al. A comparison of calcium, calcitriol, and alendronate in corticosteroid-treated premenopausal patients with systemic lupus erythematosus. J Rheumatol 2008;35(12):2344–7.

36. Wright TB, Leonard MB, Zemel BS, et al. Hypovitaminosis D is associated with greater body mass index and disease activity in pediatric systemic lupus erythematosus. J Pediatr 2009;155(2):260–5.

37. Zappitelli M, Duffy CM, Bernard C, et al. Evaluation of activity, chronicity and tubulointerstitial indices for childhood lupus nephritis. Pediatr Nephrol 2008; 23(1):83–91.

38. Marks SD, Sebire NJ, Pilkington C, et al. Clinicopathological correlations of paediatric lupus nephritis. Pediatr Nephrol 2007;22(1):77–83.

39. Brunner HI, Silverman ED, To T, et al. Risk factors for damage in childhood-onset systemic lupus erythematosus: cumulative disease activity and medication use predict disease damage. Arthritis Rheum 2002;46(2):436–44.

40. Perfumo F, Martini A. Lupus nephritis in children. Lupus 2005;14(1):83–8.

41. Steinlin MI, Blaser SI, Gilday DL, et al. Neurologic manifestations of pediatric systemic lupus erythematosus. Pediatr Neurol 1995;13(3):191–7.

42. Turkel SB, Miller JH, Reiff A. Case series: neuropsychiatric symptoms with pediatric systemic lupus erythematosus. J Am Acad Child Adolesc Psychiatry 2001; 40(4):482–5.

43. Benseler SM, Silverman ED. Neuropsychiatric involvement in pediatric systemic lupus erythematosus. Lupus 2007;16(8):564–71.

44. Olfat MO, Al-Mayouf SM, Muzaffer MA. Pattern of neuropsychiatric manifestations and outcome in juvenile systemic lupus erythematosus. Clin Rheumatol 2004;23(5):395–9.

45. Sibbitt WL Jr, Brandt JR, Johnson CR, et al. The incidence and prevalence of neuropsychiatric syndromes in pediatric onset systemic lupus erythematosus. J Rheumatol 2002;29(7):1536–42.

46. Hanly JG, Urowitz MB, Su L, et al. Short-term outcome of neuropsychiatric events in systemic lupus erythematosus upon enrollment into an international inception cohort study. Arthritis Rheum 2008;59(5):721–9.

47. Muscal E, Myones BL. The role of autoantibodies in pediatric neuropsychiatric systemic lupus erythematosus. Autoimmun Rev 2007;6(4):215–7.

48. Rivest C, Lew RA, Welsing PM, et al. Association between clinical factors, socioeconomic status, and organ damage in recent onset systemic lupus erythematosus. J Rheumatol 2000;27(3):680–4.

49. Reiff A, Miller J, Shaham B, et al. Childhood central nervous system lupus; longitudinal assessment using single photon emission computed tomography. J Rheumatol 1997;24(12):2461–5.

50. Parikh S, Swaiman KF, Kim Y. Neurologic characteristics of childhood lupus erythematosus. Pediatr Neurol 1995;13(3):198–201.

51. Avcin T, Benseler SM, Tyrrell PN, et al. A followup study of antiphospholipid antibodies and associated neuropsychiatric manifestations in 137 children with systemic lupus erythematosus. Arthritis Rheum 2008;59(2):206–13.

52. Harel L, Sandborg C, Lee T, et al. Neuropsychiatric manifestations in pediatric systemic lupus erythematosus and association with antiphospholipid antibodies. J Rheumatol 2006;33(9):1873–7.

53. Mikdashi JA, Alarcón GS, Crofford L, et al. Proposed response criteria for neuro-cognitive impairment in systemic lupus erythematosus clinical trials. Lupus 2007;16:418–25.

54. Brunner H, Levy D, Schanberg L, et al. Standardizing the neuropsychological evaluation of children with systemic lupus erythematosus. 7th European Lupus Congress, Amsterdam. Lupus 2008;17(32):467.

55. Doherty NE, Siegel RJ. Cardiovascular manifestations of systemic lupus erythe-matosus. Am Heart J 1985;110(6):1257–65.

56. Miller DJ, Maisch SA, Perez MD, et al. Fatal myocardial infarction in an 8-year-old girl with systemic lupus erythematosus, Raynaud's phenomenon, and secondary antiphospholipid antibody syndrome. J Rheumatol 1995;22(4): 768–73.

57. Asanuma Y, Oeser A, Shintani AK, et al. Premature coronary-artery atheroscle-rosis in systemic lupus erythematosus. N Engl J Med 2003;349(25):2407–15.

58. Manzi S, Meilahn EN, Rairie JE, et al. Age-specific incidence rates of myocardial infarction and angina in women with systemic lupus erythematosus: comparison with the Framingham study. Am J Epidemiol 1997;145(5):408–15.

59. Al-Abbad AJ, Cabral DA, Sanatani S, et al. Echocardiography and pulmonary function testing in childhood onset systemic lupus erythematosus. Lupus 2001;10(1):32–7.

60. Swigris JJ, Fischer A, Gillis J, et al. Pulmonary and thrombotic manifestations of systemic lupus erythematosus. Chest 2008;133(1):271–80.

61. Memet B, Ginzler EM. Pulmonary manifestations of systemic lupus erythemato-sus. Semin Respir Crit Care Med 2007;28(4):441–50.

62. Murin S, Wiedemann HP, Matthay RA. Pulmonary manifestations of systemic lupus erythematosus. Clin Chest Med 1998;19(4):641–65, viii.

63. Ferguson PJ, Weinberger M. Shrinking lung syndrome in a 14-year-old boy with systemic lupus erythematosus. Pediatr Pulmonol 2006;41(2):194–7.

64. Karim MY, Miranda LC, Tench CM, et al. Presentation and prognosis of the shrinking lung syndrome in systemic lupus erythematosus. Semin Arthritis Rheum 2002;31(5):289–98.

65. Samad AS, Lindsley CB. Treatment of pulmonary hemorrhage in childhood systemic lupus erythematosus with mycophenolate mofetil. Southampt Med J 2003;96(7):705–7.

66. Byun JY, Ha HK, Yu SY, et al. CT features of systemic lupus erythematosus in patients with acute abdominal pain: emphasis on ischemic bowel disease. Radiology 1999;211(1):203–9.

67. Lee CK, Ahn MS, Lee EY, et al. Acute abdominal pain in systemic lupus eryth-ematosus: focus on lupus enteritis (gastrointestinal vasculitis). Ann Rheum Dis 2002;61(6):547–50.

68. Richer O, Ulinski T, Lemelle I, et al. Abdominal manifestations in childhood-onset systemic lupus erythematosus. Ann Rheum Dis 2007;66(2):174–8.

69. Yu HH, Wang LC, Lee JH, et al. Lymphopenia is associated with neuropsychi-atric manifestations and disease activity in paediatric systemic lupus erythema-tosus patients. Rheumatology (Oxford) 2007;46(9):1492–4.

70. Martinez-Banos D, Crispin JC, Lazo-Langner A, et al. Moderate and severe neutropenia in patients with systemic lupus erythematosus. Rheumatology (Oxford) 2006;45(8):994–8.

71. Schmugge M, Revel-Vilk S, Hiraki L, et al. Thrombocytopenia and thromboembolism in pediatric systemic lupus erythematosus. J Pediatr 2003;143(5): 666–9.
72. Pamuk GE, Pamuk ON, Baslar Z, et al. Overview of 321 patients with idiopathic thrombocytopenic purpura. Retrospective analysis of the clinical features and response to therapy. Ann Hematol 2002;81(8):436–40.
73. Altintas A, Ozel A, Okur N, et al. Prevalence and clinical significance of elevated antinuclear antibody test in children and adult patients with idiopathic thrombocytopenic purpura. J Thromb Thrombolysis 2007;24(2):163–8.
74. Brunner HI, Freedman M, Silverman ED. Close relationship between systemic lupus erythematosus and thrombotic thrombocytopenic purpura in childhood. Arthritis Rheum 1999;42(11):2346–55.
75. Wu CY, Su YT, Wang JS, et al. Childhood hemolytic uremic syndrome associated with systemic lupus erythematosus. Lupus 2007;16(12):1006–10.
76. Musio F, Bohen EM, Yuan CM, et al. Review of thrombotic thrombocytopenic purpura in the setting of systemic lupus erythematosus. Semin Arthritis Rheum 1998;28(1):1–19.
77. Risdall RJ, McKenna RW, Nesbit ME, et al. Virus-associated hemophagocytic syndrome: a benign histiocytic proliferation distinct from malignant histiocytosis. Cancer 1979;44(3):993–1002.
78. Wong KF, Hui PK, Chan JK, et al. The acute lupus hemophagocytic syndrome. Ann Intern Med 1991;114(5):387–90.
79. Oka Y, Kameoka J, Hirabayashi Y, et al. Reversible bone marrow dysplasia in patients with systemic lupus erythematosus. Intern Med 2008;47(8):737–42.
80. Kaiser R, Cleveland CM, Criswell LA. Risk and protective factors for thrombosis in systemic lupus erythematosus: results from a large, multi-ethnic cohort. Ann Rheum Dis 2009;68(2):238–41.
81. Berube C, Mitchell L, Silverman E, et al. The relationship of antiphospholipid antibodies to thromboembolic events in pediatric patients with systemic lupus erythematosus: a cross-sectional study. Pediatr Res 1998;44(3):351–6.
82. Iwata N, Mori M, Miyamae T, et al. [Sjogren's syndrome associated with childhood-onset systemic lupus erythematosus]. Nihon Rinsho Meneki Gakkai Kaishi 2008;31(3):166–71 [in Japanese].
83. Ostuni PA, Ianniello A, Sfriso P, et al. Juvenile onset of primary Sjogren's syndrome: report of 10 cases. Clin Exp Rheumatol 1996;14(6):689–93.
84. Stiller M, Golder W, Doring E, et al. Primary and secondary Sjogren's syndrome in children–a comparative study. Clin Oral Investig 2000;4(3):176–82.
85. Chikanza IC, Kuis W, Heijnen CJ. The influence of the hormonal system on pediatric rheumatic diseases. Rheum Dis Clin North Am 2000;26(4):911–25.
86. Ilowite NT, Samuel P, Ginzler E, et al. Dyslipoproteinemia in pediatric systemic lupus erythematosus. Arthritis Rheum 1988;31(7):859–63.
87. Soep JB, Mietus-Snyder M, Malloy MJ, et al. Assessment of atherosclerotic risk factors and endothelial function in children and young adults with pediatric-onset systemic lupus erythematosus. Arthritis Rheum 2004;51(3): 451–7.
88. Compeyrot-Lacassagne S, Tyrrell PN, Atenafu E, et al. Prevalence and etiology of low bone mineral density in juvenile systemic lupus erythematosus. Arthritis Rheum 2007;56(6):1966–73.
89. Hua X, Su J, Svenungsson E, et al. Dyslipidaemia and lipoprotein pattern in systemic lupus erythematosus (SLE) and SLE-related cardiovascular disease. Scand J Rheumatol 2009;38(3):184–9.

90. Tyrrell PN, Beyene J, Benseler SM, et al. Predictors of lipid abnormalities in children with new-onset systemic lupus erythematosus. J Rheumatol 2007;34(10): 2112–9.

91. El Magadmi M, Ahmad Y, Turkie W, et al. Hyperinsulinemia, insulin resistance, and circulating oxidized low density lipoprotein in women with systemic lupus erythematosus. J Rheumatol 2006;33(1):50–6.

92. Chung CP, Avalos I, Oeser A, et al. High prevalence of the metabolic syndrome in patients with systemic lupus erythematosus: association with disease characteristics and cardiovascular risk factors. Ann Rheum Dis 2007;66(2): 208–14.

93. Appenzeller S, Pallone AT, Natalin RA, et al. Prevalence of thyroid dysfunction in systemic lupus erythematosus. J Clin Rheumatol 2009;15(3):117–9.

94. Eberhard BA, Laxer RM, Eddy AA, et al. Presence of thyroid abnormalities in children with systemic lupus erythematosus. J Pediatr 1991;119(2):277–9.

95. Athreya BH, Rafferty JH, Sehgal GS, et al. Adenohypophyseal and sex hormones in pediatric rheumatic diseases. J Rheumatol 1993;20(4):725–30.

96. Ronchezel MV, Len CA, Spinola e Castro A, et al. Thyroid function and serum prolactin levels in patients with juvenile systemic lupus erythematosus. J Pediatr Endocrinol Metab 2001;14(2):165–9.

97. Koller MD, Templ E, Riedl M, et al. Pituitary function in patients with newly diagnosed untreated systemic lupus erythematosus. Ann Rheum Dis 2004;63(12): 1677–80.

98. Silva CA, Leal MM, Leone C, et al. Gonadal function in adolescents and young women with juvenile systemic lupus erythematosus. Lupus 2002;11(7):419–25.

99. Huong DL, Amoura Z, Duhaut P, et al. Risk of ovarian failure and fertility after intravenous cyclophosphamide. A study in 84 patients. J Rheumatol 2002; 29(12):2571–6.

100. Silva CA, Hilario MO, Febronio MV, et al. Risk factors for amenorrhea in juvenile systemic lupus erythematosus (JSLE): a Brazilian multicentre cohort study. Lupus 2007;16(7):531–6.

101. Brunner HI, Bishnoi A, Barron AC, et al. Disease outcomes and ovarian function of childhood-onset systemic lupus erythematosus. Lupus 2006;15(4):198–206.

102. Silva CA, Brunner HI. Gonadal functioning and preservation of reproductive fitness with juvenile systemic lupus erythematosus. Lupus 2007;16(8):593–9.

103. Silva CA, Hallak J, Pasqualotto FF, et al. Gonadal function in male adolescents and young males with juvenile onset systemic lupus erythematosus. J Rheumatol 2002;29(9):2000–5.

104. Suehiro RM, Borba EF, Bonfa E, et al. Testicular Sertoli cell function in male systemic lupus erythematosus. Rheumatology (Oxford) 2008;47(11):1692–7.

105. Perilloux BC, Shetty AK, Leiva LE, et al. Antinuclear antibody (ANA) and ANA profile tests in children with autoimmune disorders: a retrospective study. Clin Rheumatol 2000;19(3):200–3.

106. Fox RI. Sjogren's syndrome. Lancet 2005;366(9482):321–31.

107. McGhee JL, Kickingbird LM, Jarvis JN. Clinical utility of antinuclear antibody tests in children. BMC Pediatr 2004;4:13.

108. Breda L, Nozzi M, De Sanctis S, et al. Laboratory tests in the diagnosis and follow-up of pediatric rheumatic diseases: an update. Semin Arthritis Rheum 2009. [Epub ahead of print].

109. Esdaile JM, Abrahamowicz M, Joseph L, et al. Laboratory tests as predictors of disease exacerbations in systemic lupus erythematosus. Why some tests fail. Arthritis Rheum 1996;39(3):370–8.

110. Isenberg DA, Collins C. Detection of cross-reactive anti-DNA antibody idiotypes on renal tissue-bound immunoglobulins from lupus patients. J Clin Invest 1985; 76(1):287–94.

111. Reichlin M, Broyles TF, Hubscher O, et al. Prevalence of autoantibodies to ribosomal P proteins in juvenile-onset systemic lupus erythematosus compared with the adult disease. Arthritis Rheum 1999;42(1):69–75.

112. To CH, Petri M. Is antibody clustering predictive of clinical subsets and damage in systemic lupus erythematosus? Arthritis Rheum 2005;52(12): 4003–10.

113. Jurencak R, Fritzler M, Tyrrell P, et al. Autoantibodies in pediatric systemic lupus erythematosus: ethnic grouping, cluster analysis, and clinical correlations. J Rheumatol 2009;36(2):416–21.

114. Campos LM, Kiss MH, Scheinberg MA, et al. Antinucleosome antibodies in patients with juvenile systemic lupus erythematosus. Lupus 2006;15(8): 496–500.

115. Tikly M, Gould T, Wadee AA, et al. Clinical and serological correlates of antinucleosome antibodies in South Africans with systemic lupus erythematosus. Clin Rheumatol 2007;26(12):2121–5.

116. Lettre G, Rioux JD. Autoimmune diseases: insights from genome-wide association studies. Hum Mol Genet 2008;17(R2):R116–21.

117. Pickering MC, Walport MJ. Links between complement abnormalities and systemic lupus erythematosus. Rheumatology (Oxford) 2000;39(2):133–41.

118. Kallel-Sellami M, Baili-Klila L, Zerzeri Y, et al. Hereditary complement deficiency and lupus: report of four Tunisian cases. Ann N Y Acad Sci 2007; 1108:197–202.

119. Yang Y, Lhotta K, Chung EK, et al. Complete complement components C4A and C4B deficiencies in human kidney diseases and systemic lupus erythematosus. J Immunol 2004;173(4):2803–14.

120. Reveille JD, Schrohenloher RE, Acton RT, et al. DNA analysis of HLA-DR and DQ genes in American blacks with systemic lupus erythematosus. Arthritis Rheum 1989;32(10):1243–51.

121. Barron KS, Silverman ED, Gonzales J, et al. Clinical, serologic, and immunogenetic studies in childhood-onset systemic lupus erythematosus. Arthritis Rheum 1993;36(3):348–54.

122. Baca V, Catalan T, Villasis-Keever M, et al. Effect of low-dose cyclosporine A in the treatment of refractory proteinuria in childhood-onset lupus nephritis. Lupus 2006;15(8):490–5.

123. Kyogoku C, Langefeld CD, Ortmann WA, et al. Genetic association of the R620W polymorphism of protein tyrosine phosphatase PTPN22 with human SLE. Am J Hum Genet 2004;75(3):504–7.

124. Liao CH, Yao TC, Chung HT, et al. Polymorphisms in the promoter region of RANTES and the regulatory region of monocyte chemoattractant protein-1 among Chinese children with systemic lupus erythematosus. J Rheumatol 2004;31(10):2062–7.

125. Jacob CO, Reiff A, Armstrong DL, et al. Identification of novel susceptibility genes in childhood-onset systemic lupus erythematosus using a uniquely designed candidate gene pathway platform. Arthritis Rheum 2007;56(12): 4164–73.

126. Velazquez-Cruz R, Orozco L, Espinosa-Rosales F, et al. Association of PDCD1 polymorphisms with childhood-onset systemic lupus erythematosus. Eur J Hum Genet 2007;15(3):336–41.

127. Brunner HI, Klein-Gitelman MS, Ying J, et al. Corticosteroid use in childhood-onset systemic lupus erythematosus-practice patterns at four pediatric rheumatology centers. Clin Exp Rheumatol 2009;27(1):155–62.

128. Kumar S, Benseler SM, Kirby-Allen M, et al. B-cell depletion for autoimmune thrombocytopenia and autoimmune hemolytic anemia in pediatric systemic lupus erythematosus. Pediatrics 2009;123(1):e159–63.

129. Baca V, Lavalle C, Garcia R, et al. Favorable response to intravenous methylprednisolone and cyclophosphamide in children with severe neuropsychiatric Lupus. J Rheumatol 1999;26(2):432–9.

130. Levy DM, Massicotte MP, Harvey E, et al. Thromboembolism in paediatric lupus patients. Lupus 2003;12(10):741–6.

131. Harrison MJ, Ravdin LD, Lockshin MD. Relationship between serum NR2a antibodies and cognitive dysfunction in systemic lupus erythematosus. Arthritis Rheum 2006;54(8):2515–22.

132. Bertsias G, Boumpas DT. Update on the management of lupus nephritis: let the treatment fit the patient. Nat Clin Pract Rheumatol 2008;4(9):464–72.

133. Niaudet P. Treatment of lupus nephritis in children. Pediatr Nephrol 2000;14(2): 158–66.

134. Barbano G, Gusmano R, Damasio B, et al. Childhood-onset lupus nephritis: a single-center experience of pulse intravenous cyclophosphamide therapy. J Nephrol 2002;15(2):123–9.

135. Lehman TJ, Onel K. Intermittent intravenous cyclophosphamide arrests progression of the renal chronicity index in childhood systemic lupus erythematosus. J Pediatr 2000;136(2):243–7.

136. Lehman TJ, Edelheit BS, Onel KB. Combined intravenous methotrexate and cyclophosphamide for refractory childhood lupus nephritis. Ann Rheum Dis 2004;63(3):321–3.

137. Falcini F, Capannini S, Martini G, et al. Mycophenolate mofetil for the treatment of juvenile onset SLE: a multicenter study. Lupus 2009;18(2):139–43.

138. Hagelberg S, Lee Y, Bargman J, et al. Longterm followup of childhood lupus nephritis. J Rheumatol 2002;29(12):2635–42.

139. Lionaki S, Kapitsinou PP, Iniotaki A, et al. Kidney transplantation in lupus patients: a case-control study from a single centre. Lupus 2008;17(7):670–5.

140. Cochat P, Fargue S, Mestrallet G, et al. Disease recurrence in paediatric renal transplantation. Pediatr Nephrol 2009;24(11):2097–108.

141. Ghafari A, Etemadi J, Ardalan MR. Renal transplantation in patients with lupus nephritis: a single-center experience. Transplant Proc 2008;40(1): 143–4.

142. Moroni G, Tantardini F, Gallelli B, et al. The long-term prognosis of renal transplantation in patients with lupus nephritis. Am J Kidney Dis 2005; 45(5):903–11.

143. Drenkard C, Villa AR, Garcia-Padilla C, et al. Remission of systematic lupus erythematosus. Medicine (Baltimore) 1996;75(2):88–98.

144. Urowitz MB, Feletar M, Bruce IN, et al. Prolonged remission in systemic lupus erythematosus. J Rheumatol 2005;32(8):1467–72.

145. Cook CD, Wedgwood RJ, Craig JM, et al. Systemic lupus erythematosus. Description of 37 cases in children and a discussion of endocrine therapy in 32 of the cases. Pediatrics 1960;26:570–85.

146. Glidden RS, Mantzouranis EC, Borel Y. Systemic lupus erythematosus in childhood: clinical manifestations and improved survival in fifty-five patients. Clin Immunol Immunopathol 1983;29(2):196–210.

147. Gonzalez B, Hernandez P, Olguin H, et al. Changes in the survival of patients with systemic lupus erythematosus in childhood: 30 years experience in Chile. Lupus 2005;14(11):918–23.

148. Urowitz MB, Gladman DD, Tom BD, et al. Changing patterns in mortality and disease outcomes for patients with systemic lupus erythematosus. J Rheumatol 2008;35(11):2152–8.

149. Chambers SA, Allen E, Rahman A, et al. Damage and mortality in a group of British patients with systemic lupus erythematosus followed up for over 10 years. Rheumatology (Oxford) 2009;48(6):673–5.

150. Doria A, Iaccarino L, Ghirardello A, et al. Long-term prognosis and causes of death in systemic lupus erythematosus. Am J Med 2006;119(8):700–6.

151. Moss KE, Ioannou Y, Sultan SM, et al. Outcome of a cohort of 300 patients with systemic lupus erythematosus attending a dedicated clinic for over two decades. Ann Rheum Dis 2002;61(5):409–13.

152. Cervera R, Khamashta MA, Font J, et al. Morbidity and mortality in systemic lupus erythematosus during a 5-year period. A multicenter prospective study of 1,000 patients. European Working Party on Systemic Lupus Erythematosus. Medicine (Baltimore) 1999;78(3):167–75.

153. Bernatsky S, Boivin JF, Joseph L, et al. Mortality in systemic lupus erythematosus. Arthritis Rheum 2006;54(8):2550–7.

154. Cervera R, Abarca-Costalago M, Abramovicz D, et al. Systemic lupus erythematosus in Europe at the change of the millennium: lessons from the "Euro-Lupus Project". Autoimmun Rev. 2006;5(3):180–6.

155. Bandeira M, Buratti S, Bartoli M, et al. Relationship between damage accrual, disease flares and cumulative drug therapies in juvenile-onset systemic lupus erythematosus. Lupus 2006;15(8):515–20.

156. Fernandez M, Alarcon GS, Apte M, et al. Systemic lupus erythematosus in a multiethnic US cohort: XLIII. The significance of thrombocytopenia as a prognostic factor. Arthritis Rheum 2007;56(2):614–21.

157. Mok CC, To CH, Ho LY, et al. Incidence and mortality of systemic lupus erythematosus in a southern Chinese population, 2000–2006. J Rheumatol 2008;35(10):1978–82.

158. Koneru S, Shishov M, Ware A, et al. Effectively measuring adherence to medications for systemic lupus erythematosus in a clinical setting. Arthritis Rheum 2007;57(6):1000–6.

159. Ting V, Kudalkar D, Nelson S, et al. Use of cellular text messaging to improve visit adherence in adolescents with childhood-onset Systemic Lupus Erythematosus (cSLE) [abstract]. Philadelphia; American College of Rheumatology; 2009.

160. Al Dhanhani AM, Gignac MA, Su J, et al. Work disability in systemic lupus erythematosus. Arthritis Rheum 2009;61(3):378–85.

161. Reiff A. Childhood quality of life in the changing landscape of pediatric rheumatology. J Pediatr (Rio J) 2008;84(4):285–8.

162. Becker-Merok A, Nossent HC. Damage accumulation in systemic lupus erythematosus and its relation to disease activity and mortality. J Rheumatol 2006;33(8):1570–7.

163. Gutierrez-Suarez R, Ruperto N, Gastaldi R, et al. A proposal for a pediatric version of the Systemic Lupus International Collaborating Clinics/American College of Rheumatology Damage Index based on the analysis of 1,015 patients with juvenile-onset systemic lupus erythematosus. Arthritis Rheum 2006;54(9):2989–96.

164. Brunner HI, Sherrard TM, Klein-Gitelman MS. Cost of treatment of childhood-onset systemic lupus erythematosus. Arthritis Rheum 2006;55(2):184–8.
165. Lau CS, Mak A. The socioeconomic burden of SLE. Nat Rev Rheumatol 2009; 5(7):400–4.
166. Sutcliffe N, Clarke AE, Taylor R, et al. Total costs and predictors of costs in patients with systemic lupus erythematosus. Rheumatology (Oxford) 2001; 40(1):37–47.

The Metabolic Syndrome in Systemic Lupus Erythematosus

Ben Parker, MBChB, MRCP[a], Ian N. Bruce, MD, FRCP[a,b],*

KEYWORDS

- Coronary heart disease • Inflammation
- Systemic lupus erythematosus • Metabolic syndrome

The impact of coronary heart disease (CHD) on morbidity and mortality in patients with established systemic lupus erythematosus (SLE) has assumed increasing importance in their long-term management. Classic CHD risk factors and lupus-specific factors, such as antiphospholipid antibodies, seem to be important in determining long-term cardiovascular risk, but the role of metabolic derangement, specifically the metabolic syndrome (MetS), is gaining increasing prominence in the literature. The extent to which MetS is associated with long-term CHD in the general population, and whether its presence can predict those patients at increased risk of CHD over and above existing risk scores, does remain controversial. This article considers what is known about MetS in SLE and also considers what is known about the impact of MetS on vascular risk in the lupus population.

CHD IN SLE

The bimodal mortality pattern in SLE has been recognized for over 30 years.[1] Mortality in established disease is frequently caused by manifestations of atherosclerotic disease in coronary or cerebrovascular vessels.[2,3] In a retrospective cohort study of 498 women with SLE incidence rates of myocardial infarction were found to be increased fivefold to sixfold compared with the Framingham Offspring cohort. Most strikingly, two thirds of events in the lupus cohort occurred before the age of 55 years, and the rate ratio was increased more than 50-fold in the 35- to 44-year age group.[4] Similarly, a Swedish study linking death registry data to the records of 4700 lupus patients found a standardized mortality ratio from CHD of 15.9 in SLE.[5] An increased burden of subclinical atherosclerosis has also been noted in patients with SLE. Autopsy

[a] ARC Epidemiology Unit, Manchester Academic Health Sciences Centre, The University of Manchester Stopford Building, Oxford Road, Manchester M13 9PT, UK
[b] The Kellgren Centre for Rheumatology, Manchester Royal Infirmary, Manchester, UK
* Corresponding author. ARC Epidemiology Unit, Manchester Academic Health Sciences Centre, The University of Manchester Stopford Building, Oxford Road, Manchester M13 9PT.
E-mail address: ian.bruce@manchester.ac.uk (I.N. Bruce).

Rheum Dis Clin N Am 36 (2010) 81–97
doi:10.1016/j.rdc.2009.12.004
0889-857X/10/$ – see front matter © 2010 Elsevier Inc. All rights reserved.

rheumatic.theclinics.com

studies of patients with SLE have demonstrated significant generalized atherosclerosis in approximately 50% of cases, regardless of underlying cause of death,[6] and coronary artery atherosclerosis is particularly prevalent (up to 42% of patients) in those patients who have received steroids for at least 1 year.[7] Many groups have subsequently demonstrated the presence of subclinical atherosclerosis in SLE patients in cross-sectional studies using a variety of measures, most commonly the presence of carotid plaque[8–10] but also CT detection of coronary artery calcification,[11] large artery stiffness,[12] and impaired endothelial function.[13,14]

The contribution of classic Framingham risk factors for CHD to this increased burden of cardiovascular disease has been the subject of extensive investigation. The Toronto Risk Factor Study reported that women with SLE who were free of CHD were more likely to be hypertensive, diabetic, and suffer from dyslipidemia compared with age-matched healthy controls.[15] Similarly, over half the Hopkins Lupus Cohort had three or more CHD risk factors, despite a mean age of 38.3 years.[16] Classic Framingham risk factors alone do not entirely explain the disparity in prevalence of clinical and subclinical cardiovascular disease in lupus cohorts. In a large Canadian cohort with a mean follow-up of 8.6 years, Esdaile and colleagues[17] assessed baseline classic risk factor frequency and adverse vascular outcomes. After controlling for the presence of classic risk factors, lupus patients still had a 10-fold increase in relative risk (RR) for nonfatal myocardial infarction than is expected using the Framingham model alone. Subsequent studies using measures of subclinical cardiovascular disease (eg, carotid plaque and endothelial dysfunction) have also found that after adjustment for classic risk factors, SLE remains associated with an increased burden of premature atherosclerosis.[8,13]

SLE can be considered an independent risk factor for CHD and disease-specific factors, such as antiphospholipid antibodies, renal disease, complement, and inflammatory pathways, all influence long-term cardiovascular risk.[18] The effect of metabolic derangement, and in particular the role of MetS, on cardiovascular risk in SLE has gained attention because it may also contribute to this enhanced risk.

THE MetS

Recently defined, the term "metabolic syndrome" is used to describe the presence of certain metabolic abnormalities and cardiovascular risk factors in an individual with increased adiposity. The clustering of metabolic disorders in certain individuals, however, has been recognized for much longer; as early as the 1920s the association between hyperglycemia, hypertension, and gout was described,[19] and in 1980 the association of obesity with dyslipidemia was made.[20] By 1988, Reaven[21] had coined the term "syndrome X" to describe the association between insulin-resistance, type 2 diabetes mellitus, hypertension, and cardiovascular disease and in 1998 the first formal definition of MetS was proposed by the World Health Organization (WHO).[22] Over the subsequent years the literature on MetS has expanded significantly despite, or perhaps in part because of, its controversial clinical significance and conflicting definitions.

Since first described in 1998, there have been a further four definitions of MetS published by different working groups, and one significant modification and one consensus statement. Each definition differs with regard to the most suitable measure of obesity, the thresholds used for each criterion, and most importantly in the method used to assess disordered insulin metabolism (**Table 1**). The initial WHO recommendation, published as part of wider definition and classification of diabetes, was mainly designed as a guideline and not necessarily a complete definition of MetS. This

Table 1
Summary of criteria for metabolic syndrome proposed by different bodies

	WHO 1998	EIGR 1999	NCEP ATPIII 2001	AACE 2003	IDF 2006
Essential	IR High insulin or IFG or IGT	IR Top 25% of fasting insulin values in nondiabetics		IGT	Central obesity (ethnicity specific)
Plus	Two or more of	Two or more of	Any three of	Two or more of	Two or more of
	Hypertension	Hypertension	Hypertension	Hypertension	Hypertension
	BP >140/90[a] mm Hg	BP 140/90 mm Hg	BP >130/85 mm Hg	BP 130/85 mm Hg	BP >130/85 mm Hg
	Dyslipidemia	Dyslipidemia	Dyslipidemia	Dyslipidemia	Dyslipidemia
	TG >1.7 mmol/L	TG >2 mmol/L	TG >1.7 mmol/L	TG >1.7 mmol/L	TG >1.7 mmol/L
	+/or low HDL-C	HDL-C <1 mmol/L	Low HDL-C	HDL-C	Low HDL-C
	♂ <0.9 mmol/L		♂ <1 mmol/L	♂ <1 mmol/L	♂ <1.03 mmol/L
	♀ <1 mmol/L		♀ < 1.25 mmol/L	♀ <1.25 mmol/L	♀ <1.29 mmol/L
	Central obesity	Central obesity	Central obesity		
	♂ WHR >0.9	♂ WC >94 cm	♂ WC >102 cm		
	♀ WHR >0.85	♀ WC >80 cm	♀ WC >88 cm		
	or BMI >30 kg/m²				
	Microalbuminuria		Fasting glucose >6.1 mmol/L	Fasting glucose >6.1 mmol/L	Fasting glucose >5.6 mmol/L

Abbreviations: AACE, American Association of Clinical Endocrinologists; ATPIII, Adult Treatment Panel III; BMI, body mass index; EIGR, European Group for the Study of Insulin Resistance; HDL-C, high-density lipoprotein cholesterol; IDF, International Diabetes Federation; IFG, impaired fasting glycemia; IGT, impaired glucose tolerance; NECP, National Cholesterol Education Program; TG, triglycerides; WC, waist circumference; WHR, waist-to-hip ratio; WHO, World Health Organization.
[a] Initially >160/90.

recommendation considered MetS to have at its core disordered insulin metabolism and insulin resistance (IR), and hence it is viewed as part of the diabetic spectrum.[22] It has, however, been criticized for the inclusion of microalbuminuria and its measure of IR (using a euglycemic clamp), which is not easily applicable to either routine clinical practice or large-scale research studies. In 1999, the European Group for the Study of Insulin Resistance modified this definition. They excluded diabetic subjects, used waist circumference as a measure of adiposity, and used fasting insulin levels as a surrogate for IR.[23] In contrast, the Executive Summary of the Third Report of the National Cholesterol Education Program (NCEP) Expert Panel on Detection, Evaluation and Treatment of High Blood Cholesterol in Adults (ATPIII) of 2001, modified in 2005 by the American Heart Association and National Heart, Lung, and Blood Institute (NHLBI),[24] considers MetS as a precursor to diabetes and excluded those with overt type 2 diabetes. More applicable to clinical practice, the NCEP does not include any essential criteria and does not measure IR, instead using fasting glucose levels as a surrogate.[25] Most recently, the International Diabetes Federation (IDF) definition has an essential criterion of (ethnic-specific) central obesity, removing the presence of documented IR and focusing instead on the presence of impaired glycemic control.[26] Justifying their modifications, the authors emphasize the need for a simple definition to increase the clinical applicability of the syndrome by using criteria that are easy to measure, are widely available, and are applicable to different ethic populations.

Recently, to resolve outstanding contentious issues and harmonize the criteria a Joint Interim Statement from the IDF, NHLBI, American Heart Association, World Heart Federation, International Atherosclerosis Society, and International Association for the Study of Obesity was published with agreement reached regarding a new definition of MetS (**Table 2**). Unfortunately, consensus has still to be achieved regarding thresholds for abdominal obesity until further evidence is available.[27] The lack of longer-term prospective studies on which the criteria are based is a major criticism of each definition, as is the lack of evidence to support the alteration of individual thresholds for each criterion, such as the IDF's decision to reduce the threshold for

---

Table 2
Revised criteria for clinical diagnosis of metabolic syndrome as proposed by the International Diabetes Federation Task Force on Epidemiology and Prevention; National Heart, Lung, and Blood Institute; American Heart Association; World Heart Federation; International Atherosclerosis Society; and International Association for the Study of Obesity[a]

Measure	Categorical Cut Points
Elevated waist circumference	Population and country-specific definitions
Elevated triglycerides (or drug therapy)	>1.7 mmol/L
Reduced high-density lipoprotein cholesterol (or drug therapy)	<1 mmol/L in males <1.3 mmol/L in females
Elevated blood pressure (or drug therapy)	>130/85 mm Hg
Elevated fasting glucose (or drug therapy)	>5.6 mmol/L

[a] Any three from five.
Data from Alberti KG, Eckel RH, Grundy SM, et al. Harmonizing the metabolic syndrome: a joint interim statement of the International Diabetes Federation Task Force on Epidemiology and Prevention; National Heart, Lung, and Blood Institute; American Heart Association; World Heart Federation; International Atherosclerosis Society; and International Association for the Study of Obesity. Circulation 2009;120:1640–5.

waist circumference from 102 to 94 cm. Consequently, the existence of multiple definitions has hampered comparison between studies, hence even the basic population prevalence of the syndrome is difficult to ascertain with any certainty.

EPIDEMIOLOGY OF MetS IN THE GENERAL POPULATION

The exact prevalence of MetS depends largely on the definition used and varies considerably between populations (**Table 3**). Perhaps the only certainty regarding MetS is the fact that its prevalence is increasing over time[36] in parallel with the rising prevalence of obesity.[37,38] Although an extensive review of the many studies examining the prevalence of MetS around the world is outside the scope of this article, it is worth discussing two that demonstrate several important points. First, the San Antonio Heart Study of an ethnically mixed United States population (N >2500) reported a widely variable prevalence of MetS depending on the definition used: in white males the prevalence was 18.8% using the WHO definition, 24% using the ATPIII definition, and 28% using the IDF definition.[34] The study also demonstrated a significant difference in prevalence of MetS between the two main ethnic groups (white and Hispanic), which does support the need for ethnic-specific criteria. Second, Ford and colleagues[39] demonstrate the increasing prevalence of MetS over time in two cohorts (1988–1994 and 1999–2002) of the National Health and Examination Survey from 23.1% to 26.7% using the ATPIII criteria. Much of the difference was caused by a much larger age-adjusted increase in prevalence of MetS in women (23.5%) compared with men (2.2%) because of concurrent increases in rates of obesity.

MetS AND PREDICTION OF CHD

Because the primary purpose of defining MetS is to identify those individuals at greater risk of developing CHD (and diabetes) than is otherwise predicted, it is expected that MetS is a strong predictor of cardiovascular events in the general population. Most longitudinal and prospective studies do seem to support this hypothesis and overall demonstrate that (1) the presence of MetS increases long-term CHD risk in those patients without pre-existing CHD[40–43]; (2) MetS increases the risk of CHD events in those patients with established CHD[44]; and (3) the more components of

Table 3
Worldwide prevalence (%) of the metabolic syndrome by definition

	Number	Age	ATPIII		WHO		IDF	
			M	F	M	F	M	F
Australia[28]	11,247	>25	24.4	19.9	25.4	18.2	34.4	27.2
Denmark[29]	2493	41–72	18.6	14.3			23.8	17.5
Iran[30]	10,368	>20	24	40.5	17	20	21	41
Ireland[31]	890	50–69	21.8	21.5	24.6	17.8		
Mexico[32]	2158	20–69	28.5	25.2	13.4	13.8		
Taiwan[33]	5936	20–80	18.3	13.6			16.1	13.3
United States[a34]	2559	25–64	24	16	18	12	28	24
United States[35]	8608	>20	24	23.4	27.9	22.6	—	—

Abbreviations: ATPIII, Adult Treatment Panel III; IDF, International Diabetes Federation; WHO, World Health Organization.
[a] White data only.

MetS present in an individual, the greater the risk of future CHD.[45–47] A recent meta-analysis by Gami and colleagues[44] of 37 longitudinal studies investigating MetS and CHD risk totaling more than 172,000 individuals found that the presence of MetS had a RR of CHD events or death of 1.78 (95% confidence interval [CI], 1.58–2.00). This risk was higher in women (RR 2.63) and remained even after adjusting for individual CHD risk factors (RR 1.54). The authors conclude that "the results can help clinicians counsel patients to consider lifestyle interventions and fuel research into other preventative interventions," reinforcing that MetS be viewed as a disease and not just a cluster of risk factors.

Of equal interest, however, are those studies that have not found an increased prevalence of CHD in individuals with MetS. Kragelund and colleagues[48] prospectively investigated all-cause mortality in a Danish cohort of stable CHD patients with an average follow-up period of 9.2 years. Using the WHO definition, they found that MetS was not associated with an increase in mortality overall, although it was increased in females (modified hazard ratio 2.2). The mean body mass index (BMI) was just 27 in the MetS group, compared with 25 in the control group, suggesting that many of those classified as having MetS did not have a significant increase in visceral adiposity. In a recent report on two large prospective studies Sattar and colleagues[49] investigated the extent to which MetS and its individual components were related to cardiovascular risk (and diabetes) in an elderly population. Data from the Prospective Study of Pravastatin in the Elderly at Risk study (age range, 70–82 years) were corroborated by data from the British Regional Heart Study (age range, 60–79 years), and MetS was defined using the ATPIII criteria. In the Prospective Study of Pravastatin in the Elderly at Risk study MetS was not associated with an increased CHD risk in an elderly population, and was only weakly associated with an increase in CHD risk in British Regional Heart Study (RR 1.27; 95% CI, 1.04–1.56). In contrast, both revealed a strong association between MetS and the development of type 2 diabetes. Whether this weak and negative association is caused by the lessening of the impact of MetS on cardiovascular risk as individuals age is unclear.

The mechanisms through which MetS increases CHD risk are likely to be complex but when considering SLE the interplay of chronic inflammation, obesity, and IR is of particular interest.

INFLAMMATION, CARDIOVASCULAR DISEASE, AND IR

Insulin exerts its predominantly anabolic effects by a cell-surface insulin-receptor that includes the promotion of glucose uptake by muscle and adipose tissue, the inhibition of gluconeogenesis, increased protein synthesis, and inhibition of lipolysis. Although insulin has traditionally been viewed as the hormone of glucose homeostasis, its effects on lipid metabolism are now more widely appreciated, with accumulation of lipids and free fatty acids associated with insulin-resistant states.[50] Disordered insulin metabolism is considered a key factor in the development of MetS, and the interaction between IR and chronic inflammation may provide an explanatory link between inflammatory rheumatic diseases, MetS, and CHD, and supporting the hypothesis that atherosclerosis is an inflammatory disease.[51,52]

Increased adiposity, as reflected by such measures as waist circumference and BMI, is associated with higher serum levels of tumor necrosis factor-α (TNF-α) produced by the adipose tissue itself.[53] A potent proinflammatory cytokine, TNF-α has been shown to induce IR in animal models through the inhibition of autophosphorylation of the insulin receptor.[54] Similarly, obesity and visceral adiposity are associated with higher levels of interleukin-6,[53] which inhibits insulin signal transduction in the liver, contributing to IR.[55] When applied to the general population, increased adiposity, particularly visceral adiposity, may therefore result in higher levels of inflammatory cytokines and a decrease in sensitivity to insulin, predisposing the individual to CHD. Although TNF-α may be increased as a consequence of active lupus,[56] rather than a driving force in its immunopathogenesis, higher circulating levels may adversely affect CHD risk in patients with SLE, especially in the presence of other cardiovascular risk factors.

C-reactive protein (CRP), an acute-phase protein produced by the liver in response to tissue injury and infection, is a widely used biomarker of inflammation and has recently emerged as both a marker of, and potential contributor to, long-term CHD risk. As a biomarker, elevated CRP levels (and high-sensitivity CRP) have been shown in multiple studies to be associated with the development of both CHD[57–59] and with individual components of MetS including IR.[60–63] Higher CRP levels may predate the development of both MetS and diabetes.[47,64] It has been argued that the association between CRP and CHD is so strong that an elevated high-sensitivity CRP in patients with MetS adds to the prognostic information and should be added to the clinical classification criteria.[65] CRP itself may contribute to the pathogenesis of atherosclerosis, and animal data reveal that CRP reduces the activity of endothelial nitric oxide synthase, reducing the bioavailability of nitric oxide, in turn resulting in endothelial dysfunction.[66] Other in vitro studies have demonstrated that CRP inhibits both the nitric oxide and prostacyclin pathways involved in regulating endothelial function.[67,68] The role of CRP in vascular damage and CHD risk in SLE is less clear. In general, in the absence of infection, CRP levels are significantly lower than those seen in other systemic inflammatory conditions, such as rheumatoid arthritis, and are often normal despite higher levels of disease activity.[69,70] An increase in high-sensitivity CRP does, however, seem to be associated with both increases in disease activity and disease damage indices.[71,72] The relationship between CRP, cardiovascular risk factors, and features of MetS may be of relevance in SLE. Barnes and colleagues[73] described a significant association between high-sensitivity CRP, body weight (BMI or adiposity were not measured), and hypertension, and Pons-Estel and colleagues[74] also described an association between baseline CRP levels and cardiovascular damage as defined by the SLICC-Damage Index (SLICC-DI) cardiovascular domain in the LUMINA lupus cohort.

The adipose-derived hormone adiponectin may provide further evidence for the link between IR, obesity, and inflammation. Adiponectin increases peripheral sensitivity to insulin but its levels decline with increasing adiposity,[75] and it has been implicated in the development of MetS.[76] Animal models demonstrate that a lack of adiponectin contributes to IR in nutritionally overloaded states[77] and in vitro studies have demonstrated that adiponectin has beneficial effects on endothelial function through nitric oxide pathways and endothelial repair.[78,79] Surprisingly, adiponectin levels seem to be higher in patients with SLE compared with controls, possibly because of coexistent renal impairment and the potential anti-inflammatory role of the hormone. The inverse relationship with MetS remains, however, suggesting that a relative reduction in adiponectin within SLE patients is associated with increased IR.[80,81] Following treatment of patients with lupus nephritis using mycophenolate mofetil, Clancy and colleagues[82] described an increase in serum adiponectin levels suggesting that improving disease control in patients with active SLE may provide a beneficial effect on CHD risk, perhaps through the mechanism of reduced IR.

Current evidence suggests that the increased CHD risk associated with features of MetS, particularly IR and increased adiposity, may relate to a chronic inflammatory state adversely affecting the endothelium. Two key questions therefore arise: what is the prevalence of MetS in SLE and does it influence cardiovascular risk?

PREVALENCE OF MetS IN SLE

Several studies have examined the prevalence of MetS in cross-sectional lupus cohorts from around the world (**Table 4**), mostly using the NCEP ATPIII definition. As seen in the larger studies of nonlupus patients already discussed, using ATPIII the prevalence of the syndrome in SLE varies significantly, from 18% in the United Kingdom[83] to almost 30% in the United States,[84] possibly reflecting the background population prevalence of MetS. Examining individual MetS components, the presence of hypertension is consistently higher in lupus cohorts compared with controls; however, measures of increased adiposity are not, suggesting different clinical sub-phenotypes of MetS in the lupus population. In a United States cohort, for example, 51% of lupus patients were hypertensive, compared with 34% of controls (P = .05)[84] and in the United Kingdom the proportions were 36.4% and 9.4% (P = .01), respectively.[83] Sabio and colleagues[89] report an almost identical (nonobese) mean BMI of 25.9 in both their SLE and control groups, whereas more control subjects had an elevated waist circumference than SLE patients. Similar findings have been reported from both Argentina and the United Kingdom.[83,87] In contrast, Vadacca and colleagues[86] and Chung and colleagues[84] both report statistically significant higher waist circumference in lupus patients compared with controls.

FACTORS ASSOCIATED WITH MetS IN SLE

A key theme of all the studies investigating MetS in SLE has been the assessment of the potential impact of disease-specific factors on the likelihood of fulfilling the criteria for MetS. El-Magadmi and colleagues[83] did not find any association between SLE factors (eg, disease activity and steroid usage) and MetS in their cohort of 61 consecutive female patients with SLE from the United Kingdom. This is likely to reflect the small numbers of patients who fulfilled the ATPIII criteria for MetS (N = 11), however, rather than a real lack of any association. In a Spanish cohort of 160 patients with SLE (18 of whom were male), Sabio and colleagues[89] confirmed the increased rate of

Table 4
Prevalence of MetS in SLE

Location	References	Number of SLE Patients	Prevalence in SLE (%)	Prevalence Controls (%)	Definition
United Kingdom	83	61	18	2.5	NCEP ATPIII
United States	84	102	32.4	10.9[a]	WHO
Brazil	85	86	20	5.4[a]	NCEP ATPIII
Italy	86	50	28	7.7[a]	WHO
Argentina	87	147	28.6	16[a]	NCEP ATPIII
Puerto Rico	88	204	38.2	n/a	AHA/NHLBI[b]
Spain	89	160	20	13	NCEP ATPIII

Abbreviations: AHA, American Heart Association; ATPIII, Adult Treatment Panel III; MetS, metabolic syndrome; NCEP, National Cholesterol Education Program; NHLBI, National Heart, Lung, and Blood Institute; SLE, systemic lupus erythematosus; WHO, World Health Organization.
[a] Association reached statistical significance.
[b] 2005 AHA/NHLBI modification of ATPIII.
Data from Grundy SM, Cleeman JI, Daniels SR, et al. Diagnosis and management of the metabolic syndrome: an American Heart Association/National Heart, Lung, and Blood Institute Scientific Statement. Circulation 2005;112:2735–52.

established CHD in SLE with rates increased 28-fold in the lupus group compared with age- and gender-matched controls. The presence of MetS in SLE was also associated with a threefold increase in established CHD, compared with the group without MetS. Univariate analysis of a range of factors suggested that both higher damage (SLICC-DI) and higher erythrocyte sedimentation rate (ESR) and CRP were associated with the presence of MetS in SLE. The current use of hydroxychloroquine (HCQ) seemed to be protective against MetS, which remained significant in a multivariate analysis (OR 0.192; 95% CI, 0.061–0.605). Both disease activity (as measured by SLEDAI) and average prednisolone dosage were not associated with MetS, despite the higher ESR and CRP. This may be caused by the relatively low SLEDAI in the cohort (mean = 3.6) and low average daily dose of prednisolone (4.1 mg/day), suggesting most patients had mild-moderate disease. In a subsequent study of a slightly smaller cohort (N = 128) the same group found a significant increase in pulse wave velocity (PWV) in those lupus patients with MetS, compared with those without (OR 4.36; 95% CI, 1.70–10.9) and MetS was again associated with higher CRP levels. Again, however, no relationship was found between disease activity and damage and MetS or measures of disease activity and PWV.[90] On the basis of these two studies, it seems that the presence of MetS is an additional factor in predisposing patients with SLE to both clinical and subclinical atherosclerosis; however, confirmation from other centers is necessary to establish whether this is a generalizable conclusion. A similarly sized study from Argentina reports similar findings with regard to factors associated with SLE and the presence of MetS. In this cohort of 147 patients (including 16 males) only an increased SLICC-DI was associated with MetS (OR 1.98; 95% CI, 1.11–3.55). Again, HCQ use seemed to be protective against developing MetS (OR 0.13; 95% CI, 0.03–0.68), but both disease activity and mean cumulative dose of prednisolone were not associated with MetS.[87] It is notable that the prevalence of MetS was higher in the SLE cohort compared with controls despite the fact that the lupus patients were significantly younger. In a cross-sectional study of 204 patients with SLE (eight of whom were male) from Puerto Rico, Negron and colleagues[88] found that a higher ESR was associated with MetS, as were disease activity (using the SLAM-R; OR 1.14; 95% CI, 1.00–1.33) and ever-use of higher doses of prednisolone (>10 mg/day; OR 3.69; 95% CI, 1.22–11.11). In contrast, HCQ use was not found to be protective against MetS in this cohort, although not surprisingly higher levels of self-reported exercise were (OR 0.33; 95% CI, 0.14–0.92). Finally, Chung and colleagues[84] evaluated the relationship of MetS to cardiovascular risk factors and inflammation in 102 patients with SLE (nine of who were male). Using the ATPIII definition, in the 30 patients with MetS only higher CRP levels seemed to be associated with the presence of the syndrome and no associations were noted between disease activity, damage, current steroid dose, or current HCQ use, although those with MetS had a nonsignificant higher cumulative steroid dose (18.2 versus 9.8 g; $P = .10$) than those without.

It seems that no single disease-specific factor predisposes patients with SLE to developing MetS, although higher levels of disease-related damage and inflammatory markers may increase the risk. The use of HCQ may be protective against MetS, but whether this is reflective of a beneficial effect of the drug on metabolic derangement or reflects confounding related to patients with more mild disease is unclear. Surprisingly, the association between steroids and MetS is weak in most studies and this may in part be caused by limited power. It may, however, give clues to how inflammation and metabolic factors interact in SLE patients and is a subject worthy of further study. As already discussed, MetS is broadly associated with IR and several studies have also specifically examined the relation of disordered insulin metabolism in SLE to both disease-specific factors and CHD risk.

INSULIN RESISTANCE IN SLE

The association between atherosclerosis and chronic inflammation may in part be caused by IR and increased adiposity is associated with both IR and markers of inflammation. Not all subjects with IR fulfill criteria for MetS, however, and certainly more recent definitions have removed the need to demonstrate IR. In the context of SLE, mouse models of SLE have shown that lupus-prone mice are more likely to be hypertensive and overweight than controls, with higher fasting insulin levels and impaired glycemic control.[91] In contrast, clinical studies have not consistently demonstrated increased adiposity in SLE cohorts. This raises the possibility that the IR seen in SLE may be caused by the presence of chronic inflammation in addition to obesity, and may explain why despite a higher cardiovascular risk, lupus cohorts are not consistently more obese than controls.

Using the homeostatic model assessment equations El Magadmi and colleagues[83] compared insulin sensitivity (HOMA-S) with secretion (HOMA-B) in 44 female patients with SLE and 45 healthy control subjects. Patients with SLE had higher fasting insulin levels and lower insulin sensitivity, compared with controls, which correlated with measures of adiposity, lower high-density lipoprotein, and increased oxidized low-density lipoprotein. No correlation was found, however, between IR and disease activity (as measured by SLEDAI; $r = 0.15$, $P = NS$) or average steroid dose ($r = -0.24$, $P = NS$). In a larger study of 87 female patients with SLE Tso and Huang[92] investigated the relationship between insulin metabolism and cardiovascular risk factors, including brachial-ankle PWV. Again, SLE patients had higher fasting insulin levels, HOMA-IR, and HOMA-B measures than age-matched controls, and when stratified according to fasting insulin levels, those lupus patients with the highest insulin levels had significantly higher BMI and brachial-ankle PWV than SLE controls. No correlation, however, was found with SLEDAI or prednisolone usage, but again other inflammatory markers, such as ESR and CRP, were not recorded.[92] More recently, Chung and colleagues[93] noted that the HOMA-IR was increased in their cohort, and that this increase was associated with higher BMI and ESR, but not SLEDAI, CRP, TNF-α, or steroid use.

Box 1
Summary of concerns regarding MetS from American Diabetes Association and European Association for the Study of Diabetes

- Criteria are ambiguous or incomplete and rationale for thresholds is ill-defined
- Value of including diabetes in the definition of MetS is questionable
- IR as the unifying etiology is uncertain
- No clear basis for including or excluding other cardiovascular risk factors
- CHD risk associated with MetS is variable and dependent on the specific risk factors present
- The CHD risk associated with the syndrome seems to be no greater than the sum of its parts
- Treatment of the syndrome is no different than the treatment for each of its components
- The medical value of diagnosing MetS is unclear

Data from Kahn R, Buse J, Ferrannini E, et al. The metabolic syndrome: time for a critical appraisal: joint statement from the American Diabetes Association and the European Association for the Study of Diabetes. Diabetes Care 2005;28:2289–304.

SUMMARY AND FUTURE RESEARCH

Despite most studies reporting an association of MetS with increased CHD risk in the general population substantial controversy continues to surround MetS. The MetS has been shown to be inferior to existing CHD risk scores, such as the Framingham Risk Score in middle-aged men,[94] and whether the presence of MetS adds to CHD prediction gained from existing and widely used risk prediction formulas is hotly debated.[95,96] Other criticisms of the syndrome include the use of discrete variables rather than continuous variables resulting in a loss of predictive power[97] and the absence of other factors associated with CHD and metabolic derangement, such as age, CRP, and renal impairment. In 2005 a joint statement from the American Diabetes Association and European Association for the Study of Diabetes (**Box 1**) strongly criticized MetS, questioned its designation as a syndrome, and urged clinicians to focus on the individual components present in each patient instead.[96]

Many questions also remain unanswered in the context of SLE. As in the general population, it remains unclear whether the presence of MetS or IR adds to the ability to predict those at increased risk of CHD. It is also unclear if the metabolic derangements seen with MetS in lupus are the same as those observed in MetS in the general population who do not have a chronic inflammatory condition. Surprisingly, it still remains unclear what role steroids play. It may be that their anti-inflammatory effects balance their adverse metabolic effects. Alternatively and more likely, there may be interindividual variation in sensitivity to steroid side effects that cannot be identified from the cross-sectional studies performed to date. Further research is required to specifically address if MetS contributes to long-term cardiovascular risk in SLE, and key to this may be the role of inflammatory pathways not assessed in current risk scores.

It seems unlikely that MetS will be used ahead of established CHD risk factor screening in SLE; instead, it is likely to act as an adjunct to current screening strategies.[98] As in the general population the major benefit of identifying MetS in patients with SLE is likely to be from highlighting the risk factor that is most amenable to patient-led lifestyle interventions: obesity. To focus the attention of both the clinician and patient on a clustering of metabolic abnormalities that influence long-term cardiovascular risk can only result in an increased likelihood of addressing each component. It is also likely to prompt caution with corticosteroid doses, and in the longer-term support the development of individualized therapeutic regimes that take into account CHD risk.

REFERENCES

1. Urowitz MB, Bookman AA, Koehler BE, et al. The bimodal mortality pattern of systemic lupus erythematosus. Am J Med 1976;60(2):221–5.
2. Nossent J, Cikes N, Kiss E, et al. Current causes of death in systemic lupus erythematosus in Europe, 2000–2004: relation to disease activity and damage accrual. Lupus 2007;16(5):309–17.
3. Ward MM. Premature morbidity from cardiovascular and cerebrovascular diseases in women with systemic lupus erythematosus. Arthritis Rheum 1999; 42(2):338–46.
4. Manzi S, Meilahn EN, Rairie JE, et al. Age-specific incidence rates of myocardial infarction and angina in women with systemic lupus erythematosus: comparison with the Framingham Study. Am J Epidemiol 1997;145(5):408–15.

5. Bjornadal L, Yin L, Granath F, et al. Cardiovascular disease a hazard despite improved prognosis in patients with systemic lupus erythematosus: results from a Swedish population based study 1964–95. J Rheumatol 2004;31(4):713–9.
6. Abu-Shakra M, Urowitz MB, Gladman DD, et al. Mortality studies in systemic lupus erythematosus: results from a single center. I. Causes of death. J Rheumatol 1995; 22(7):1259–64.
7. Bulkley BH, Roberts WC. The heart in systemic lupus erythematosus and the changes induced in it by corticosteroid therapy: a study of 36 necropsy patients. Am J Med 1975;58(2):243–64.
8. Ahmad Y, Shelmerdine J, Bodill H, et al. Subclinical atherosclerosis in systemic lupus erythematosus (SLE): the relative contribution of classic risk factors and the lupus phenotype. Rheumatology 2007;46(6):983–8.
9. de Leeuw K, Freire B, Smit AJ, et al. Traditional and non-traditional risk factors contribute to the development of accelerated atherosclerosis in patients with systemic lupus erythematosus. Lupus 2006;15(10):675–82.
10. Roman MJ, Shanker BA, Davis A, et al. Prevalence and correlates of accelerated atherosclerosis in systemic lupus erythematosus. N Engl J Med 2003;349(25): 2399–406.
11. Asanuma Y, Oeser A, Shintani AK, et al. Premature coronary-artery atherosclerosis in systemic lupus erythematosus. N Engl J Med 2003;349(25):2407–15.
12. Selzer F, Sutton-Tyrrell K, Fitzgerald S, et al. Vascular stiffness in women with systemic lupus erythematosus. Hypertension 2001;37(4):1075–82.
13. El-Magadmi M, Bodill H, Ahmad Y, et al. Systemic lupus erythematosus: an independent risk factor for endothelial dysfunction in women. Circulation 2004;110(4): 399–404.
14. Wright SA, O'Prey FM, Rea DJ, et al. Microcirculatory hemodynamics and endothelial dysfunction in systemic lupus erythematosus. Arterioscler Thromb Vasc Biol 2006;26(10):2281–7.
15. Bruce IN, Urowitz MB, Gladman DD, et al. Risk factors for coronary heart disease in women with systemic lupus erythematosus: the Toronto risk factor study. Arthritis Rheum 2003;48(11):3159–67.
16. Petri M, Spence D, Bone LR, et al. Coronary artery disease risk factors in the Johns Hopkins Lupus Cohort: prevalence, recognition by patients, and preventive practices. Am J Med 1992;71(5):291–302.
17. Esdaile JM, Abrahamowicz M, Grodzicky T, et al. Traditional Framingham risk factors fail to fully account for accelerated atherosclerosis in systemic lupus erythematosus. Arthritis Rheum 2001;44(10):2331–7.
18. Bruce IN. Not only but also: factors that contribute to accelerated atherosclerosis and premature coronary heart disease in systemic lupus erythematosus. Rheumatology 2005;44(12):1492–502.
19. Sarafidis PA, Nilsson PM. The metabolic syndrome: a glance at its history. J Hypertens 2006;24(4):621–6.
20. Albrink MJ, Krauss RM, Lindgrem FT, et al. Intercorrelations among plasma high density lipoprotein, obesity and triglycerides in a normal population. Lipids 1980; 15(9):668–76.
21. Reaven GM. Banting Lecture 1988. Role of insulin resistance in human disease. Diabetes 1988;37(12):1595–607.
22. Alberti KG, Zimmet PZ. Definition, diagnosis and classification of diabetes mellitus and its complications. Part 1: diagnosis and classification of diabetes mellitus provisional report of a WHO consultation. Diabet Med 1998;15(7): 539–53.

23. Balkau B, Charles MA. Comment on the provisional report from the WHO consultation. European Group for the Study of Insulin Resistance (EGIR). Diabet Med 1999;16(5):442–3.
24. Grundy SM, Cleeman JI, Daniels SR, et al. Diagnosis and management of the metabolic syndrome: an American Heart Association/National Heart, Lung, and Blood Institute Scientific Statement. Circulation 2005;112(17):2735–52.
25. Executive summary of the third report of the National Cholesterol Education Program (NCEP) expert panel on detection, evaluation, and treatment of high blood cholesterol in adults (Adult Treatment Panel III). JAMA 2001;285(19):2486–97.
26. Alberti KG, Zimmet P, Shaw J. Metabolic syndrome: a new world-wide definition. A consensus statement from the International Diabetes Federation. Diabet Med 2006;23(5):469–80.
27. Alberti KG, Eckel RH, Grundy SM, et al. Harmonizing the metabolic syndrome: a joint interim statement of the International Diabetes Federation task force on epidemiology and prevention; National Heart, Lung, and Blood Institute; American Heart Association; World Heart Federation; International Atherosclerosis Society; and International Association for the Study of Obesity. Circulation 2009;120(16):1640–5.
28. Cameron AJ, Magliano DJ, Zimmet PZ, et al. The metabolic syndrome in Australia: prevalence using four definitions. Diabetes Res Clin Pract 2007; 77(3):471–8.
29. Jeppesen J, Hansen TW, Rasmussen S, et al. Insulin resistance, the metabolic syndrome, and risk of incident cardiovascular disease: a population-based study. J Am Coll Cardiol 2007;49(21):2112–9.
30. Zabetian A, Hadaegh F, Azizi F. Prevalence of metabolic syndrome in Iranian adult population, concordance between the IDF with the ATPIII and the WHO definitions. Diabetes Res Clin Pract 2007;77(2):251–7.
31. Villegas R, Creagh D, Hinchion R, et al. Prevalence and lifestyle determinants of the metabolic syndrome. Ir Med J 2004;97(10):300–3.
32. Aguilar-Salinas CA, Rojas R, Gomez-Perez FJ, et al. High prevalence of metabolic syndrome in Mexico. Arch Med Res 2004;35(1):76–81.
33. Hwang LC, Bai CH, Chen CJ. Prevalence of obesity and metabolic syndrome in Taiwan. J Formos Med Assoc 2006;105(8):626–35.
34. Lorenzo C, Williams K, Hunt KJ, et al. The National Cholesterol Education Program - Adult Treatment Panel III, International Diabetes Federation, and World Health Organization definitions of the metabolic syndrome as predictors of incident cardiovascular disease and diabetes. Diabetes Care 2007;30(1):8–13.
35. Ford ES, Giles WH. A comparison of the prevalence of the metabolic syndrome using two proposed definitions. Diabetes Care 2003;26(3):575–81.
36. Grundy SM. Metabolic syndrome pandemic. Arterioscler Thromb Vasc Biol 2008; 28(4):629–36.
37. Hillier TA, Fagot-Campagna A, Eschwege E, et al. Weight change and changes in the metabolic syndrome as the French population moves towards overweight: the D.E.S.I.R. cohort. Int J Epidemiol 2006;35(1):190–6.
38. Hollman G, Kristenson M. The prevalence of the metabolic syndrome and its risk factors in a middle-aged Swedish population: mainly a function of overweight? Eur J Cardiovasc Nurs 2008;7(1):21–6.
39. Ford ES, Giles WH, Mokdad AH. Increasing prevalence of the metabolic syndrome among U.S. Adults. Diabetes Care 2004;27(10):2444–9.
40. Dekker JM, Girman C, Rhodes T, et al. Metabolic syndrome and 10-year cardiovascular disease risk in the Hoorn Study. Circulation 2005;112(5):666–73.

41. Lakka HM, Laaksonen DE, Lakka TA, et al. The metabolic syndrome and total and cardiovascular disease mortality in middle-aged men. JAMA 2002;288(21): 2709–16.

42. Malik S, Wong ND, Franklin SS, et al. Impact of the metabolic syndrome on mortality from coronary heart disease, cardiovascular disease, and all causes in United States adults. Circulation 2004;110(10):1245–50.

43. McNeill AM, Rosamond WD, Girman CJ, et al. The metabolic syndrome and 11-year risk of incident cardiovascular disease in the atherosclerosis risk in communities study. Diabetes Care 2005;28(2):385–90.

44. Gami AS, Witt BJ, Howard DE, et al. Metabolic syndrome and risk of incident cardiovascular events and death: a systematic review and meta-analysis of longitudinal studies. J Am Coll Cardiol 2007;49(4):403–14.

45. Hong Y, Jin X, Mo J, et al. Metabolic syndrome, its preeminent clusters, incident coronary heart disease and all-cause mortality: results of prospective analysis for the Atherosclerosis Risk in Communities Study. J Intern Med 2007;262(1): 113–22.

46. Klein BE, Klein R, Lee KE. Components of the metabolic syndrome and risk of cardiovascular disease and diabetes in Beaver Dam. Diabetes Care 2002; 25(10):1790–4.

47. Sattar N, Gaw A, Scherbakova O, et al. Metabolic syndrome with and without C-reactive protein as a predictor of coronary heart disease and diabetes in the West of Scotland Coronary Prevention Study. Circulation 2003;108(4):414–9.

48. Kragelund C, Kober L, Faber J, et al. Metabolic syndrome and mortality in stable coronary heart disease: relation to gender. Int J Cardiol 2007;121(1):62–7.

49. Sattar N, McConnachie A, Shaper AG, et al. Can metabolic syndrome usefully predict cardiovascular disease and diabetes? Outcome data from two prospective studies. Lancet 2008;371(9628):1927–35.

50. Shulman GI. Cellular mechanisms of insulin resistance. J Clin Invest 2000;106(2): 171–6.

51. Hansson GK. Immune mechanisms in atherosclerosis. Arterioscler Thromb Vasc Biol 2001;21(12):1876–90.

52. Libby P. Inflammation in atherosclerosis. Nature 2002;420(6917):868–74.

53. Kern PA, Ranganathan S, Li C, et al. Adipose tissue tumor necrosis factor and interleukin-6 expression in human obesity and insulin resistance. Am J Physiol Endocrinol Metab 2001;280(5):E745–51.

54. Uysal KT, Wiesbrock SM, Marino MW, et al. Protection from obesity-induced insulin resistance in mice lacking TNF-alpha function. Nature 1997;389(6651): 610–4.

55. Senn JJ, Klover PJ, Nowak IA, et al. Interleukin-6 induces cellular insulin resistance in hepatocytes. Diabetes 2002;51(12):3391–9.

56. Smolen JS, Steiner G, Aringer M. Anti-cytokine therapy in systemic lupus erythematosus. Lupus 2005;14(3):189–91.

57. Ford ES. The metabolic syndrome and C-reactive protein, fibrinogen, and leukocyte count: findings from the Third National Health and Nutrition Examination Survey. Atherosclerosis 2003;168(2):351–8.

58. Ridker PM, Buring JE, Cook NR, et al. C-reactive protein, the metabolic syndrome, and risk of incident cardiovascular events: an 8-year follow-up of 14 719 initially healthy American women. Circulation 2003;107(3):391–7.

59. Yudkin JS, Juhan-Vague I, Hawe E, et al. Low-grade inflammation may play a role in the etiology of the metabolic syndrome in patients with coronary heart disease: the HIFMECH study. Metabolism 2004;53(7):852–7.

60. Frohlich M, Imhof A, Berg G, et al. Association between C-reactive protein and features of the metabolic syndrome: a population-based study. Diabetes Care 2000;23(12):1835–9.
61. Guerrero-Romero F, Rodriguez-Moran M. Relation of C-reactive protein to features of the metabolic syndrome in normal glucose tolerant, impaired glucose tolerant, and newly diagnosed type 2 diabetic subjects. Diabete Metab 2003; 29(1):65–71.
62. Mendall MA, Patel P, Ballam L, et al. C reactive protein and its relation to cardiovascular risk factors: a population based cross sectional study. BMJ 1996; 312(7038):1061–5.
63. Yudkin JS, Stehouwer CD, Emeis JJ, et al. C-reactive protein in healthy subjects: associations with obesity, insulin resistance, and endothelial dysfunction: a potential role for cytokines originating from adipose tissue? Arterioscler Thromb Vasc Biol 1999;19(4):972–8.
64. Han TS, Sattar N, Williams K, et al. Prospective study of C-reactive protein in relation to the development of diabetes and metabolic syndrome in the Mexico City Diabetes Study. Diabetes Care 2002;25(11):2016–21.
65. Ridker PM, Wilson PW, Grundy SM. Should C-reactive protein be added to metabolic syndrome and to assessment of global cardiovascular risk? Circulation 2004;109(23):2818–25.
66. Teoh H, Quan A, Lovren F, et al. Impaired endothelial function in C-reactive protein overexpressing mice. Atherosclerosis 2008;201(2):318–25.
67. Venugopal SK, Devaraj S, Jialal I. C-reactive protein decreases prostacyclin release from human aortic endothelial cells. Circulation 2003;108(14):1676–8.
68. Venugopal SK, Devaraj S, Yuhanna I, et al. Demonstration that C-reactive protein decreases eNOS expression and bioactivity in human aortic endothelial cells. Circulation 2002;106(12):1439–41.
69. ter Borg EJ, Horst G, Limburg PC, et al. C-reactive protein levels during disease exacerbations and infections in systemic lupus erythematosus: a prospective longitudinal study. J Rheumatol 1990;17(12):1642–8.
70. Zein N, Ganuza C, Kushner I. Significance of serum C-reactive protein elevation in patients with systemic lupus erythematosus. Arthritis Rheum 1979;22(1):7–12.
71. Bertoli AM, Fernandez M, Alarcon GS, et al. Systemic lupus erythematosus in a multiethnic US cohort LUMINA (XLI): factors predictive of self-reported work disability. Ann Rheum Dis 2007;66(1):12–7.
72. Lee SS, Singh S, Link K, et al. High-sensitivity C-reactive protein as an associate of clinical subsets and organ damage in systemic lupus erythematosus. Semin Arthritis Rheum 2008;38(1):41–54.
73. Barnes EV, Narain S, Naranjo A, et al. High sensitivity C-reactive protein in systemic lupus erythematosus: relation to disease activity, clinical presentation and implications for cardiovascular risk. Lupus 2005;14(8):576–82.
74. Pons-Estel GJ, Gonzalez LA, Zhang J, et al. Predictors of cardiovascular damage in patients with systemic lupus erythematosus: data from LUMINA (LXVIII), a multiethnic US cohort. Rheumatology 2009;48(7):817–22.
75. Arita Y, Kihara S, Ouchi N, et al. Paradoxical decrease of an adipose-specific protein, adiponectin, in obesity. Biochem Biophys Res Commun 1999;257(1): 79–83.
76. Yang WS, Chuang LM. Human genetics of adiponectin in the metabolic syndrome. J Mol Med 2006;84(2):112–21.
77. Maeda N, Shimomura I, Kishida K, et al. Diet-induced insulin resistance in mice lacking adiponectin/ACRP30. Nat Med 2002;8(7):731–7.

78. Chen H, Montagnani M, Funahashi T, et al. Adiponectin stimulates production of nitric oxide in vascular endothelial cells. J Biol Chem 2003;278(45):45021–6.

79. Okamoto Y, Arita Y, Nishida M, et al. An adipocyte-derived plasma protein, adiponectin, adheres to injured vascular walls. Horm Metab Res 2000;32(2): 47–50.

80. Chung CP, Long AG, Solus JF, et al. Adipocytokines in systemic lupus erythematosus: relationship to inflammation, insulin resistance and coronary atherosclerosis. Lupus 2009;18(9):799–806.

81. Sada KE, Yamasaki Y, Maruyama M, et al. Altered levels of adipocytokines in association with insulin resistance in patients with systemic lupus erythematosus. J Rheumatol 2006;33(8):1545–52.

82. Clancy RM, Kim M, Ginzler E. Contribution of vascular well being to the therapeutic response in the induction phase of a randomised multicentre trial comparing MMF to IVC. Arthritis Rheum 2008;58(Suppl 9):925.

83. El-Magadmi M, Ahmad Y, Turkie W, et al. Hyperinsulinemia, insulin resistance, and circulating oxidized low density lipoprotein in women with systemic lupus erythematosus. J Rheumatol 2006;33(1):50–6.

84. Chung CP, Avalos I, Oeser A, et al. High prevalence of the metabolic syndrome in patients with systemic lupus erythematosus: association with disease characteristics and cardiovascular risk factors. Ann Rheum Dis 2007;66(2):208–14.

85. Vilar MJ, Azevedo GD, Gadelha RG, et al. Prevalence of metabolic syndrome and its components in Brazilian women with systemic lupus erythematosus: implications for cardiovascular risk. Ann Rheum Dis 2006;65(Suppl 2):362.

86. Vadacca M, Margiotta D, Rigon A, et al. Adipokines and systemic lupus erythematosus: relationship with metabolic syndrome and cardiovascular disease risk factors. J Rheumatol 2009;36(2):295–7.

87. Bellomio V, Spindler A, Lucero E, et al. Metabolic syndrome in Argentinean patients with systemic lupus erythematosus. Lupus 2009;18(11):1019–25.

88. Negron AM, Molina MJ, Mayor AM, et al. Factors associated with metabolic syndrome in patients with systemic lupus erythematosus from Puerto Rico. Lupus 2008;17(4):348–54.

89. Sabio JM, Zamora-Pasadas M, Jimenez-Jaimez J, et al. Metabolic syndrome in patients with systemic lupus erythematosus from Southern Spain. Lupus 2008; 17(9):849–59.

90. Sabio JM, Vargas-Hitos J, Zamora-Pasadas M, et al. Metabolic syndrome is associated with increased arterial stiffness and biomarkers of subclinical atherosclerosis in patients with systemic lupus erythematosus. J Rheumatol 2009;36(10): 2204–11.

91. Ryan MJ, McLemore GR Jr, Hendrix ST. Insulin resistance and obesity in a mouse model of systemic lupus erythematosus. Hypertension 2006;48(5):988–93.

92. Tso TK, Huang WN. Elevation of fasting insulin and its association with cardiovascular disease risk in women with systemic lupus erythematosus. Rheumatol Int 2009;29(7):735–42.

93. Chung CP, Oeser A, Solus JF, et al. Inflammation-associated insulin resistance: differential effects in rheumatoid arthritis and systemic lupus erythematosus define potential mechanisms. Arthritis Rheum 2008;58(7):2105–12.

94. Wannamethee SG, Shaper AG, Lennon L, et al. Metabolic syndrome vs Framingham Risk Score for prediction of coronary heart disease, stroke, and type 2 diabetes mellitus. Arch Intern Med 2005;165(22):2644–50.

95. Grundy SM. Does the metabolic syndrome exist? Diabetes Care 2006;29(7): 1689–92.

96. Kahn R, Buse J, Ferrannini E, et al. The metabolic syndrome: time for a critical appraisal: joint statement from the American Diabetes Association and the European Association for the Study of Diabetes. Diabetes Care 2005;28(9):2289–304.
97. de Zeeuw D, Bakker SJ. Does the metabolic syndrome add to the diagnosis and treatment of cardiovascular disease? Nat Clin Pract Cardiovasc Med 2008; 5(Suppl 1):S10–4.
98. Wajed J, Ahmad Y, Durrington PN, et al. Prevention of cardiovascular disease in systemic lupus erythematosus: proposed guidelines for risk factor management. Rheumatology 2004;43(1):7–12.

Gonadal Failure with Cyclophosphamide Therapy for Lupus Nephritis: Advances in Fertility Preservation

Jennifer Mersereau, MD[a], Mary Anne Dooley, MD, MPH[b],*

KEYWORDS

- Intravenous cyclophosphamide therapy
- Systemic lupus erythematosus • Lupus nephritis
- Gonadotropin-releasing hormone agonist

Intravenous cyclophosphamide (IVC) remains an important therapy for patients with severe systemic lupus erythematosus (SLE) including lupus nephritis (LN). Given the striking female predominance in SLE (9:1 in reproductive years) and greater risk of nephritis with younger age at onset, women with LN in their reproductive years comprise the largest group of rheumatic disease patients receiving this therapy. As prognosis in SLE improves, the chronic toxicity of this therapy assumes greater importance. Among the devastating complications of IVC therapy for young patients is the high rate of gonadal failure. The risk of premature ovarian failure with sterility, menopausal symptoms, and increased long-term risks of osteoporosis and coronary artery disease may delay physicians and young women with SLE from undertaking IVC therapy, despite the risks of poor long-term renal outcome.[1]

CYCLOPHOSPHAMIDE USE IN LN

Despite widespread use of IVC therapy for proliferative LN, few studies have formally evaluated the ovarian toxicity of this regimen in humans without malignancy. The

[a] Department of Obstetrics and Gynecology, Division of Reproductive Endocrinology and Infertility, University of North Carolina at Chapel Hill, CB #7570, 4001 Old Clinic Building, Chapel Hill, NC 27599-7570 , USA
[b] Department of Medicine, Division of Rheumatology and Immunology, CB#7289, 3330 Thurston Building, University of North Carolina at Chapel Hill, Chapel Hill, NC 27599-7280, USA
* Corresponding author.
E-mail address: Mary_dooley@med.unc.edu (M.A. Dooley).

Rheum Dis Clin N Am 36 (2010) 99–108
doi:10.1016/j.rdc.2009.12.010
0889-857X/10/$ – see front matter © 2010 Elsevier Inc. All rights reserved.

National Institutes of Health (NIH) IVC regimen evolved to include 6 monthly doses of IVC followed by quarterly doses to complete 2 years; patients with inadequate response could "recycle" for additional monthly dosing as needed.[2] The ovarian toxicity of this regimen has been reported in several retrospective studies.[3–15] One was a retrospective, nested cohort study of 39 women with either LN or neuropsychiatric lupus receiving either short (7 doses) or long (at least 15 doses) courses of pulse IVC as compared with women receiving pulse intravenous methylprednisolone.[7] Subjects were followed for up to 4 years and those with cessation of menses had a full gynecologic evaluation. As shown in **Table 1**, there was an increased risk of sustained amenorrhea in women who were older at the time of treatment and in those receiving a higher cumulative dose of IVC. No patients treated with methylprednisolone had amenorrhea. This study is limited by its small sample size, lack of information regarding use of gonadotropin-releasing hormone agonist (GnRHa), and relatively short duration of follow-up. Ioannidis and colleagues[3] found that 21 out of 67 (31%) receiving pulse IVC had sustained amenorrhea and, in women greater than 32-years of age, the risk of amenorrhea increased rapidly and linearly with the adjusted cumulative dose of IVC. The dose at which 50% of the women age 32 or more developed amenorrhea was about $8gm/m^2$, and the dose at which 90% had amenorrhea was $12gm/m^2$. They also noted that there was an increased prevalence of premature amenorrhea in women with longer prior SLE disease duration (over 5 years), anti-Ro antibodies, and anti-U1RNP antibodies. Mok and colleagues[5] demonstrated a similar trend regarding increasing age and risk of ovarian failure, but also noted that women with IVC-induced amenorrhea had significantly fewer severe flares of SLE during the 5-year follow-up period as compared with those who continued to menstruate. While no studies were designed to assess fecundity after IVC treatment, Wang and colleagues[10] observed that 14 of the 23 (60%) IVC-treated women who desired conception after cessation of treatment were able to conceive, resulting in 20 live births and 2 abortions. Unfortunately, the current data does not demonstrate an absolute threshold dose of IVC by age to maintain ovarian function, nor does it provide data on fecundity in women who do maintain menstrual function after IVC treatment.

EFFECT OF CYCLOPHOSPHAMIDE ON OVARIAN FUNCTION
Pathophysiology

Traditionally it was believed that women are born with their lifetime supply of oocytes, with approximately 2 million resting oocytes present at birth. At menarche, there are approximately 300,000 to 400,000 oocytes, and there was thought to be a steady decline in the number of oocytes, both via ovulation and atresia, throughout a woman's

Table 1
Rate of sustained amenorrhea in patients treated with pulse IVC according to age and duration of therapy

Age	All Subjects	Short-course IVC	Long-course IVC
<25	2/16 (12)	0/4 (0)	2/12 (17)
26–30	4/15 (27)	1/8 (12)	3/7 (43)
>31	5/8 (62)	1/4 (25)	4/4 (100)
All ages	11/39 (28)	2/16 (12)	9/23 (39)

Data from Boumpas DT, Austin 3rd HA, Vaughan EM, et al. Risk for sustained amenorrhea in patients with systemic lupus erythematosus receiving intermittent pulse cyclophosphamide therapy. Ann Intern Med 1993;119(5):366–9.

reproductive life. In a series of studies in mice, Tilley and colleagues[16] recently challenged the dogma that there is a fixed and nonrenewing pool of oocytes, demonstrating a return of fertility after bone-marrow transplantation in mice treated with chemotherapy.[17] These studies suggest that a bone marrow transplant may restore lost or damaged germ cells in the ovary, though further research needs to be completed to test this hypothesis and assess these results in a human population. Neither rat nor human granulosa cells metabolize IVC in vitro under varying concentrations of luteinizing hormone.[18] Whereas previous research suggested that IVC exerts its greatest toxicity to primordial follicles in the rat and human ovary,[19] more recently researchers have found greater toxicity to growing or antral follicles in rat models.[20,21] In a study with immature rats treated with IVC (100 mg/kg) as compared with control rats, the number of granulosa cells decreased, the mean follicular diameter decreased, and the granulosa nuclear size increased.[20] In another study with mature cycling rats, there was a significant reduction in the number of ovarian follicles (especially medium and large follicles) after a 21-day course of IVC (5 mg/kg/d).[22]

Cyclophosphamide Effects on Human Gonadal Function

Females

Chemotherapy can affect a woman's reproductive function, though the exact mechanism is unclear. One theory is that chemotherapy causes injury to rapidly dividing granulosa cells that normally provide hormonal support to developing follicles and oocytes, and that damage to these cells causes loss of ovarian function. Another theory is that oocytes, both in the resting and developing stages, are damaged by chemotherapy, perhaps because of their unique situation in which the chromosomes are arrested in meiosis I and perhaps more vulnerable to damage. The degree of damage to the ovary by chemotherapy depends on several factors, including the agent used, cumulative dose, and the age of the patient. Unfortunately, to date, nearly all of the prior studies related to chemotherapy and ovarian function use premature ovarian failure (POF) as the primary outcome. One of the largest studies looks at POF in childhood cancer survivors.[23] This study involves a retrospective cohort of 5-year survivors of childhood cancer diagnosed before the age of 21 who were given a survey about late adverse outcomes, including a menstrual history. Of a total of 3390 survivors studied, 215 developed POF (incidence of 6.7%) with a slightly older mean age of diagnosis in the POF group versus the nonaffected survivors (9.8 ± 6 years vs 8.3 ± 6 years). Multivariate logistic regression found that the independent risk factors included older age at diagnosis, exposure of the ovaries to radiotherapy, and exposure to IVC and procarbazine. The risk of POF with IVC was only significant in older girls (age 13–20) as compared with the cohort treated before the age of 12.

Ovarian pathology in prepubertal girls receiving IVC in combination with other chemotherapeutic regimens reveals ovarian tissue depleted of ova at any stage.[24,25] In contrast, studies evaluating ovarian outcome following treatment of childhood disorders employing IVC as a single chemotherapeutic agent suggest maintained ovarian function with high rates of normal pubertal development and onset of menses.[8,26,27] However, the primary concern for many patients is the effect of chemotherapy on future fertility potential—there have been no studies to date on risk of infertility or subfertility after chemotherapy in women who continue to have menstrual cycles.

Males

Traditionally, prepubertal children have been thought to be at relatively low risk of gonadal toxicity from IVC. Unfortunately, boys receiving IVC treatment before puberty are not protected from gonadal dysfunction. Prepubertal age has been classically characterized as a quiet period. However, during this period, there is active proliferation of Sertoli and Leydig cells in the testes, which may account for the damage from IVC.[28,29] Unlike females, the risk of infertility after IVC in boys is independent of age and pubertal stage. Cyclophosphamide is among the most damaging chemotherapeutic agents impacting the testes; prolonged or permanent azoospermia has been seen in boys who received IVC.[30,31]

Recently, 248 adult male long-term survivors of childhood cancer were assessed for IVC gonadal toxicity.[32] Approximately 70% of male patients who had received less than 7.5 g/m^2 (median 4.1 g/m^2) of IVC regained fertility, but only 10% recovered when doses exceeded 7.5 g/m^2. Almost all survivors who received IVC of 10 g/m^2 or more were at risk for severe spermatogenic dysfunction. Testosterone levels were slightly lower than the controls; however, only 7% of the survivors had low testosterone values and all patients had achieved adult secondary sex characteristics. In a group of 33 young, male survivors of childhood cancer, IVC treatment caused severe gonadal failure with reduced testicular size, low sperm counts, and impairment of Leydig cell function.[33] Testicular biopsy specimens from 19 of these patients showed germinal aplasia in all cases.

In a pilot study of 15 males receiving IVC, 5 patients who were randomized to receive depot testosterone therapy showed higher sperm counts and testosterone levels after chemotherapy than the remaining 10 patients.[34] Given the lack of research that supports the use of a concurrent protective therapy in males, young men should continue to be counseled about gamete storage before IVC treatment.

Techniques to store gametes before chemotherapy are both more readily available and more technically successful for spermatozoa than for oocytes. Unfortunately, prevention of sterility by sperm banking is not possible in prepubertal boys, as active spermatogenesis does not occur at this age. Artificial procedures including electroejaculation methods may be considered. New techniques, including intrauterine insemination, intracytoplasmic sperm injection, and testicular sperm extraction have improved fertility outcomes for men with low sperm counts or motility defects, both of which can be caused by IVC.

PROTECTING OVARIAN RESERVE DURING IVC THERAPY
Use of GnRHa to Protect Ovarian Function?

Strategies to prevent ovarian toxicity from chemotherapeutic agents focus on preventing ovulation, decreasing ovarian metabolic activity and blood flow, hence IVC dose to the ovary. GnRHa act to suppress pituitary release of gonadotropins, therefore creating a temporary "prepubertal" state. In theory, this prepubertal state could help protect ovarian function during IVC therapy. Proposed mechanisms of action include centrally mediated suppression of gonadotropins, direct suppression of gonadotropin receptors on ovaries, or reduction of biologic activity of gonadotropins.

Data from animal models support this premise. Ataya and colleagues[22] found that rats treated with IVC and luteinizing hormone-releasing hormone agonist (LHRHa) had an increased number of small follicles and overall follicles as compared with rats treated with IVC alone. They theorize that treatment with LHRHa inhibits the recruitment of small follicles into the pool of medium or large follicles that are more susceptible to damage by IVC, thus minimizing the number of follicles damaged by chemotherapy. In another study, female rats treated with both IVC and LHRHa increased the future pregnancy rate as compared with rats treated with IVC alone (9:10 vs 4:11, $P<.05$).[35] Of course, there are differences between rats and humans that make it difficult to extrapolate these findings to humans. For example, it is possible that human ovaries have a different susceptibility to damage from chemotherapy and radiation as compared with rats. In addition, rats have a very different reproductive cycle compared with women. Therefore, studies in nonhuman primates and humans are crucial to confirm the efficiency of GnRHa before widespread use is recommended.

The majority of human studies that evaluate the efficacy of GnRHa with respect to protecting ovarian reserve are nonrandomized observational studies with premature ovarian failure as the primary outcome. A recent meta-analysis concluded that the use of a GnRHa during chemotherapy was associated with a 68% increase in the rate of preserved ovarian function compared with women not receiving a GnRHa (summary relative risk = 1.68, 95% CI 1.34–2.1).[36] However, only 2 of 9 studies included in the meta-analysis were randomized-controlled trials and these two trials included only 37 patients collectively. Also, the authors note that included studies have varying intensities and types of chemotherapy, making comparisons between studies difficult. There are very few reported studies of GnRHa use in women with rheumatologic disease.[37,38] One was a prospective, nonrandomized trial involving women receiving IVC for LN and a depot GnRHa was associated with a significant reduction of POF; 5% in the GnRHa-treated group compared with 30% of controls.[38] The study included add-back estradiol therapy, demonstrating that the benefit was not the result of a hypoestrogenemia. Recently, Blumenfeld and Eckman[39] reported in a prospective nonrandomized study that less than 7% of 125 young women exposed to gonadotoxic chemotherapy for malignant or nonmalignant diseases while receiving GnRHa therapy developed POF. However, the use of GnRHa to prevent POF was shown ineffective in a recent cancer trial.[40] Differences in age distribution and the doses of IVC employed may explain the widely differing results observed. Given the conflicting results regarding efficacy of GnRHa at preventing diminished ovarian reserve, it is difficult to advise patients about the use of this treatment. Large randomized controlled trials are currently underway and will, hopefully, provide definitive data about this treatment.

Potential Adverse Effects of Gonadotropin-releasing Hormone Suppression During Cyclophosphamide

In addition to the routine risks to young women receiving GnRHa, 2 potentially disastrous risks are important in the LN population. If GnRHa are started in the follicular phase of the cycle, the initial ovarian upregulation within the first days following therapy increases estrogen levels. The majority of LN patients are hypertensive and nephrotic and a substantial minority may have antiphospholipid antibodies—all increased risks for potential thrombotic events. Physicians should evaluate the individual patient's risk for thrombosis to assess the need to treat with anticoagulation until downregulation is documented. The risk for pregnancy with failure to employ effective contraception is a concern, especially during the first month of therapy and if ovarian suppression is interrupted during therapy. The potential for a multiple pregnancy is increased if conception occurs during initial upregulation following dosing.

General risks from GnRHa include menopausal symptoms such as hot flashes, decreased libido, emotional lability, headaches, acne, decreased breast size, or vaginal dryness. Ovarian hyperstimulation with GnRHa has been described: a woman receiving the medication during hemodialysis and a woman receiving subcutaneous GnRHa.[41,42] The hyperstimulation was attributed to possible intermittent dosing and has not been described with intramuscular depot administration. In each case, hyperstimulation resolved with continued therapy. Dual energy x-ray absorptiometry performed to assess bone mineral density in women receiving GnRHa for treatment of endometriosis has raised concern for bone loss.[43,44]

GnRHa is associated with an increase in blood cholesterol and triglycerides in 9% and 12% of women receiving this therapy, however, HDL/LDL ratios are not altered.[45] The effects of GnRHa are short term and resolve in 4 to 12 weeks after stopping the drug. In addition to potential central nervous system effects of high-dose corticosteroids that may be given at the same time, GnRHa has potential risk of mood alteration or depression.[46]

EGG, EMBRYO, OR OVARIAN TISSUE CRYOPRESERVATION

Egg, embryo, or ovarian cryopreservation techniques remain potential options for women with LN seeking to preserve reproductive potential. Individual patient preferences must be taken into consideration when deciding about appropriate fertility preservation options. To preserve gametes from their own germ line, some patients may opt to undergo 1 cycle of ovarian stimulation with subsequent cryopreservation of either oocytes or embryos.[46] This may take between 2 and 4 weeks, depending on whether the woman is in her follicular or luteal phase when deciding to proceed with ovarian stimulation. Ovarian stimulation involves daily injections with follicle-stimulating hormone for approximately 10 to 15 days, with subsequent oocyte retrieval via trans-vaginal, ultrasound-guided needle aspiration. Freezing embryos is the most mature technology available, and is routinely performed in an infertility population. Future pregnancy rates vary based on the age of the woman at the time of banking, but can be as high as 40% to 60% in a younger population.[47] Of course, freezing embryos requires a sperm source—either the patient must have a male partner or opt to use anonymous donor sperm. Alternately, ovarian stimulation with oocyte cryopreservation is an option for single women, but success rates are likely significantly lower.[48,49] To date, there have been only approximately 1000 babies born worldwide from this technique; therefore, future pregnancy rates are difficult to predict. The best available data suggests estimating a 4% future pregnancy rate per oocyte frozen, though a majority of this data comes from young egg donors and may not be applicable in an older population.[50] Whereas some recent studies have indicated a similar delivery rate with cryopreserved oocytes as compared with traditional in vitro fertilization,[51] currently the American Society of Reproductive Medicine advises offering oocyte cryopreservation only in a research setting with appropriate Institutional Review Board-approved consent.[48]

Ovarian stimulation does result in supraphysiologic serum estradiol levels as ovarian follicles mature, which may be a concern for women with rheumatologic disease who are already at risk for thromboembolic events. In women with hormone-sensitive breast cancers, some researchers advocate a modified ovarian stimulation protocol using aromatase inhibitors to mitigate the peak levels of estradiol. Oktay and colleagues[52] found that the peak estradiol levels were significantly lower in women on the letrozole protocol as compared with women on standard ovarian stimulation protocols (484 ± 278 pg/mL vs 1464 ± 644 pg/mL), with no compromise in the number of oocytes retrieved. This protocol that minimizes peak estradiol levels may be safer in the rheumatologic population than traditional stimulation protocols, though there have been no studies evaluating this theory. One published case-series involved 7 patients with rheumatologic disease undergoing fertility preservation before chemotherapy.[53] Five patients underwent in vitro maturation of immature oocytes aspirated during a natural menstrual cycle and 2 underwent ovarian stimulation, all with subsequent frozen oocytes or embryos. No adverse events occurred. In vitro maturation is a relatively new procedure and should only be offered on research protocols.

Ovarian tissue cryopreservation is an option for women who want to preserve gametes, but do not have time or the inclination to undergo ovarian stimulation for embryo or oocyte cryopreservation. Without any hormonal stimulation, ovarian tissue freezing involves an outpatient laparoscopic oophorectomy. Subsequently, depending on where the woman is in her cycle, maturing oocytes may be aspirated and matured in vitro, and frozen as mature oocytes. Alternately, ovarian cortical tissue can be cut into strips and frozen. In the future, this tissue could be thawed and undergo in vitro follicular maturation or tissue transplantation. Ovarian tissue freezing is currently only available through research protocols as fewer than 10 babies have been born worldwide using this technology.

In women who do not undergo fertility preservation techniques before IVC use, they may have limited options for family building in the future if they undergo premature ovarian failure or significantly diminished ovarian reserve. One option is the use of donor eggs with in vitro fertilization using her partner's sperm. This technology is used routinely in an infertility population, and pregnancy rates are greater than 60% per cycle, regardless of the recipient's age. Ideally, all interested women should undergo a consultation appointment with a reproductive specialist before beginning IVC treatment to discuss the range of options available to her (GnRHa therapy, ovarian stimulation with egg or embryo cryopreservation, ovarian tissue freezing, future pregnancy with egg donor and IVF, adoption, etc).

ALTERNATIVE THERAPEUTIC STRATEGIES FOR LN TO AVOID IVC-INDUCED OVARIAN TOXICITY

Alternative therapeutic strategies for LN include pulse methylprednisolone or short course IVC (6 months), though the limited 6-month course of IVC was associated with greater risks of doubling serum creatinine or relapsing nephritis than in patients receiving a 2-year course.[54] Contreras and colleagues[55] showed superior renal response to 6 monthly doses of IVC followed by mycophenolate mofetil (MMF) or azathioprine (AZA) compared with the traditional 2-year NIH IVC therapy. Among predominately Caucasian patients, the Euro-lupus Nephritis Trial has shown similar efficacy between 500 mg doses of IVC given at 2-week intervals over 3 months followed by azathioprine maintenance to the 2-year NIH regimen.[56] The reproductive rate of this regimen did not differ between the low-dose and high-dose arms of the trial at 10 years.[57] This approach is presently in trial in the United States. Other strategies include completely avoiding therapy with IVC, and employing AZA or MMF alone. Recent concern about the efficacy of long-term AZA versus ICP has been raised by a Dutch study, noting increased chronicity on repeat renal biopsy in patients receiving AZA alone, despite similar clinical endpoints.[58] Despite the continuing search for a more effective, less toxic therapy for LN, the recent Aspreva Lupus Management trial, including more than 350 patients with LN, did not show superiority of induction therapy with MMF compared with IVC in efficacy or toxicity.[59] Additionally, the long-term outcome of MMF therapy has not been well-defined, with the longest follow-up report of less than 5 years.

REFERENCES

1. Fraenkel L, Bogardus S, Concato J. Patient preferences for treatment of lupus nephritis. Arthritis Rheum 2002;47(4):421–8.

2. Gourley MF, Austin HA 3rd, Scott D, et al. Methylprednisolone and cyclophospha-mide, alone or in combination, in patients with lupus nephritis. A randomized, controlled trial. Ann Intern Med 1996;125(7):549–57.

3. Ioannidis JP, Katsifis GE, Tzioufas AG, et al. Predictors of sustained amenorrhea from pulsed intravenous cyclophosphamide in premenopausal women with systemic lupus erythematosus. J Rheumatol 2002;29(10):2129–35.

4. McDermott EM, Powell RJ. Incidence of ovarian failure in systemic lupus erythe-matosus after treatment with pulse cyclophosphamide. Ann Rheum Dis 1996; 55(4):224–9.

5. Mok CC, Wong RW, Lau CS. Ovarian failure and flares of systemic lupus erythe-matosus. Arthritis Rheum 1999;42(6):1274–80.

6. Belmont HM, Storch M, Buyon J, et al. New York University/Hospital for Joint Diseases experience with intravenous cyclophosphamide treatment: efficacy in steroid unresponsive lupus nephritis. Lupus 1995;4(2):104–8.

7. Boumpas DT, Austin HA 3rd, Vaughan EM, et al. Risk for sustained amenorrhea in patients with systemic lupus erythematosus receiving intermittent pulse cyclo-phosphamide therapy. Ann Intern Med 1993;119(5):366–9.

8. Kumar R, Biggart JD, McEvoy J, et al. Cyclophosphamide and reproductive func-tion. Lancet 1972;1(7762):1212–4.

9. Uldall PR, Kerr DN, Tacchi D. Sterility and cyclophosphamide. Lancet 1972; 1(7752):693–4.

10. Wang CL, Wang F, Bosco JJ. Ovarian failure in oral cyclophosphamide treatment for systemic lupus erythematosus. Lupus 1995;4(1):11–4.

11. Warne GL, Fairley KF, Hobbs JB, et al. Cyclophosphamide-induced ovarian failure. N Engl J Med 1973;289(22):1159–62.

12. Langevitz P, Klein L, Pras M, et al. The effect of cyclophosphamide pulses on fertility in patients with lupus nephritis. Am J Reprod Immunol 1992;28(3–4):157–8.

13. Park MC, Park YB, Jung SY, et al. Risk of ovarian failure and pregnancy outcome in patients with lupus nephritis treated with intravenous cyclophosphamide pulse therapy. Lupus 2004;13(8):569–74.

14. Huong DL, Amoura Z, Duhaut P, et al. Risk of ovarian failure and fertility after intra-venous cyclophosphamide. A study in 84 patients. J Rheumatol 2002;29(12): 2571–6.

15. Medeiros MM, Silveira VA, Menezes AP, et al. Risk factors for ovarian failure in patients with systemic lupus erythematosus. Braz J Med Biol Res 2001;34(12): 1561–8.

16. Johnson J, Canning J, Kaneko T, et al. Germline stem cells and follicular renewal in the postnatal mammalian ovary. Nature 2004;428(6979):145–50.

17. Lee HJ, Selesniemi K, Niikura Y, et al. Bone marrow transplantation generates immature oocytes and rescues long-term fertility in a preclinical mouse model of chemotherapy-induced premature ovarian failure. J Clin Oncol 2007;25(22): 3198–204.

18. Ataya K, Pydyn E, Young J, et al. The uptake and metabolism of cyclophospha-mide by the ovary. Sel Cancer Ther 1990;6(2):83–92.

19. Jarrell J, Lai EV, Barr R, et al. Ovarian toxicity of cyclophosphamide alone and in combination with ovarian irradiation in the rat. Cancer Res 1987;47(9):2340–3.

20. Ataya KM, Valeriote FA, Ramahi-Ataya AJ. Effect of cyclophosphamide on the immature rat ovary. Cancer Res 1989;49(7):1660–4.

21. Delrio G, De Placido S, Pagliarulo C, et al. Hypothalamic-pituitary-ovarian axis in women with operable breast cancer treated with adjuvant CMF and tamoxifen. Tumori 1986;72(1):53–61.

22. Ataya KM, McKanna JA, Weintraub AM, et al. A luteinizing hormone-releasing hormone agonist for the prevention of chemotherapy-induced ovarian follicular loss in rats. Cancer Res 1985;45(8):3651–6.
23. Chemaitilly W, Mertens AC, Mitby P, et al. Acute ovarian failure in the childhood cancer survivor study. J Clin Endocrinol Metab 2006;91(5):1723–8.
24. Nicosia SV, Matus-Ridley M, Meadows AT. Gonadal effects of cancer therapy in girls. Cancer 1985;55(10):2364–72.
25. Stillman RJ, Schinfeld JS, Schiff I, et al. Ovarian failure in long-term survivors of childhood malignancy. Am J Obstet Gynecol 1981;139(1):62–6.
26. Callis L, Nieto J, Vila A, et al. Chlorambucil treatment in minimal lesion nephrotic syndrome: a reappraisal of its gonadal toxicity. J Pediatr 1980;97(4):653–6.
27. Parra A, Santos D, Cervantes C, et al. Plasma gonadotropins and gonadal steroids in children treated with cyclophosphamide. J Pediatr 1978;92(1):117–24.
28. Chemes HE. Infancy is not a quiescent period of testicular development. Int J Androl 2001;24(1):2–7.
29. Thomson AB, Campbell AJ, Irvine DC, et al. Semen quality and spermatozoal DNA integrity in survivors of childhood cancer: a case-control study. Lancet 2002;360(9330):361–7.
30. Kuhajda FP, Haupt HM, Moore GW, et al. Gonadal morphology in patients receiving chemotherapy for leukemia. Evidence for reproductive potential and against a testicular tumor sanctuary. Am J Med 1982;72(5):759–67.
31. Meistrich ML. Male gonadal toxicity. Pediatr Blood Cancer 2009;53(2):261–6.
32. van Casteren NJ, van der Linden GH, Hakvoort-Cammel FG, et al. Effect of childhood cancer treatment on fertility markers in adult male long-term survivors. Pediatr Blood Cancer 2009;52(1):108–12.
33. Meistrich ML, Wilson G, Brown BW, et al. Impact of cyclophosphamide on long-term reduction in sperm count in men treated with combination chemotherapy for Ewing and soft tissue sarcomas. Cancer 1992;70(11):2703–12.
34. Masala A, Faedda R, Alagna S, et al. Use of testosterone to prevent cyclophosphamide-induced azoospermia. Ann Intern Med 1997;126(4):292–5.
35. Ataya K, Ramahi-Ataya A. Reproductive performance of female rats treated with cyclophosphamide and/or LHRH agonist. Reprod Toxicol 1993;7(3):229–35.
36. Clowse ME, Behera MA, Anders CK, et al. Ovarian preservation by GnRH agonists during chemotherapy: a meta-analysis. J Womens Health (Larchmt) 2009;18(3):311–9.
37. Blumenfeld Z, Shapiro D, Shteinberg M, et al. Preservation of fertility and ovarian function and minimizing gonadotoxicity in young women with systemic lupus erythematosus treated by chemotherapy. Lupus 2000;9(6):401–5.
38. Somers EC, Marder W, Christman GM, et al. Use of a gonadotropin-releasing hormone analog for protection against premature ovarian failure during cyclophosphamide therapy in women with severe lupus. Arthritis Rheum 2005;52(9): 2761–7.
39. Blumenfeld Z, Eckman A. Preservation of fertility and ovarian function and minimization of chemotherapy-induced gonadotoxicity in young women by GnRH-a. J Natl Cancer Inst Monographs 2005;34:40–3.
40. Ismail-Khan R, Minton S, Cox C, et al. Preservation of ovarian function in young women treated with neoadjuvant chmotherapy for breast cancer: a randomized trial using the GnRH agonist (triptorelin) during chemotherapy [abstract]. J Clin Oncol 2008;26:54.
41. Barbieri R, Yeh J, Ravnikar VA. GnRH agonists and ovarian hyperstimulation. Fertil Steril 1991;56(2):376–7.

42. Hampton HL, Whitworth NS, Cowan BD. Gonadotropin-releasing hormone agonist (leuprolide acetate) induced ovarian hyperstimulation syndrome in a woman undergoing intermittent hemodialysis. Fertil Steril 1991;55(2):429–31.

43. Johansen JS, Riis BJ, Hassager C, et al. The effect of a gonadotropin-releasing hormone agonist analog (nafarelin) on bone metabolism. J Clin Endocrinol Metab 1988;67(4):701–6.

44. Matta WH, Shaw RW, Hesp R, et al. Reversible trabecular bone density loss following induced hypo-oestrogenism with the GnRH analogue buserelin in premenopausal women. Clin Endocrinol (Oxf) 1988;29(1):45–51.

45. Gerhard I, Schindler AE, Buhler K, et al. Treatment of endometriosis with leuprorelin acetate depot: a German multicentre study. Clin Ther 1992;14(Suppl A):3–16.

46. Roberts JE, Oktay K. Fertility preservation: a comprehensive approach to the young woman with cancer. J Natl Cancer Inst Monogr 2005;34:57–9.

47. Veeck LL, Bodine R, Clarke RN, et al. High pregnancy rates can be achieved after freezing and thawing human blastocysts. Fertil Steril 2004;82(5):1418–27.

48. Practice Committee of the Society for Assisted Reproductive Technology, Practice Committee of the American Society for Reproductive Medicine. Essential elements of informed consent for elective oocyte cryopreservation: a Practice Committee opinion. Fertil Steril 2007;88(6):1495–6.

49. Stachecki JJ, Cohen J. An overview of oocyte cryopreservation. Reprod Biomed Online 2004;9(2):152–63.

50. Oktay K, Cil AP, Bang H. Efficiency of oocyte cryopreservation: a meta-analysis. Fertil Steril 2006;86(1):70–80.

51. Grifo JA, Noyes N. Delivery rate using cryopreserved oocytes is comparable to conventional in vitro fertilization using fresh oocytes: potential fertility preservation for female cancer patients. Fertil Steril 2010;93(2):391–6.

52. Oktay K, Hourvitz A, Sahin G, et al. Letrozole reduces estrogen and gonadotropin exposure in women with breast cancer undergoing ovarian stimulation before chemotherapy. J Clin Endocrinol Metab 2006;91(10):3885–90.

53. Elizur SE, Chian RC, Pineau CA, et al. Fertility preservation treatment for young women with autoimmune diseases facing treatment with gonadotoxic agents. Rheumatology (Oxford) 2008;47(10):1506–9.

54. Boumpas DT, Austin HA 3rd, Vaughn EM, et al. Controlled trial of pulse methylprednisolone versus two regimens of pulse cyclophosphamide in severe lupus nephritis. Lancet 1992;340(8822):741–5.

55. Contreras G, Pardo V, Leclercq B, et al. Sequential therapies for proliferative lupus nephritis. N Engl J Med 2004;350(10):971–80.

56. Houssiau FA, Vasconcelos C, D'Cruz D, et al. Immunosuppressive therapy in lupus nephritis: the Euro-Lupus Nephritis Trial, a randomized trial of low-dose versus high-dose intravenous cyclophosphamide. Arthritis Rheum 2002;46(8):2121–31.

57. Houssiau FA, Vasconcelos C, D'Cruz D, et al. The 10-year follow-up data of the Euro-Lupus Nephritis Trial comparing low-dose versus high-dose intravenous cyclophosphamide. Ann Rheum Dis 2010;69(1):61–4.

58. Grootscholten C, Bajema IM, Florquin S, et al. Treatment with cyclophosphamide delays the progression of chronic lesions more effectively than does treatment with azathioprine plus methylprednisolone in patients with proliferative lupus nephritis. Arthritis Rheum 2007;56(3):924–37.

59. Appel GB, Contreras G, Dooley MA, et al. Mycophenolate mofetil versus cyclophosphamide for induction treatment of lupus nephritis. J Am Soc Nephrol 2009;20(5):1103–12.

B-cell Biology and Related Therapies in Systemic Lupus Erythematosus

Sadia Ahmed, MD, Jennifer H. Anolik, MD, PhD*

KEYWORDS

- B lymphocytes • Systemic lupus erythematosus
- Anti-CD20 • Rituximab • Belimumab • Atacicept

Systemic lupus erythematosus (SLE) is a complex autoimmune disease with considerable heterogeneity in clinical manifestations and disease course, characterized by pathogenic autoantibody formation, immune complex deposition, and end-organ damage. The mortality and morbidity of patients with SLE has significantly improved during the last few decades. In the 1950s, the 4-year survival rate for lupus was approximately 50%; more recent series estimate 5-year and 10-year survival rates of 96% and 85%, respectively.[1] Despite these improvements, SLE continues to be associated with significant morbidity and a three- to fivefold increased mortality compared with the general population. Moreover, there is a group of patients with SLE who continue to suffer from aggressive disease that does not respond to conventional treatments.

The continuing need for more effective therapies with less toxic side effects has led to the interest in targeted biologic therapies for severely affected patients who are refractory to or cannot tolerate traditional therapies. However, major obstacles in finding efficacious therapies for SLE include the challenges of clinical trial design given the low prevalence of disease, great clinical heterogeneity, relapsing-remitting course, and lack of well-established end points.[2–4] Partly because of these challenges, no new drugs have been approved for the treatment of SLE in more than 50 years. Despite these difficulties there is reason for optimism, including concerted efforts toward improving lupus clinical trial methodology[4] that have recently led to a successful outcome in 2 clinical trials of a B-cell targeted biologic in SLE. Moreover, our

Dr Anolik has been supported by several grants including U19 Autoimmunity Center of Excellence AI56390, R01 AI077674-01A1, the Lupus Foundation of American, and the Lupus Research Institute. Dr Anolik has received grants from Amgen Pharmaceuticals, Genentech, Proteolix, and Vaccinex. She has served as a consultant for Genentech and Roche.
Division of Allergy Immunology Rheumatology, Department of Medicine, University of Rochester Medical Center, 601 Elmwood Avenue, Box 695, Rochester, NY 14642, USA
* Corresponding author.
E-mail address: jennifer_anolik@urmc.rochester.edu (J.H. Anolik).

understanding about the pathogenesis of SLE has grown substantially in the past decade, leading to an increase in promising biologic therapies. This article reviews the state-of-the-art pathophysiology of SLE, providing the rationale for B-cell targeted therapies, followed by a critical evaluation of the efficacy and safety of B-cell depletion (BCD) with anti-CD20 monoclonal antibody therapy in the management of the disease, and other promising B-cell targeted approaches.

ROLE OF B CELLS IN SLE

Although multiple immunologic abnormalities are important for the development and clinical expression of SLE, a large body of evidence strongly points to the B cell as a critical player in the pathogenesis of this disease.[5]

B-cell Tolerance Loss

As SLE is characterized by the generation of large amounts of autoantibodies directed against chromatin and various other self-antigens the loss of B-cell tolerance is believed to play a key role in the disease. Evidence that the breakdown of B-cell tolerance likely occurs early in SLE and may precede or trigger other immune abnormalities is provided by the demonstration that patients with SLE express antinuclear antibodies (ANAs) several years before the onset of clinical disease. The lag time observed between the appearance of ANAs and clinical expression of SLE may be explained by the need for epitope spreading and generation of increasingly pathogenic autoantibodies.[6]

Numerous single gene defects affecting the B-cell compartment can lead to lupus-like disease in murine models, and many of these defects share a common end point, the loss of B-cell tolerance. At least 3 broad categories of defects that can lead to a lupus like phenotype have been defined in the mouse and are instructive for thinking about B-cell abnormalities in SLE. These defects may affect (1) B-cell activation thresholds (eg, Fc receptor [FcR]), (2) B-cell longevity (eg, B-cell activator of the tumor necrosis factor [TNF] family [BAFF] transgenics), or (3) apoptotic cell/autoantigen processing (eg, mer knockout). Although many alterations in B-cell signaling or costimulatory molecules that may alter (1) or (2) have been shown to lead to a lupus like phenotype in the mouse, their relevance for human SLE and even spontaneous murine models of SLE is not well defined. Kumar and colleagues have recently elucidated the mechanism by which the Sle1 susceptibility locus derived from lupus-prone New Zealand Mixed (NZM2410) mice contributes to the development of autoimmunity. A gene within this locus encoding a member of the signaling lymphocyte activation molecule (SLAM) family was found to be highly expressed in immature B cells and altered in these lupus-prone mice in such a way as to impair signaling and impede antigen-driven negative selection (B-cell deletion, receptor revision, and anergy induction).[7] This finding suggests that some of the genes that contribute to lupus may function by downregulating B-cell receptor (BCR) signaling at the immature stage and impairing B-cell tolerance.

In contrast, other B-cell signaling defects may cause upregulated signaling, as exemplified by loss of inhibitory FcR function. Thus, FcγRIIb deficiency leads to a lupus like phenotype in mice, although with different penetrance depending on mouse strain.[8] Moreover, deficiency of the inhibitory FcγRIIb reduces the threshold for autoreactive B-cell activation,[9] and restoration of proper FcγRIIb expression on B cells in lupus-prone mice prevents the expansion and accumulation of autoantibody-producing plasma cells (PCs).[10] These findings are even more meaningful given that polymorphisms in FcγRIIb are associated with human SLE and have a direct functional consequence on B-cell signaling.[11,12] Thus, an FcγRIIb membrane spanning Ile232 to Thr232 substitution associated with lupus in Asian populations caused decreased FcR lipid raft association and greater, more sustained calcium mobilization and downstream biochemical signaling events on B-cell receptor engagement.[11] Moreover, other defects may lead to decreased expression of FcgRIIb as recently demonstrated in human lupus memory B cells.[12] Such alterations in B-cell signaling proteins could explain earlier observations of increased calcium responses to BCR ligation in SLE B cells.[13] Olferiev and Crow[14] recently approached this question in human lupus by comparing the gene-expression signatures specifically in memory B cells and found the underexpression of several inhibitory receptors including CD22 and CD72, and the overexpression of type I interferon (IFN) inducible genes. Overall, such defects in B-cell signaling pathways are important because they may contribute to the loss of peripheral B-cell tolerance in SLE.

Alterations in B-cell longevity also can lead to lupuslike phenotypes, as exemplified by transgenic expression of BAFF, a key cytokine that promotes B-cell survival. These mice develop a lupuslike phenotype with excessive numbers of mature B cells, spontaneous germinal center (GC) reactions, autoantibodies, high PC numbers, and immunoglobulin (Ig) deposition in the kidney.[15] Moreover, lupus-prone mice have elevated levels of circulating BAFF, and administration of soluble BAFF receptor ameliorates disease progression and improves survival.[16] The importance of BAFF in human SLE has been demonstrated by the finding of increased serum levels in patients with SLE and the correlation with serum IgG and autoantibody levels.[17] Excessive BAFF may be another factor that promotes the survival of autoreactive B cells in the periphery.[18,19] Thus, 2 recent reports have shown that BAFF is a key limiting resource for early (transitional) B-cell survival, with autoreactive B cells surviving selection into the mature pool only when BAFF was in excess.[18,19] Miller and colleagues[20] have proposed a model of B-cell selection and tolerance induction that postulates that the number of cells entering the transitional B-cell pool must exceed the available space if appropriately stringent negative selection is to occur. Events that compromise this rule, including a decrease in incoming cell numbers or increases in BAFF, may circumvent negative selection of autoreactivity (**Fig. 1**).

The impaired clearance of apoptotic debris may also lead to SLE and may do so in part by providing large amounts of self-antigen and immune complexes that deliver stimulatory signals to autoreactive B cells. Several publications in recent years indicate that such apoptotic blebs and immune complexes contain ligands for toll-like receptors (TLR), including RNA or DNA, which can provide costimulatory signals for autoreactive B cells,[21–24] as further described later.

Abnormalities in the B-cell Compartment in Human SLE

Recent work has demonstrated the role of the breakdown of peripheral B-cell tolerance mechanisms in human SLE.[25,26] Thus, Pugh-Bernard and colleagues[27] have shown that an important tolerance checkpoint operates in healthy subjects to censor autoreactive (9G4) B cells in the mature naive compartment, thereby preventing the expansion of these cells into the memory compartment, a checkpoint recently corroborated by others[28] and further shown by the authors to be faulty in SLE.[26] Other work by Wardemann and colleagues[29] has shown that 50% to 75% of newly produced human B cells are autoreactive and must be silenced by tolerance mechanisms. Key checkpoints to censor autoreactive B-cell clones occur at the immature B-cell stage in the bone marrow (BM) and between new transitional emigrants and mature B cells in the periphery. In this system up to 20% of mature naive B cells were self-reactive, indicating the need for additional censoring mechanisms at this stage,

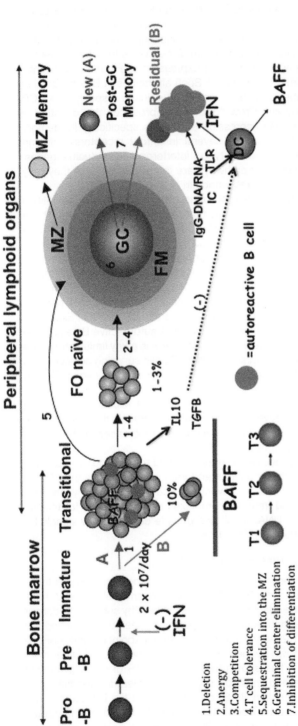

Fig. 1. A model for B-cell development, selection, and function after BCD therapy. The outcome of BCD depends on how well established autoimmunity is eradicated and how the immune system reconstitutes. B cells are continually generated in the BM, and once rituximab is cleared can develop through well-recognized stages (T, transitional; FO, follicular naive; FM, follicular mantle; MZ, marginal zone; GC, germinal center) with defined tolerance checkpoints as shown. Autoreactive B cells (depicted in pink) are deleted in the BM immature subsets, and cells in the transitional subsets undergo further selection, the stringency of which is determined in part by available BAFF (BAFF excess caused by overproduction, peripheral lymphopenia, or reduced BM output reduces selective stringency). A favorable reconstitution profile (denoted A) is characterized by an abundance of newly emerging transitional B cells in an environment that favors stringent negative selection of autoreactivity (high numbers of transitional B cells relative to BAFF). A nonfavorable reconstitution profile (B in red) will be characterized by a higher fraction of residual memory B cells induced by an environment of TLR activation (via DNA and RNA containing immune complex activation of plasmacytoid DC), yielding large quantities of IFN and inhibition of new BM B-cell lymphopoiesis. The outcome of BCD also depends on the balance between protective (regulatory, antiinflammatory) B cells and pathogenic (effector, proinflammatory) B cells and their corresponding cytokines. The authors postulate that physiologically, transitional cells predominantly produce IL-10 (or TGF-β), which in a normal environment exerts antiinflammatory actions. This situation would be altered in autoimmune disease. BCD therapy may restore the physiologic balance between protective and pathogenic B-cell functions by creating an environment dominated by transitional cells with antiinflammatory and tolerogenic functions and Treg-inducing activity.

as suggested by Pugh-Bernard and colleagues and recently shown in the transition to the IgM memory compartment.[28] Wardemann and colleagues have also studied a small number of patients with SLE (n = 3) and found the transitional B-cell checkpoint to be defective although with some heterogeneity, with 41% to 50% of antibodies from the mature naive compartment retaining autoreactivity with HEp-2 cell lysates. These data are intriguing, although the precise point of tolerance breakdown, the variability in this finding in different patient subsets, and the cause of this tolerance checkpoint defect remain to be defined.

A large body of additional evidence indicates that B cells are abnormal in human SLE, with defects ranging from increased calcium flux on signaling through the BCR to high or aberrant expression of costimulatory molecules such as CD80, CD86, and CD40 ligand.[30] B-cell alterations in SLE peripheral blood seem to be more prominent and fluid than in other autoimmune diseases. A range of abnormalities in B-cell homeostasis in SLE have been observed, including a naive B-cell lymphopenia, expansion of peripheral blood plasma cells, increased transitional B cells, and expansion of activated memory B-cell subsets.[31–34] The authors surmise that this reflects the systemic nature of the autoimmune process with frequent cycles of activation, differentiation, and traffic between secondary lymphoid organs and target tissues. The frequency and absolute number of PCs in peripheral blood has correlated with disease activity and antidouble-stranded DNA (anti-dsDNA) titers.[35] More recent studies have begun to refine subsets of PCs, including a human leukocyte antigen (HLA) dopamine receptor high fraction, that may better delineate plasmablasts enriched for autoreactivity and correlating with disease activity.[36] Similarly, the authors' group has elucidated the heterogeneity that exists in human B-cell memory and found that active patients with SLE have an expansion of effector memory B-cell populations positive for markers of homing to sites of systemic inflammation (CXCR3+) and negative for lymphoid homing markers (CD62L−).[33,37] Other groups have found a subset of CD27-IgD-CD95+ memory B cells with an activated phenotype that correlated with disease activity and serologic abnormality.[34] Abnormal expansion of peripheral blood B cells with a pre-GC phenotype has also been reported and proposed to indicate exuberant or abnormally regulated GC reactions in SLE.[38] However, in many cases these cells may actually represent immature transitional B cells as opposed to pre-GC cells.[39]

Overall, the frequency of these diverse B-cell subset abnormalities, their association with each other and other immunologic abnormalities, and relationship with disease activity and disease subsets remain to be better elucidated in larger longitudinal cohorts of patients with SLE. However, several of the B-cell targeted therapies have been shown to reverse at least some of these peripheral B-cell abnormalities. For example, the authors have shown that CD20 targeted BCD normalizes naive lymphopenia, effector memory B-cell expansion (CD27-IgD- double-negative B cells), the presence of PC precursors, and expansion of autoreactive memory B-cell populations.[32] In other studies, BAFF blockade has also been shown to alter peripheral B-cell homeostasis in SLE with decreases in transitional B cells, naive B cells, and plasmablasts, but with less significant effects on the memory B-cell compartment at least at early time points.[40]

The Diverse Role of B Cells in the Initiation and Propagation of Autoimmunity

B cells may participate in the immune dysregulation of SLE at multiple levels by: (1) serving as the precursors of antibody-secreting cells, (2) taking up and presenting autoantigens to T cells, (3) helping to regulate and organize inflammatory responses through cytokine and chemokine secretion (such as interleukin 10 [IL-10], IL-6, IFN-γ, and lymphotoxin-α), and (4) regulating other immune cells (5) (**Fig. 2**). The importance of these latter functions has been demonstrated in murine SLE, in which B cells

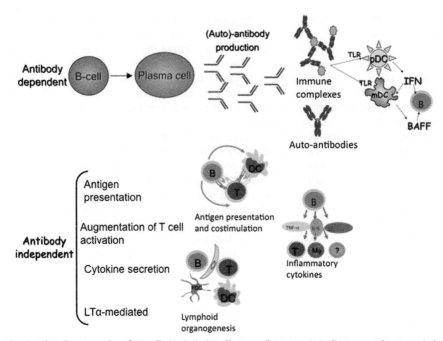

Fig. 2. The diverse role of B cells in SLE. B cells contribute to SLE disease pathogenesis by antibody-dependent and -independent mechanisms. In addition to direct binding of auto-antibodies to target antigens on cells, which can lead to cellular cytotoxicity and complement activation, immune complexes can also activate complement and cause TLR activation. Antibody-independent functions for B cells include antigen presentation and costimulation to T cells, such that B cells can affect T-cell function in diverse ways, contributing to T-cell activation, polarization, and even recruitment of follicular T helper cells to the GC. Other antibody-independent functions for B cells include proinflammatory and anti-inflammatory cytokine secretion and chemokine secretion, including LTα which affects lymphoid organogenesis.

have been found to be critical to the development of disease even when they are unable to secrete autoantibodies. Thus, genetically B-cell deficient J_H knockout MRL/lpr lupus-prone mice have strikingly attenuated disease, with the expected absence of autoantibodies but also the surprising lack of T-cell activation.[41] Chan and colleagues[5] used a novel approach to further elucidate the role of B cells in SLE by generating MRL/lpr mice that express a mutant transgene encoding surface Ig that cannot be secreted. These mice have B cells, but no circulating Ig, yet develop T-cell activation and nephritis. This landmark study was the first to highlight that B cells can play a pathogenic role in lupus independent of serum autoantibody and has been recently supported by the authors' observations that BCD with anti-CD20 has robust effects in the treatment of murine lupus without changes in autoantibodies.[42] This notion has also been corroborated in humans by the authors' own and others' findings that clinical improvement in patients with SLE treated with rituximab correlates with BCD and precedes by several months any decline in serum levels of relevant autoantibodies.[43]

Autoantibody-independent Functions for B Cells in SLE

There has been much speculation about what the key autoantibody-independent functions of B cells are in SLE (**Fig. 2**). A particularly novel function may be direct effects on lymphoid neogenesis through the production of lymphotoxin α (LTα). The formation of tertiary or ectopic lymphoid tissue formation is a process that may lead to dysregulated B-/T-cell interactions and local amplification of autoimmune responses in multiple autoimmune diseases, including rheumatoid arthritis (RA), Sjögren syndrome, type I diabetes, multiple sclerosis, inflammatory bowel disease, Hashimoto thyroditis, and SLE.[44,45] For example, recent reports suggest the importance of this process in human lupus nephritis (LN).[46]

Moreover, B cells can produce numerous other cytokines and may do so in a polarized fashion, mimicking Th1/Th2 cells. So-called effector B cells (Be1 and Be2) can participate in feedback regulation of T helper cells,[47] although the relevance of these mechanisms for SLE have yet to be demonstrated. Along similar lines, B cells play a key role in the recruitment of CXCR5+ follicular T helper (T$_{FH}$) cells to the germinal center.[48] T$_{FH}$ cells provide critical assistance for follicular and GC B cells, inducing activation, differentiation, and antibody production. Recent data indicate that T$_{FH}$ cells and a newly defined population of extrafollicular helper T cells are dependent on B cells for development.[49] The influence of B cells on T$_{FH}$ cells via ICOSL and OX40L costimulation may be important in SLE as excessive activity of T$_{FH}$ cells induces hyperactive GC, breakdown of B-cell tolerance, autoantibody production, and a lupus-like phenoytype in sanroque mice.[50]

From an autoimmunity standpoint, B cells may either stimulate or inhibit pathogenic responses (**Table 1**). Thus, evidence is accumulating for regulatory B cells capable of preventing or suppressing autoimmunity in different mouse models.[51,52] This protective role can be mediated by inducing T-cell anergy during antigen presentation or inducing Treg expansion or activity.[52] B cells may also directly suppress Th1- and Th17-mediated diseases.[53] These activities are mediated, at least in part, by the production of IL-10 or transforming growth factor β (TGF-β) and may control various autoinflammatory diseases, including inflammatory arthritis, inflammatory bowel disease, autoimmune diabetes, experimental autoimmune encephalitis, and contact hypersensitivity.[54–57] Understanding the imbalance between these opposing B-cell functions in disease and how this imbalance may be restored after targeted biologic therapy is an important area of ongoing research.

The Interface Between Innate and Adaptive Immunity: Autoantibodies, IFN, and TLR Activation

Once B-cell tolerance is broken, autoantibodies can contribute to disease pathogenesis in SLE through several classic effector roles, including the formation of damaging

Table 1
The balance between proinflammatory and protective B-cell functions

Induce Autoimmunity	Suppress Autoimmunity
• T-cell activation	• T-cell anergy
• Th1 cytokines (Be1)	• Th2 cytokines (Be2)
• Treg inhibition	• Treg priming/expansion
• DC recruitment	• DC inhibition (IL-10)
• Pathogenic autoantibody	• Protective antibody
• Proinflammatory cytokines TNF, IFN$_\gamma$, IL-12p40, IL-6 • Formation of ectopic lymphoid tissue	• Antiinflammatory cytokines IL-10, TGF-β

immune complexes (immune complex mediated type III hypersensitivity reactions) and direct pathogenesis (type II antibody-dependent cytotoxicity) (**Fig. 2**).[58] However, as alluded to earlier, evidence has emerged that autoantibodies can play an active role in propagating the autoimmune process in SLE, through immune cell activation involving RNA- or DNA-containing autoantigens and TLRs.[21–24,59,60] Plasmacytoid dendritic cells (DCs) may be activated by costimulation of TLRs (TLR-7, -8, or -9) and FcRs via immune complex binding, stimulating the secretion of large quantities of IFN-α,[61] a cytokine with important immunomodulatory functions that include activation and maturation of DCs and stimulation of T and B cells. In combination with TLR-7 and -9 activation of myeloid DCs to produce BAFF, a feedback loop is generated that triggers more B-cell activation (**Fig. 1**). Moreover, by binding to cell surface autoantibodies and subsequently to TLR-7 or -9 within B cells, RNA- or DNA-containing autoantigens or immune complexes can directly trigger activation and proliferation of autoantibody-producing B cells.[21,62,63] In support of the importance of TLR signaling to lupus disease pathogenesis and B-cell activation, deficiency of TLR-7 or -9 can prevent autoantibody production in various mouse models.[62,64] It was recently shown that the murine autoimmune Yaa locus represents a TLR-7 duplication that increases the responsiveness of B cells to TLR-7 ligands, thus contributing to a break in B-cell tolerance.[65] One of the mechanisms by which antimalarials likely exert their effect in SLE is via inhibition of TLR signaling.

As reviewed elsewhere, recent evidence suggests a prominent role for IFN-α activation in SLE. IFN-α may contribute to B-cell abnormalities in SLE, promoting the differentiation of activated B cells into plasmablasts[66] and in conjunction with TLR stimulation triggering B-cell expansion[67] and a lowered activation threshold for autoreactive B cells.[68] The authors have also recently reported a novel role for IFN-α activation in the BM of patients with SLE by decreasing B-cell lymphopoeisis, contributing to B-cell lymphopenia, and theoretically decreasing the stringency of B-cell negative selection.[69]

Although the relative importance of autoantibody-dependent versus -independent roles of B cells in human SLE pathogenesis remains to be defined, given the multiple pathogenic roles of autoantibodies in SLE enumerated earlier, it could be postulated that the most effective therapeutic interventions might decrease autoantibody levels, which may require targeting of the PC compartment directly or indirectly. To do so effectively, it is important to understand the nuances of PC biology. In particular, the premise that autoreactive PCs are short-lived and continually replenished from ongoing immune responses has recently been called into question. There is accumulating evidence that some autoreactive PC populations may be long-lived and resistant to conventional therapies.[70]

THERAPEUTIC TARGETING OF THE B-CELL COMPARTMENT

Several different approaches to targeting B cells have been used: (1) BCD with monoclonal antibodies against B-cell–specific molecules (eg, anti-CD20), (2) induction of negative signaling in B cells (eg, anti-CD22); (3) blocking B-cell survival and activation factors (eg, anti-BAFF), and (4) blocking costimulatory interactions between B and T cells. Many of these agents are currently undergoing formal testing in clinical trials or are under development (**Table 2**).

BCD
Anti-CD20 Monoclonal Antibody

The largest body of clinical data regarding BCD involves anti-CD20 targeted therapy with the monoclonal antibody rituximab. CD20 is a member of the tetraspan family of

Table 2
Approaches to target B cells

Compound	Description	Stage of Development
BCD		
• Rituximab	Chimeric anti-CD20 monoclonal antibody	Phase III SLE
• Ocrelizumab	Humanized anti-CD20 monoclonal antibody	Phase III SLE
• TRU-015	Anti-CD20 SMIP (small modular immunopharmaceutical)	Phase III RA
• Ofatumumab	Fully human anti-CD20 monoclonal antibody	Phase III RA
Inhibitory signaling		
• Epratuzumab	Humanized anti-CD22 monoclonal antibody	Phase II in SLE
Costimulatory blockade		
• Anti-CD40L	Monoclonal antibody against CD40L	No longer in development
• CTLA4-Ig	Fusion protein of CTLA4: blocks B7-CD28 costimulation	Phase II SLE
Cytokine blockade		
• Belimumab/Benlysta	Fully human anti-BAFF monoclonal antibody	Advanced development in SLE
• BR3-Fc	Fusion protein of the BR3 BAFF receptor	Phase II RA
• Anti-BR3	Fully human antibody against BR3	Phase II RA
• Atacicept	Fusion protein of the TACI receptor blocks BAFF/APRIL	Phase I, II RA, SLE

integral membrane proteins[71] and is specifically expressed on immature, naive, memory, and GC B cells, but not on early pre-B cells or PCs. In vitro rituximab can kill B cells by complement-mediated cytotoxicity, antibody-dependent cell-mediated cytotoxicity, and induction of apoptosis.[72] Studies in a murine model of human CD20 expression have demonstrated that different B-cell subsets may be more dependent on certain mechanisms of depletion than others because of tissue microenvironment effects.[73] The kinetics of BCD in tissues is slower than that in the peripheral blood, and certain tissue-bound subsets may be incompletely depleted. The latter point may be particularly relevant for human autoimmune diseases in which complete depletion of autoreactive B-cell clones may be critical for full therapeutic potential. Although anti-CD20 is usually effective in depleting B cells from peripheral blood, success in depleting B cells from other sites such as lymph nodes or tertiary lymphoid tissues may be highly variable.[74,75] Failure to deplete in these tissue sites may lead to nonresponse or early relapse.

Clinical Data on BCD in SLE

Approved by the US Food and Drug Administration for lymphoma in 1997 and rheumatoid arthritis refractory to antitumor necrosis factor in 2006, BCD with rituximab has also shown benefit in open-label studies and case series for many other autoimmune diseases.[76] Initial evidence for the potential benefit of BCD in SLE has been gathered from the combination of the original dose escalation trials of rituximab performed by the authors' group at the University of Rochester[43] and by Albert and colleagues[77] at the University of Pennsylvania and from several open-label series and numerous published and unpublished case reports.[78–80]

Recently, Lu and colleagues[81] published an update of their large single-center experience with rituximab use in 50 patients with SLE with severe refractory disease to conventional immunosuppressives, the longest follow-up to date. Six months after the initial treatment, 42% and 47% of patients showed complete and partial remissions, respectively. Among the patients followed for 7.5 years, 1 remained B-cell depleted for more than 7 years and 53% had experienced a disease flare. Three-quarters of flares occurred within a year of initial treatment, and 80% of these patients were re-treated with good effect. Similarly, in an article reviewing the worldwide experience, Sfikakis and colleagues[82] reported that rituximab was well tolerated in a total of 100 patients with severe, refractory SLE. Ramos-Casals and colleagues[83] also recently reported favorable results through a systematic review of off-label use in 188 cases from the literature between 2002 and 2007. In this latter review 52% of patients received concomitant cyclophosphamide, and a higher rate of therapeutic response was observed in those patients (98% vs 82%, $P<.001$). The University of California at Los Angeles group recently reported their experience with rituximab in 35 Hispanic and African American patients with refractory SLE.[84] These investigators observed significant clinical and immunologic responses, with particular benefit in arthritis and nephritis. In addition, in data from the Autoimmunity and Rituximab French registry, 104 patients with SLE were treated with rituximab (largely without cyclophosphamide) for various indications (including cutaneous/articular involvement in 41%, renal involvement in 30%, and autoimmune cytopenia in 23%) and had an overall clinician-observed efficacy of 73%.[85]

These results support the conclusion that BCD therapy may be effective for patients with active SLE that is refractory to standard immunosuppression. Moreover, the combination of rituximab and cyclophosphamide may offer synergy because both agents can target B cells (even if not used in direct combination, refractory patients have often received cyclophosphamide in the recent past). Although most studies have found adequate peripheral blood BCD, as noted earlier, depletion may be less complete in tissue sites. In SLE this is suggested by the finding of residual circulating B cells by high-sensitivity flow cytometry, predominantly of a memory phenotype, and a reconstitution in poor responders that is dominated by memory B cells.[32,86] The problem of incomplete BCD is highlighted by the authors' original open-label dose escalation phase I/II trial of rituximab in 17 moderately active patients with SLE.[43] In most patients with effective BCD (11/17), the SLAM score was significantly improved at 2 and 3 months, respectively ($P = .0016$ and $P = .0022$), an improvement that persisted for at least 12 months. Six patients in this study had incomplete BCD (including 1 of 4 in the high-dose group) and no clinical improvement. These results highlight that BCD can be effective in a nonrefractory group of patients with SLE as monotherapy when high-dose steroids and other treatments do not confound the results. Incomplete BCD was associated with certain FcR genotypes,[21] African American ancestry, lower serum rituximab levels,[22] and the development of human antichimeric antibodies (HACAs). Another phase I/II prospective open-label study also found that a third of patients developed HACAs, which tended to correlate with less complete BCD, as measured by early B-cell return or ability to respond to vaccinations.[77] The results raise the concern that rituximab may be more immunogenic in active SLE.

Despite considerable enthusiasm for rituximab in SLE based on this open-label experience, 2 recent placebo-controlled trials in nonrenal lupus (EXPLORER) and renal lupus (LUNAR) failed to meet primary end points. At the 2008 American College of Rheumatology (ACR) meeting, Merrill and colleagues[87] reported the EXPLORER trial, a randomized, double-blind, placebo-controlled phase II/III multicenter trial comparing rituximab to placebo in a 2:1 randomization in 257 active patients with SLE. Both groups had significant and sustained decreases in global British Isles Lupus Assessment Group (BILAG) and Systemic Lupus Erythematosus Disease Activity Index (SLE-DAI) scores over time, but with no differences in primary and secondary end points. In a prespecified subgroup analysis of black and Hispanic subjects, who overall had lower placebo responses (15.7% partial clinical response [PCR] including major clinical response [MCR]), there was a statistically significant difference with the addition of rituximab (33.8% PCR including MCR).

Although most lupus manifestations have been reported to respond to BCD in case series and open-label studies, there have been no organ-specific clinical trials with the exception of the recently completed LUNAR study in LN. Organ-specific trials may be advantageous because of less disease heterogeneity and possibly better outcome measures. Moreover, patients can theoretically be selected based on a pathophysiology that might be particularly responsive to BCD. For example, rituximab treatment may be particularly efficacious for disease manifestations predominantly mediated by B cells (directly or indirectly) or short-lived PCs (for example, cytopenias) but not those mediated by antibodies produced by long-lived PCs.

Recent data from small open-label studies have supported the benefit of rituximab in LN. Gunnarsson and colleagues[88] evaluated a combination of cyclophosphamide and rituximab in 18 patients with active nephritis (10 class III/IV, 7 class V, 1 unknown). On repeat renal biopsy, improvement in the histopathologic class of nephritis and a decrease in the renal activity index occurred in most patients. Moreover, a reduction in the number of CD3, CD4, and CD20 cells in the renal interstitium was noted in 50% of the patients on repeat biopsy (updated results at the 2008 ACR meeting). In a similarly small study of 10 patients with LN treated with rituximab and oral prednisolone (at 0.5 mg/kg/d for 10 weeks then tapered by 4 mg every 2 weeks), Sfikakis and colleagues[89] found a complete renal response in 5 and a partial response in another 3. T-cell activation as measured by CD40 ligand on CD4 cells decreased significantly. The effect on T-cell activation was greatest when complete response was attained and remained low in patients who maintained a complete response. Other retrospective studies,[90] prospective cohorts,[91] and open-label studies[92] have suggested similar benefit.

Thus, there was great hope for the phase III, randomized, double blind, placebo-controlled, multicenter study (LUNAR) evaluating the efficacy and safety of rituximab plus mycophenolate in patients with SLE with active proliferative nephritis (types III/IV) (n = 144), which was recently reported at the 2009 ACR meeting.[93] Rituximab was administered as in EXPLORER using RA dosing at baseline and 6 months, with the primary end point the fraction of patients achieving a complete or partial renal response at 52 weeks. Although there were numerically more responders in the rituximab group (57% vs 46%), the study did not show a statistically significant difference in primary or clinical secondary end points. Black and Hispanic patients randomized to rituximab had greater responses compared with placebo than White patients, but statistical significance was not achieved. Rituximab did have a greater effect on levels of anti-dsDNA ($P = .007$) and complement ($P = .025$) at week 52. Adverse events were similar between groups with no new or unexpected safety signals. Overall, this study failed to indicate that the addition of rituximab to mycophenolate and steroids provides additional benefit, at least at 52 weeks, which some may argue is a short follow-up in a nephritis study.

Summary and Perspectives: Does BCD Work in SLE?

Given that there have been notable examples of therapeutics that appeared effective in open-label studies until well-controlled studies provided contrary evidence, the results of the 2 recent randomized trials of rituximab in SLE should give us pause. Two alternative explanations are possible: either BCD is not effective in SLE or trial design was suboptimal for demonstrating clinical efficacy. Because of the large body of preclinical and open-label data in refractory disease suggesting efficacy, the authors favor the latter explanation. Several recent articles have addressed the formidable challenges of trial design in SLE.[3,94–96] As different manifestations of SLE may result from different mechanisms, 1 targeted therapy is unlikely to be effective for all patients. Additionally the most impressive open-label results with rituximab for SLE have been observed in (1) refractory patients (often previously receiving cyclophosphamide) and (2) those treated with 1 or 2 low doses of cyclophosphamide in combination with rituximab, an approach not used in either EXPLORER or LUNAR.

How Does BCD Work in SLE?

BCD has the potential to induce disease amelioration by inhibiting autoantibody production or by interfering with other B-cell pathogenic functions. In some diseases at least (RA, antineutrophil cytoplasmic antibody [ANCA] vasculitis, and IgM antibody-associated polyneuropathy) autoantibody decline seems to be associated with clinical improvement.[97,98] The autoantibody decline suggests that the autoreactive PCs are short-lived and thus disappear if their B-cell precursors are eliminated. Conversely, subsequent increases in autoantibody titers (rheumatoid factor, ANCA) seem to be closely associated with B-cell repopulation and sometimes may even precede the expansion of B cells.[97] Collectively, the data suggest that at least in some patients repopulation may be dominated by the preferential expansion of residual autoreactive B cells perhaps because of a competitive advantage (or lack of competition) in a depleted peripheral compartment.[32,86,99] The picture seems to be more complicated in SLE, in which total IgM and IgG antibody levels and disease-specific autoantibodies remain relatively stable for at least 1 year, particularly when cyclophosphamide is not coadministered, which implicates the importance of the autoantibody-independent role of B cells in ongoing disease. Limited studies of the effects of BCD on other immune cells have demonstrated decreases in T-cell activation[100] and increases in T-regulatory cell numbers and function.[101]

The authors have found that on longer follow-up, however, patients with SLE with good BCD could be split into those whose anti-dsDNA levels progressively declined after 1 year and eventually normalized and those whose levels failed to diminish.[32] As a group, serologic responders experienced dramatic and sustained clinical responses. Patients in this subset have a robust B-cell reconstitution, with up to 80% of all peripheral blood B cells displaying a transitional phenotype (B cells intermediate between immature and mature naive).[32,86] The authors speculate that the reconstitution phenotype observed in long-term responders is the consequence of profound BCD induced by rituximab and the ensuing BM-derived repopulation and suggests the potential emergence of a protective, regulatory B-cell population (**Fig. 1**). In addition, it seems likely that tissue depletion of autoreactive B cells that may continue to generate PCs of heterogeneous life span may have been less successful in patients with good blood depletion but poor serologic response. Expansion of transitional cells also correlates with prevention of diabetes after BCD in NOD mice.[102] Overall, these studies raise critical questions regarding the factors that influence depletion, the kinetics and quality of repopulation, and the mechanisms responsible for long-term remission in a subset of patients.

Potential Complications of BCD Therapy

Given that primary and secondary immune responses may be compromised even a year after BCD therapy[103–105] it is recommended that immunizations be given 1 month before starting rituximab, and yearly influenza vaccine given as late as possible after the last dose. More careful studies of humoral immune responses after rituximab and the correlation with B-cell subset recovery are necessary, however. The authors predict that primary immune responses may be impaired post rituximab even after recovery of normal absolute B-cell counts if the B cells are predominantly immature transitional cells, given the hyporesponsiveness of transitional B cells.[39]

Because of the lack of expression of CD20 on PCs (the major antibody-producing cells) it has been long appreciated that Ig levels are not significantly affected in patients who are treated with rituximab, at least not in the short-term after a single course of therapy. Preexisting antitetanus toxoid and antipneumococcal polysaccharide antibodies remain stable for prolonged periods of time in SLE and RA.[106] However, hypogammaglobulinemia with low IgG levels has been observed in children treated with rituximab,[107] and intravenous Ig has been advocated in this group and prophylactically in infants.[108] With repeated BCD, development of low Ig levels is more common, although not clearly associated with increased infectious complications. A recent meta-analysis supports prior literature regarding the safety of BCD in that treatment of RA patients with rituximab was not associated with an increased incidence of serious infections,[109] even after repeated courses[110] or with TNF blockade after BCD.[111] The caveat here is that the database is small for RA and even smaller for SLE. Moreover, there have been reports of fulminant hepatitis B reactivation and rare cases of progressive multifocal leukoencephalopathy (PML).[103] Thus, patients should be screened for hepatitis B before the use of rituximab and viral prophylaxis considered in high-risk patients.

There are no screening methods to identify patients at risk for development of PML. A recent article reported on 57 cases of PML occurring in the setting of rituximab, 52 in the patients with lymphoproliferative disease, 2 for SLE, and 1 for RA, with a mortality of 89%.[112] Many of these patients were heavily immunosuppressed with medications in addition to rituximab currently or historically. Although the frequency of PML in patients with RA receiving rituximab is rare (3/100,000), the incidence may be higher in SLE, which is independently associated with PML.[103] Overall, the data suggest that patients who receive rituximab have an increased risk of PML. Calabrese and Molloy[113] recently provided a cogent discussion of this topic and made several important points: (1) PML is a risk associated with all immunosuppressive therapies; (2) as PML has been observed in SLE in the absence of exposure to rituximab, it is unclear how much additional risk is imparted by BCD; and (3) given that PML is a devastating complication and the risk of it occurring is not zero, a risk-benefit discussion should take place with patients.

OTHER AGENTS THAT TARGET B CELLS
Other B-cell Depleting Antibodies

Other monoclonal antibodies that target CD20 are in various phases of development, including ocrelizumab (humanized anti-CD20) (**Table 2**). Theoretically, a fully human antibody may be better tolerated during infusions because of less immunogenicity. This could translate into more complete BCD especially in SLE, in which HACAs are more common after rituximab. The trial of ocrelizumab in lupus nephritis may answer the question of synergy with cyclophosphamide given that a subset of patients will receive BCD in combination.

Epratuzumab is a humanized anti-CD22 that also induces BCD although less pronounced than with anti-CD20 and preferentially of naive and transitional B cells. However, anti-CD22 also blocks the activation and proliferation of B cells, possibly acting as a negative regulator of B-cell function. A recent press release regarding a phase IIb trial of epratuzumab in SLE reported superior response rates compared with placebo at week 12. Other approaches to BCD under development include anti-bodies against CD19, which is expressed on virtually all B cells and is lost at a later stage than CD20 as B cells differentiate into PCs. In animal models of autoimmunity, anti-CD19 depletes a wider spectrum of B cells than anti-CD20, for example, perito-neal B cells including B1 B cells are depleted with anti-CD19 but spared with anti-CD20.[114] Moreover, treatment with anti-CD19 in these models was associated with a decrease in total Igs, indicating an effect on PCs.

Inhibition of Costimulation

As an alternative to selective BCD, there has been interest in targeting costimulatory signaling pathways. Direct inhibition of B-/T-cell collaboration through inhibition of the CD40-CD40L pathway has been shown to be effective in mouse models of lupus.[115] Two studies of anti-CD40L antibodies in SLE have been reported,[116,117] but either failed to show clinical efficacy over placebo or were complicated by unexpected thromboembolic events.[117] Two small mechanistic studies demonstrated beneficial immune effects (n = 5 for each), including a marked reduction in autoreactive anti-dsDNA producing B cells[118] and substantial reductions in abnormal B-cell popula-tions.[30] These reports suggest that anti-CD40L can interfere with aberrant GC reactions in SLE and translate into clinical benefit, if administered with the proper pharmacokinetics for adequate costimulatory blockade.

An alternative costimulatory target in SLE includes the CD28 and cytotoxic T lymphocyte antigen 4 (CTLA4) receptors and their B-cell coligands B7-1 and B7-2. Blockade of B7 stimulation on B cells with a fusion protein of the extracellular domain of CTLA and Ig constant regions has yielded promising results in murine SLE.[119] A double blind, placebo-controlled phase II trial evaluated the efficacy of abatacept (CTLA4-Ig) in reducing BILAG flares in 180 patients with nonrenal SLE with active poly-arthritis, serositis, or discoid lesions. Although primary and secondary end points were not met, post hoc analyses suggested that the outcome measures used may have been suboptimal and also that there may be greater efficacy of abatacept in the poly-arthritis subset of disease.

Inhibition of Cytokines with B-cell Effects

There has been active interest in developing antagonists of BAFF in the treatment of SLE. Belimumab (fully human monoclonal antibody against BAFF) for SLE has now been evaluated in multiple double blind, placebo-controlled trials. Although the orig-inal phase II study did not meet its primary efficacy end point, when only the serolog-ically active subjects were analyzed post hoc there was a statistically significant improvement in disease activity using a novel responder index. During long-term open treatment, the frequency of Safety of Estrogen in Lupus Erythematosus National. Assessment (SELENA)-SLEDAI flares declined to 7% at 3 years, suggestive of sus-tained improvement of disease activity with long-term therapy. After these initial encouraging results in phase II trials, 2 large phase III trials were initiated and have recently reported favorable clinical responses compared with placebo. The first of these studies BLISS-52 was presented at the 2009 ACR meeting, and the second BLISS-72 was reported in November 2009 to have also met its primary efficacy end point. Given these initial reports, it is important to consider whether BAFF blockade would be expected to yield different results compared with anti-CD20. This would be surprising given that both agents deplete B cells, with anti-CD20 causing even more pronounced BCD and likely better depletion of memory B-cell subsets. On the other hand, BAFF blockade may have additional effects on other immune cells important in SLE including T cells and DC.[120] Moreover, rituximab causes a compensatory increase in BAFF, which may theoretically have adverse effects on B-cell selection. Despite these speculations, it is likely that the distinct trial results with BAFF blockade versus anti-CD20 in SLE are more related to trial design than biologic differences between the 2 therapies.

Additional agents neutralizing BAFF are in various active stages of development, including fusion proteins of Ig Fc and the BAFF receptors, either BAFF-R (BR3) or transmembrane activation and calcium modulating cyclophilin ligand interactor (TACI) (atacicept). Atacicept blocks BAFF and its related cytokine proliferation inducing ligand (APRIL) and was well tolerated in an SLE phase I study, with reductions in total IgG, IgM, and autoantibodies.[121] However, a phase II study of atacicept in combination with mycophenolate mofetil for lupus nephritis was terminated because of infections. A phase II/III trial of atacicept for nonrenal lupus is ongoing and still recruiting. Because of its effects on PCs TACI-Ig seems to have potential in autoantibody-mediated diseases. Another potential explanation for the disappointing results of BCD in SLE is the lack of effect on autoantibodies and long-lived PCs.[122] However, a challenge will be to eliminate autoantibody-producing PCs without increasing the risk of infection caused by adverse effects on protective antibodies.

SUMMARY

Recent controlled clinical trials of B-cell targeting agents in SLE have had variable benefit but have contributed to our understanding of how to conduct trials in lupus and have recently shown promise. New agents capable of affecting long-lived PCs are now being developed.[123] These agents should allow eradication of autoantibodies, but will need to be used carefully to prevent infectious complications and to ensure that autoimmune PCs do not repopulate the long-lived PC compartment. The effect of these emerging targeted therapies on patient survival is likely to be dramatic, and studies on the immune system of patients in ongoing clinical trials should continue to provide invaluable insight into the pathogenesis of human SLE.

ACKNOWLEDGMENTS

The authors thank Andreea Coca for expert review of the manuscript and Inaki Sanz and Gregg Silverman for input on figures. The collaborations and thoughtful discussions with colleagues, especially Inaki Sanz and John Looney, are gratefully noted.

REFERENCES

1. Bongu A, Chang E, Ramsey-Goldman R. Can morbidity and mortality of SLE be improved? Best Pract Res Clin Rheumatol 2002;16:313–32.

2. Gordon C, Bertsias GK, Ioannidis JP, et al. EULAR recommendations for points to consider in conducting clinical trials in systemic lupus erythematosus (SLE) [review]. Ann Rheum Dis 2009;68(4):470–6.

3. Dall'Era M, Wofsy D. Clinical trial design in systemic lupus erythematosus. Curr Opin Rheumatol 2006;18(5):476–80.

4. Bertsias G, Gordon C, Boumpas DT. Clinical trials in systemic lupus erythematosus (SLE): lessons from the past as we proceed to the future–the EULAR recommendations for the management of SLE and the use of end-points in clinical trials. Lupus 2008;17(5):437–42.

5. Chan OT, Hannum LG, Haberman AM, et al. A novel mouse with B cells but lacking serum antibody reveals an antibody-independent role for B cells in murine lupus. J Exp Med 1999;189(10):1639–48.

6. Arbuckle M, McClain M, Rubertone M, et al. Development of autoantibodies before the clinical onset of systemic lupus erythematosus. N Engl J Med 2003;349(16):1526–33.

7. Kumar KR, Li L, Yan M, et al. Regulation of B cell tolerance by the lupus susceptibility gene Ly108. Science 2006;312(5780):1665–9.

8. Bolland S, Ravetch JV. Spontaneous autoimmune disease in Fc(gamma)RIIB-deficient mice results from strain-specific epistasis. Immunity 2000;13(2):277–85.

9. Fukuyama H, Nimmerjahn F, Ravetch JV. The inhibitory Fcgamma receptor modulates autoimmunity by limiting the accumulation of immunoglobulin G+ anti-DNA plasma cells. Nat Immunol 2005;6(1):99–106.

10. McGaha TL, Sorrentino B, Ravetch JV. Restoration of tolerance in lupus by targeted inhibitory receptor expression. Science 2005;307(5709):590–3.

11. Floto RA, Clatworthy MR, Heilbronn KR, et al. Loss of function of a lupus-associated FcgammaRIIb polymorphism through exclusion from lipid rafts. Nat Med 2005;11(10):1056–8.

12. Mackay M, Stanevsky A, Wang T, et al. Selective dysregulation of the FcgammaIIB receptor on memory B cells in SLE. J Exp Med 2006;203(9):2157–64.

13. Liossis SN, Kovacs B, Dennis G, et al. B cells from patients with systemic lupus erythematosus display abnormal antigen receptor-mediated early signal transduction events. J Clin Invest 1996;98(11):2549–57.

14. Olferiev M, Crow M. Activation of interferon and ubiquitin pathways in lupus memory B cells. Arthritis Rheum 2009;60(Suppl 10):S744.

15. Mackay F, Woodcock S, Lawton P, et al. Mice transgenic for BAFF develop lymphocytic disorders along with autoimmune manifestations. J Exp Med 1999;190:1697–710.

16. Gross J, Johnston J, Mudri S. TACI and BCMA are receptors for a TNF homologue implicated in B cell autoimmune disease. Nature 2000;404:995–9.

17. Stohl W, Metyas S, Tan SM, et al. B lymphocyte stimulator overexpression in patients with systemic lupus erythematosus: longitudinal observations. Arthritis Rheum 2003;48(12):3475–86.

18. Lesley R, Xu Y, Kalled SL, et al. Reduced competitiveness of autoantigen-engaged B cells due to increased dependence on BAFF [comment]. Immunity 2004;20(4):441–53.

19. Thien M, Phan TG, Gardam S, et al. Excess BAFF rescues self-reactive B cells from peripheral deletion and allows them to enter forbidden follicular and marginal zone niches. Immunity 2004;20(6):785–98.

20. Miller J, Stadanlick JE, Cancro MP. Space, selection, and surveillance: setting boundaries with BLyS. J Immunol 2006;176:6405–10.

21. Leadbetter EA, Rifkin IR, Hohlbaum AM, et al. Chromatin-IgG complexes activate B cells by dual engagement of IgM and Toll-like receptors [comment]. Nature 2002;416(6881):603–7.
22. Viglianti GA, Lau CM, Hanley TM, et al. Activation of autoreactive B cells by CpG dsDNA. Immunity 2003;19(6):837–47.
23. Boule MW, Broughton C, Mackay F, et al. Toll-like receptor 9-dependent and -independent dendritic cell activation by chromatin-immunoglobulin G complexes. J Exp Med 2004;199(12):1631–40.
24. Means TK, Latz E, Hayashi F, et al. Human lupus autoantibody-DNA complexes activate DCs through cooperation of CD32 and TLR9. J Clin Invest 2005;115(2):407–17.
25. Yurasov S, Wardemann H, Hammersen J, et al. Defective B cell tolerance checkpoints in systemic lupus erythematosus. J Exp Med 2005;201(5):703–11.
26. Cappione A 3rd, Anolik JH, Pugh-Bernard A, et al. Germinal center exclusion of autoreactive B cells is defective in human systemic lupus erythematosus. J Clin Invest 2005;115(11):3205–16.
27. Pugh-Bernard AE, Silverman GJ, Cappione AJ, et al. Regulation of inherently autoreactive VH4-34 B cells in the maintenance of human B cell tolerance. J Clin Invest 2001;108(7):1061–70.
28. Tsuiji M, Yurasov S, Velinzon K, et al. A checkpoint for autoreactivity in human IgM+ memory B cell development. J Exp Med 2006;203(2):393–400.
29. Wardemann H, Yurasov S, Schaefer A, et al. Predominant autoantibody production by early human B cell precursors. Science 2003;301:1374–7.
30. Grammer A, Lipsky PE. B cell abnormalities in systemic lupus erythematosus. Arthritis Res Ther 2003;5:S22–7.
31. Odendahl M, Jacobi A, Hansen A, et al. Disturbed peripheral B lymphocyte homeostasis in systemic lupus erythematosus. J Immunol 2000;165:5970–9.
32. Anolik J, Barnard J, Cappione A, et al. Rituximab improves peripheral B cell abnormalities in human systemic lupus erythematosus. Arthritis Rheum 2004;50:3580–90.
33. Wei C, Anolik J, Cappione A, et al. A new population of cells lacking expression of CD27 represents a notable component of the B cell memory compartment in systemic lupus erythematosus. J Immunol 2007;178(10):6624–33.
34. Jacobi AM, Reiter K, Mackay M, et al. Activated memory B cell subsets correlate with disease activity in systemic lupus erythematosus: delineation by expression of CD27, IgD, and CD95. Arthritis Rheum 2008;58(6):1762–73.
35. Jacobi AM, Odendahl M, Reiter K, et al. Correlation between circulating CD27high plasma cells and disease activity in patients with systemic lupus erythematosus. Arthritis Rheum 2003;48(5):1332–42.
36. Jacobi AM, Mei H, Hoyer BF, et al. HLA-DRhigh/CD27high plasmablasts indicate active disease in patients with SLE. Ann Rheum Dis 2010;69(1):305–8.
37. Wei C, Palanichamy A, Jenks S, et al. B Cell signatures as biomarkers in SLE. Arthritis Rheum 2009;60(Suppl 10):1764.
38. Arce E, Jackson DG, Gill MA, et al. Increased frequency of pre-germinal center B cells and plasma cell precursors in the blood of children with systemic lupus erythematosus. J Immunol 2001;167(4):2361–9.
39. Palanichamy A, Barnard J, Zheng B, et al. Novel human transitional B cell populations revealed by B cell depletion therapy. J Immunol 2009;182(10):5982–93.
40. Sabahi R, Owen T, Barnard J, et al. Immunologic effects of BAFF antagonism in the treatment of human SLE. Arthritis Rheum 2007;56:S566.

41. Shlomchik MJ, Madaio MP, Ni D, et al. The role of B cells in lpr/lpr-induced auto-immunity. J Exp Med 1994;180(4):1295–306.
42. Bekar K, Owen T, Dunn R, et al. Prolonged effects of short-term anti-CD20 B cell depletion therapy in murine systemic lupus erythematosus [abstract]. Arthritis Rheum 2009;60(Suppl 10):677.
43. Looney RJ, Anolik JH, Campbell D, et al. B cell depletion as a novel treatment for systemic lupus erythematosus: a phase I/II dose-escalation trial of rituximab. Arthritis Rheum 2004;50(8):2580–9.
44. Lorenz RG, Chaplin DD, McDonald KG, et al. Isolated lymphoid follicle formation is inducible and dependent upon lymphotoxin-sufficient B lymphocytes, lymphotoxin beta receptor, and TNF receptor I function. J Immunol 2003;170(11):5475–82.
45. Ware CF. Network communications: lymphotoxins, LIGHT, and TNF. Annu Rev Immunol 2005;23:787–819.
46. Chang A, Henderson S, Liu N, et al. In situ B cell mediated immune responses and tubulointerstitial inflammation in human lupus nephritis. 2010.
47. Harris D, Haynes L, Sayles P, et al. Reciprocal regulation of polarized cytokine production by effector B and T cells. Nat Immunol 2000;1:475–81.
48. Ebert LM, Horn MP, Lang AB, et al. B cells alter the phenotype and function of follicular-homing CXCR5+ T cells. Eur J Immunol 2004;34(12):3562–71.
49. Odegard JM, Marks BR, DiPlacido LD, et al. ICOS-dependent extrafollicular helper T cells elicit IgG production via IL-21 in systemic autoimmunity. J Exp Med 2008;205(12):2873–86.
50. Vinuesa CG, Cook MC, Angelucci C, et al. A RING-type ubiquitin ligase family member required to repress follicular helper T cells and autoimmunity. Nature 2005;435(7041):452–8.
51. Lund FE. Cytokine-producing B lymphocytes – key regulators of immunity. Curr Opin Immunol 2008;20(3):332–8.
52. Fillatreau S, Gray D, Anderton SM. Not always the bad guys: B cells as regulators of autoimmune pathology. Nat Rev Immunol 2008;8(5):391–7.
53. Lampropoulou V, Hoehlig K, Roch T, et al. TLR-Activated B cells suppress T cell-mediated autoimmunity. J Immunol 2008;180(7):4763–73.
54. Fillatreau S, Sweenie CH, McGeachy MJ, et al. B cells regulate autoimmunity by provision of IL-10. Nat Immunol 2002;3(10):944–50.
55. Mauri C, Gray D, Mushtaq N, et al. Prevention of arthritis by interleukin 10-producing B cells. J Exp Med 2003;197(4):489–501.
56. Chen X, Jensen PE. Cutting edge: primary B lymphocytes preferentially expand allogeneic FoxP3+ CD4 T cells. J Immunol 2007;179(4):2046–50.
57. Mann MK, Maresz K, Shriver LP, et al. B cell regulation of CD4+CD25+ T regulatory cells and IL-10 via B7 is essential for recovery from experimental autoimmune encephalomyelitis. J Immunol 2007;178(6):3447–56.
58. Martin F, Chan AC. B cell immunobiology in disease: evolving concepts from the clinic. Annu Rev Immunol 2006;24:467–96.
59. Bave U, Alm GV, Ronnblom L. The combination of apoptotic U937 cells and lupus IgG is a potent IFN-alpha inducer. J Immunol 2000;165(6):3519–26.
60. Bave U, Magnusson M, Eloranta M, et al. Fc gamma RIIa is expressed on natural IFN-alpha producing cells (plasmacytoid dendritic cells) and is required for the IFN-alpha production induced by apoptotic cells combined with lupus IgG. J Immunol 2003;171:3296–302.
61. Ronnblom L, Alm GV. A pivotal role for the natural interferon alpha-producing cells (plasmacytoid dendritic cells) in the pathogenesis of lupus [comment]. J Exp Med 2001;194(12):F59–63.

62. Christensen SR, Shupe J, Nickerson K, et al. Toll-like receptor 7 and TLR9 dictate autoantibody specificity and have opposing inflammatory and regulatory roles in a murine model of lupus [comment]. Immunity 2006;25(3):417–28.

63. Herlands RA, Christensen SR, Sweet RA, et al. T cell-independent and toll-like receptor-dependent antigen-driven activation of autoreactive B cells. Immunity 2008;29(2):249–60.

64. Ehlers M, Fukuyama H, McGaha TL, et al. TLR9/MyD88 signaling is required for class switching to pathogenic IgG2a and 2b autoantibodies in SLE. J Exp Med 2006;203(3):553–61.

65. Pisitkun P, Deane JA, Difilippantonio MJ, et al. Autoreactive B cell responses to RNA-related antigens due to TLR7 gene duplication. Science 2006;312(5780): 1669–72.

66. Jego G, Palucka AK, Blanck JP, et al. Plasmacytoid dendritic cells induce plasma cell differentiation through type I interferon and interleukin 6. Immunity 2003;19(2):225–34.

67. Bekeredjian-Ding IB, Wagner M, Hornung V, et al. Plasmacytoid dendritic cells control TLR7 sensitivity of naive B cells via type I IFN. J Immunol 2005;174(7): 4043–50.

68. Uccellini MB, Busconi L, Green NM, et al. Autoreactive B cells discriminate CpG-rich and CpG-poor DNA and this response is modulated by IFN-alpha. J Immunol 2008;181(9):5875–84.

69. Barnard J, Palanichamy A, Bauer J, et al. Interferon activation in human SLE bone marrow inhibits B cell lymphopoeisis. Arthritis Rheum 2008;10(11).

70. Hoyer B, Moser K, Hauser A, et al. Short-lived plasmablasts and long-lived plasma cells contribute to chronic humoral autoimmunity in NZB/W mice. J Exp Med 2004;199:1577.

71. Tedder TF, Engel P. CD20: a regulator of cell-cycle progression of B lympho-cytes. Immunol Today 1994;15(9):450–4.

72. Maloney DG, Smith B, Rose A. Rituximab: mechanism of action and resistance. Semin Oncol 2002;29(1 Suppl 2):2–9.

73. Gong Q, Ou Q, Ye S, et al. Importance of cellular microenvironment and circu-latory dynamics in B cell immunotherapy. J Immunol 2005;174:817–26.

74. Mamani-Matsuda M, Cosma A, Weller S, et al. The human spleen is a major reservoir for long-lived vaccinia virus-specific memory B cells. Blood 2008; 111(9):4653–9.

75. Vos K, Thurlings RM, Wijbrandts CA, et al. Early effects of rituximab on the synovial cell infiltrate in patients with rheumatoid arthritis. Arthritis Rheum 2007;56(3):772–8.

76. Levesque MC. Translational Mini-Review Series on B Cell-Directed Therapies: Recent advances in B cell-directed biological therapies for autoimmune disor-ders. Clin Exp Immunol 2009;157(2):198–208.

77. Albert D, Dunham J, Khan S, et al. Variability in the biological response to anti-CD20 B cell depletion in systemic lupus erythaematosus. Ann Rheum Dis 2008; 67(12):1724–31.

78. Lindholm C, Borjesson-Asp K, Zendjanchi K, et al. Longterm clinical and immu-nological effects of anti-CD20 treatment in patients with refractory systemic lupus erythematosus. J Rheumatol 2008;35(5):826–33.

79. Jonsdottir T, Gunnarsson I, Risselada A, et al. Treatment of refractory SLE with rituximab plus cyclophosphamide: clinical effects, serological changes, and predictors of response. Ann Rheum Dis 2008;67(3):330–4.

80. Amoura Z, Mazodier K, Michel M, et al. Efficacy of rituximab in systemic lupus erythematosus: a series of 22 cases. Arthritis Rheum 2007;56(9):S458.

81. Lu TY, Ng KP, Cambridge G, et al. A retrospective seven-year analysis of the use of B cell depletion therapy in systemic lupus erythematosus at University College London Hospital: the first fifty patients. Arthritis Rheum 2009;61(4): 482–7.

82. Sfikakis PP, Boletis JN, Tsokos GC. Rituximab anti-B-cell therapy in systemic lupus erythematosus: pointing to the future. Curr Opin Rheumatol 2005;17(5):550–7.

83. Ramos-Casals M, Soto MJ, Cuadrado MJ, et al. Rituximab in systemic lupus erythematosus: a systematic review of off-label use in 188 cases. Lupus 2009; 18(9):767–76.

84. Karpouzas G, Gogia M, Moran R, et al. Rituximab therapy induces durable remissions in Hispanic and African American patients with refractory systemic lupus erythematosus (SLE). Arthritis Rheum 2009;60(Suppl 10):274.

85. Terrier B, Hachulla E, Pallot-Prades B. Tolerance and efficacy of rituximab (RTX) in systemic lupus erythematosus (SLE): data of 104 patients from the AIR (Autoimmunity and Rituximab) Registry. Arthritis Rheum 2009;60(Suppl 10):272.

86. Anolik JH, Barnard J, Owen T, et al. Delayed memory B cell recovery in peripheral blood and lymphoid tissue in systemic lupus erythematosus after B cell depletion therapy. Arthritis Rheum 2007;56(9):3044–56.

87. Merrill J, Neuwelt C, Wallace D, et al. Efficacy and safety of rituximab in patients with moderately to severely active systemic lupus erythematosus: results from the randomized, double-blind phase II/III study EXPLORER. American College of Rheumatology Annual Meeting. October 29, 2008. Available at: www. abstractsonline.com.

88. Gunnarsson I, Sundelin B, Jonsdottir T, et al. Histopathologic and clinical outcome of rituximab treatment in patients with cyclophosphamide-resistant proliferative lupus nephritis. Arthritis Rheum 2007;56(4):1263–72.

89. Sfikakis PP, Boletis JN, Lionaki S, et al. Remission of proliferative lupus nephritis following B cell depletion therapy is preceded by down-regulation of the T cell costimulatory molecule CD40 ligand: an open-label trial. Arthritis Rheum 2005;52(2):501–13.

90. Melander C, Sallee M, Trolliet P, et al. Rituximab in severe lupus nephritis: early B-cell depletion affects long-term renal outcome. Clin J Am Soc Nephrol 2009; 4(3):579–87.

91. Pepper R, Griffith M, Kirwan C, et al. Rituximab is an effective treatment for lupus nephritis and allows a reduction in maintenance steroids. Nephrol Dial Transplant 2009;24(12):3717–23.

92. Li EK, Tam LS, Zhu TY, et al. Is combination rituximab with cyclophosphamide better than rituximab alone in the treatment of lupus nephritis? Rheumatology (Oxford) 2009;48(8):892–8.

93. Furie R, Looney J, Rovin B, et al. Efficacy and safety of rituximab in subjects with active proliferative lupus nephritis (LN): results from the randomized, double-blind phase III LUNAR study. Arthritis Rheum 2009;60(Suppl 10):1149.

94. Isenberg D, Gordon C, Merrill J, et al. New therapies in systemic lupus erythematosus – trials, troubles and tribulations. Working towards a solution. Lupus 2008;17(11):967–70.

95. Looney J, Anolik J, Sanz I. A perspective on B-cell targeting therapy for SLE. Mod Rheumatol 2009. [Epub ahead of print].

96. Coca A, Anolik J. Two negative randomized controlled trials in lupus: now what? F1000 Medicine Reports 2009;1:28.

97. Cambridge G, Stohl W, Leandro M, et al. Circulating levels of B lymphocyte stimulator in patients with rheumatoid arthritis following rituximab treatment: relationships

with B cell depletion, circulating antibodies, and clinical relapse. Arthritis Rheum 2006;54(3):723–32.

98. Keogh KA, Wylam ME, Stone JH, et al. Induction of remission by B lymphocyte depletion in eleven patients with refractory antineutrophil cytoplasmic antibody-associated vasculitis. Arthritis Rheum 2005;52(1):262–8.

99. Rouziere A-S, Kneitz C, Palanichamy A, et al. Regeneration of the immunoglobulin heavy-chain repertoire after transient B-cell depletion with an anti-CD20 antibody. Arthritis Res Ther 2005;7(4):R714–24.

100. Sfikakis P, Boletis J, Lionaki S, et al. Remission of proliferative lupus nephritis following anti-B cell therapy is preceded by downregulation of the T cell costimulatory molecule CD40 ligand. Arthritis Rheum 2004;50:S227.

101. Vigna-Perez M, Hernandez-Castro B, Paredes-Saharopulos O, et al. Clinical and immunologic effects of rituximab in patients with lupus nephritis refractory to conventional therapy: a pilot study. Arthritis Res Ther 2006;8:R83.

102. Hu Cy, Rodriguez-Pinto D, Du W, et al. Treatment with CD20-specific antibody prevents and reverses autoimmune diabetes in mice. J Clin Invest 2007; 117(12):3857–67.

103. Looney RJ, Srinivasan R, Calabrese LH. The effects of rituximab on immunocompetency in patients with autoimmune disease. Arthritis Rheum 2008;58(1):5–14.

104. van der Kolk L, Baars J, Prins M, et al. Rituximab treatment results in impaired secondary humoral immune responsiveness. Blood 2002;100:2257–9.

105. Bearden CM, Agarwal A, Book BK, et al. Rituximab inhibits the in vivo primary and secondary antibody response to a neoantigen, bacteriophage phiX174. Am J Transplant 2005;5(1):50–7.

106. Cambridge G, Leandro MJ, Edwards JC, et al. Serologic changes following B lymphocyte depletion therapy for rheumatoid arthritis. Arthritis Rheum 2003; 48(8):2146–54.

107. Willems M, Haddad E, Niaudet P, et al. Rituximab therapy for childhood-onset systemic lupus erythematosus. J Pediatr 2006;148(5):623–7.

108. Zecca M, Nobili B, Ramenghi U, et al. Rituximab for the treatment of refractory autoimmune hemolytic anemia in children. Blood 2003;101(10):3857–61.

109. Salliot C, Dougados M, Gossec L. Risk of serious infections during rituximab, abatacept and anakinra treatments for rheumatoid arthritis: meta-analyses of randomised placebo-controlled trials. Ann Rheum Dis 2009;68(1):25–32.

110. Keystone E, Fleischmann R, Emery P, et al. Safety and efficacy of additional courses of rituximab in patients with active rheumatoid arthritis: an open-label extension analysis. Arthritis Rheum 2007;56(12):3896–908.

111. Genovese MC, Breedveld FC, Emery P, et al. Safety of biologic therapies following rituximab treatment in rheumatoid arthritis patients. Ann Rheum Dis 2009;68:1894–7.

112. Carson KR, Focosi D, Major EO, et al. Monoclonal antibody-associated progressive multifocal leucoencephalopathy in patients treated with rituximab, natalizumab, and efalizumab: a Review from the Research on Adverse Drug Events and Reports (RADAR) Project. Lancet Oncol 2009;10(8):816–24.

113. Calabrese LH, Molloy ES. Therapy: rituximab and PML risk-informed decisions needed! Nat Rev Rheumatol 2009;5(10):528–9.

114. Yazawa N, Hamaguchi Y, Poe JC, et al. Immunotherapy using unconjugated CD19 monoclonal antibodies in animal models for B lymphocyte malignancies and autoimmune disease. Proc Natl Acad Sci U S A 2005;102(42):15178–83.

115. Wang X, Huang W, Schiffer LE, et al. Effects of anti-CD154 treatment on B cells in murine systemic lupus erythematosus. Arthritis Rheum 2003;48(2):495–506.

116. Kalunian KC, Davis JC Jr, Merrill JT, et al. Treatment of systemic lupus erythematosus by inhibition of T cell costimulation with anti-CD154: a randomized, double-blind, placebo-controlled trial. Arthritis Rheum 2002;46(12):3251–8.

117. Boumpas DT, Furie R, Manzi S, et al. A short course of BG9588 (anti-CD40 ligand antibody) improves serologic activity and decreases hematuria in patients with proliferative lupus glomerulonephritis. Arthritis Rheum 2003; 48(3):719–27.

118. Huang W, Sinha J, Newman J, et al. The effect of anti-CD40 ligand antibody on B cells in human systemic lupus erythematosus. Arthritis Rheum 2002;46: 1554–62.

119. Daikh DI, Wofsy D. Cutting edge: reversal of murine lupus nephritis with CTLA4Ig and cyclophosphamide. J Immunol 2001;166(5):2913–6.

120. Chang SK, Mihalcik SA, Jelinek DF. B lymphocyte stimulator regulates adaptive immune responses by directly promoting dendritic cell maturation. J Immunol 2008;180(11):7394–403.

121. Dall'Era M, Chakravarty E, Wallace D, et al. Reduced B lymphocyte and immunoglobulin levels after atacicept treatment in patients with systemic lupus erythematosus: results of a multicenter, phase Ib, double-blind, placebo-controlled, dose-escalating trial. Arthritis Rheum 2007;56(12):4142–50.

122. Munafo A, Priestley A, Nestorov I, et al. Safety, pharmacokinetics and pharmacodynamics of atacicept in healthy volunteers. Eur J Clin Pharmacol 2007;63(7): 647–56.

123. Neubert K, Meister S, Moser K, et al. The proteasome inhibitor bortezomib depletes plasma cells and protects mice with lupus-like disease from nephritis. Nat Med 2008;14(7):748–55.

Biomarkers in Lupus Nephritis

Anup Manoharan, MBBS*, Michael P. Madaio, MD

KEYWORDS

- Serologic markers • Urinary markers • Indicators of Renal flare
- Assessment of renal functional activity
- Noninvasive biomarkers

Although biomarkers have high utility for the diagnosis of systemic lupus erythematosus (SLE), current serologic and urinary markers do not correlate well with nephritic activity. This has led to a search for better indicators of renal flare (or lack thereof). In this context, assessment of renal functional activity (eg, markers of glomerular filtration rate [GFR]), such as serum creatinine, has limitations. For example, the GFR may be still preserved while there is severe inflammation thus making it difficult to assess its true changes. For example, in a 25-year-old, 50-kg woman with lupus nephritis, an increase in the serum creatinine from 0.6 mg/dL to 0.9 mg/dL (estimated GFR change from 114 to 75 mL/min), with both levels in the normal laboratory range, represents a 35% reduction in function. Although this example seems obvious, in practice less evident changes are often missed. Such a delay in recognition may lead to a delay in treatment and irreversible scarring in the kidney. Urine protein quantization also has its own limitations. For instance, resolution of proteinuria may take weeks to months to normalize, or not normalize at all, irrespective of immunologic or inflammatory activity. Immunosuppressive therapy in this situation will not be effective.

In other situations, even with the pathology in hand, it is difficult to ascertain the extent of disease activity. Distinguishing the relative extent of ongoing inflammation from chronic fibrotic disease may be especially difficult. Thus, it would be extremely useful to identify either inflammatory or other renal functional signals in blood or urine that are indicative of inflammation and ongoing autoimmune activity (ie, with flares). Similarly, better markers of irreversible damage would also be helpful. To address this problem, researchers began looking for better urinary and serum biomarkers.

For purposes of this discussion, the potential use of urine and serum markers will be considered separately. Although the American College of Rheumatology criteria and other criteria (eg, systemic lupus erythematosus disease activity index 2000 [SLEDAI-2K], systemic lupus activity measure [SLAM]) have diagnostic utility, they do not accurately assess either severity or changes in nephritic activity, and serologic

Department of Medicine, Nephrology and Kidney Transplantation Section, Medical College of Georgia, 1120 15th Street, BA 9413, Augusta, GA 30912-3140, USA
* Corresponding author.
E-mail address: AMANOHARAN@mail.mcg.edu (A. Manoharan).

Rheum Dis Clin N Am 36 (2010) 131–143
doi:10.1016/j.rdc.2009.12.009
0889-857X/10/$ – see front matter. Published by Elsevier Inc.
rheumatic.theclinics.com

evaluations alone are insufficient. Ideally, biomarkers should indicate the severity of nephritis and guide therapy at various stages of disease.

Biomarkers are defined as a genetic, biologic, biochemical, or event, whose alterations correlate with disease pathogenesis or manifestations, and can be evaluated qualitatively and/or quantitatively in laboratories.[1,2] Biomarkers should (1) be biologically active and pathophysiologically relevant, (2) be simple to use in routine practice, and (3) accurately and sensitively change with disease activity.[1,2] In lupus nephritis, biomarkers should identify patients at risk for flare so that therapy can be tailored to individual situations and duration of treatment can be precisely determined. Biomarkers should also provide surrogate end points for evaluating the efficacy of new therapies. In the paragraphs below, serum and urine biomarkers are considered. The authors do not consider the utility of renal biopsy, although it is anticipated that combining information from biomarkers and renal pathology may lead to a more precise determination of the most rationale therapy for an individual patient. The authors' focus is on the use of noninvasive biomarkers that complement the use of pathologic evaluation during the course of disease (**Box 1**). It is anticipated that in some situations, fluctuations in activity in one or more of these parameters will lead to renal biopsy, whereas in others, the levels alone may obviate the procedure.

BIOMARKERS
Nonspecific Biomarkers

Nonspecific biomarkers occur in many inflammatory states and are not disease specific. For example, prolactin and ferritin serum levels may be elevated in autoimmune diseases like SLE.[3] Similarly, erythrocyte sedimentation rate, C-reactive protein, and resistin are not lupus specific.[4]

Genetic Markers

Genetic markers typically identify patients at risk for disease (eg, lupus or specific disease manifestations). They are useful for early diagnosis and monitoring patients at risk (eg, family members) (**Box 1**).

Protein tyrosine phosphatase 22
Protein tyrosine phosphatase 22 (PTPN22) is a tyrosine-specific phosphotase in T cell signaling, expressed preferentially in memory and effector T cells. Expression of this lymphoid specific protein was predictive in Caucasians and Europeans for increased risk of developing autoimmune diseases, including lupus.[5]

Interferon regulatory factor-5
Interferon regulatory factor-5 (IRF-5), which encodes a transcription factor regulating interferon α (IFN-α), may be a useful diagnostic marker.[6] A single-nucleotide polymorphism was associated with disease susceptibility and SLE activity. However, it was also elevated in other autoimmune diseases.

STAT 4
STAT 4, a transcription factor that regulates cytokine production, is helpful in early detection of SLE, although increased protein levels (rs7574865) were present with other autoimmune diseases (eg, rheumatoid arthritis, inflammatory bowel disease, type 1 diabetes mellitus).[6]

Type I interferons

Type I interferons have also been studied as potential biomarkers of disease activity (eg, $IFIT_1$, OAS1, LY6E, ISG15, and MX^7). $IFIT_1$ correlated with active lupus but lagged behind clinical remission.

Other candidates

Other candidates under evaluation include poly–adenosine diphosphate-ribose polymerase (PARP), B lymphoid tyrosine kinase (BLK), *ITGAM*, LYN, and intergrin alpha X (ITGAX), and they await validation.

Serologic Diagnosis

Anti–double-stranded DNA (anti-dsDNA), anti-Ro, anti-La, anti-Sm and antiribonucleoprotein antibodies remain useful for diagnosis, although limited for monitoring activity. By flow cytometry, erythrocyte-bound complement-activation product C4d (E-C4d) was higher, and complement receptor C1 (E-CR1) was lower when compared with healthy patients.[8] The sensitivity and specificity of the ratio was 81% and 94 %, respectively, compared with healthy controls, and 72% and 79%, respectively, compared with inactive patients. In other studies, platelet-bound C4d (P-C4d) was 98% specific in diagnosing lupus,[9] although its utility requires further validation. Anti-guanosine antibodies distinguished active lupus from inactive disease. However, they were not predictive of organ involvement.[10]

Overall Disease Activity

Reticulocyte-C4d has promise. Reticulocytes have a short half-life (120 days), and during active autoimmunity and complement activation, C4d binds to them. Manzi and colleagues[8] correlated reticulocyte-C4d levels with disease activity, and also correlated the combination of decreased E-CR-1 and decreased E-C4d, with enhanced sensitivity and specificity (83% and 89%, respectively). During active disease with C3 and C4 levels decreasing, E-C4d increased.[11] CD27 levels on B cells also correlate with disease activity.[12]

Type I interferons (ie, IFN-α) may help distinguish the severe form of such disease as cerebritis, nephritis, and hematological pathologies from other forms.[13] Type I interferons were shown to be associated with anti-Ro, U1-RNP, and Smith antibodies, although their utility has been disputed.

B-lymphocyte stimulator (BLyS), a transmembrane protein located on monocytes, macrophages, and dendritic cells, is crucial for B cell growth and survival.[6] In animal models, overexpression of this protein and lupus activity has been linked. However, in humans, BLyS levels have been variable and not useful in monitoring either disease activity or specific organ involvement.[14] Nevertheless, in a comparison of rheumatoid arthritis and SLE patients, the lupus patients had higher levels, and they correlated better with overall disease activity.[15]

Cytokines

Serum levels of IL-17 and IL-23 were increased in both active and inactive SLE patients, whereas IL-22 levels were decreased in patients with active lupus.[16] Chun and colleagues found that IL-6, IL-10, IL-12, and IFN-γ levels were higher in the SLE patients, while IL-2 levels were lower. IL-6 and IL-10 levels correlated with some aspects of disease activity but not with lupus nephritis. In separate studies, IL-6 elevations and tumor necrosis factor α levels were found to correlate with active disease.[16] By contrast, although IL-12 and IL-18 were elevated in lupus patients, the levels did not correlate with activity.[17,18] IL-2Rα levels were found to be increased,

Box 1
Biomarkers in lupus nephritis

Overall disease activity

Genes

    PTPN22 (protein tyrosine phosphatase 22)

    IRF-5 (interferon regulatory factor–5)

    STAT-4

    Type I interferon

    $IFIT_1$

    OAS1

    LY6E

    ISG15

    MX1

    FCγIIa polymorphism

Interleukins

    IL-22

    IL-6

    IL-10

    IL-12

    IL-18

    IL-2 receptor α

Chemokines

    RANTES (regulated on activation, normal T expressed and secreted)

    CXCL-11 (C-X-C chemokine ligand 11)

    CCL-19 (C-C chemokine ligand 19)

    MCP-1 (monocyte chemoattractant protein–1)

    CXCL-13 (C-X-C chemokine ligand 13)

    IP-10 (interferon inducible protein 10)

Other molecules

    CD27

    Reticulocyte-C4d

    BLyS (B-lymphocyte stimulator)

Lupus diagnosis

    E-C4d (erythrocyte-bound complement-activation product C4d)

    Anti-DsDNA (anti–double-stranded DNA)

    ANA (antinuclear antibody)

    Antinucleosome

Organ specific

Renal involvement

    Serum

Antinucleosome

Anti-Clq

α-actinin

Anti–α-actinin

Adrenomedullin

Urine

Endothelial-1

Lipocalin-2 (neutrophil gelatinase-associated lipocalin)

U-MCP-1 (urinary monocyte chemoattractant protein–1)

Migration inhibition factor

Adiponectin

VCAM-1 (vascular cell adhesion molecule-1)

P-selectin

CXCL-16 (C-X-C chemokine ligand 16)

FOXP3 (forkhead family transcription factor 3)

TWEAK (tumor necrosis factor–like weak inducer of apoptosis)

Osteoprotegerin

Neural

Antihistone

Anti-N

AECA (antiendothelial cell antibodies)

MMP-9 (matrix metalloproteinase 9)

Anti-NMDA (anti–N-methyl-D-asapartate)

Anti-NR2 (anti–N-methyl-D-asapartate receptor subunit NR2)

Anti-P ribosome

Skin

Anticyclic citrullinated peptide Ab

especially in those with severe lupus nephritis, and this biomarker may prove to be useful if confirmed.[19]

Chemokines

Fu and colleagues[20] measured IFN-inducible chemokines (RANTES [regulated on activation, normal T expressed and secreted], CXCL-11 [C-X-C chemokine ligand 11]), IP-10 (IFN inducible protein 10), MIG (monokine induced by IFN-γ), CCL-19 (C-C chemokine ligand 19), monocyte chemoattractant protein-1 (MCP-1), and IL-8 as biomarkers for disease activity. An IFN score was created from measuring the gene expression, a chemokine score was created by measuring chemokine serum levels, and the results were compared with those of patients with rheumatoid arthritis and those of healthy controls. The chemokine score correlated with disease activity compared with C3 levels and SLEDAI-2K. As the disease activity improved with treatment, the score decreased.

CXCL-13 (B cell attractant to areas of inflammation) levels were increased in lupus sera. Active nephritic patients had higher levels. However, CXCL-13 levels were not useful in determining histologic class.[21]

Type I interferon-inducible protein-10 (IP-10, a chemokine produced by peripheral mononuclear cells) was elevated in chronic inflammatory diseases and SLE. However, it was associated more closely with mucocutaneous disease and hematological manifestations but not nephritis.[22]

BIOMARKERS FOR RENAL INVOLVEMENT

Most lupus nephritis patients have antichromatin/nucleosome antibodies (specificity ~98%; sensitivity 69%),[23] and they may be positive when the anti-dsDNA antibodies are negative.[24] Similar findings were observed with anti-C1q antibodies,[25] especially with nephritic flares (negative positive predictive value of 97%–100%,)[26–30] although their precise role has been debated.

Anti-α actinin antibodies are prevalent in patients with active lupus nephritis, and they may be more predictive of nephritis than anti-dsDNA antibodies, although larger studies are needed for confirmation. Anti-Sc-70 (topoisomerase) antibodies have also had mixed results.[29] Adrenomedullin released from macrophages and smooth muscle cells is elevated in SLE, pregnancy, hypertension with left ventricular hypertrophy, diabetes, and other chronic diseases, and it appears to be elevated in active lupus nephritis, although its specificity needs to be determined.[30]

URINE BIOMARKERS

Urine biomarkers are influenced by urine concentration, breakdown in the urine, protein binding, interpretation, and other factors. Nevertheless, they have the advantage of being noninvasive and easily obtainable. Their utility is discussed below.

Endothelial-1 (ET-1) is a 21–amino acid peptide produced in the vasculature, and it participates in cell proliferation, inflammation, vasoconstriction, and fibrosis. Urinary ET-1 reflects both renal and extrarenal production. In one study, serum ET-1, urinary ET-1, and the fractional excretion of ET-1 (feEt-1) were evaluated as biomarkers for chronic kidney disease, rheumatoid arthritis, and SLE. FeET-1 increased during progression of both chronic kidney disease and lupus nephritis.[31] FeET-1 decreased after therapy in lupus nephritis, so it may have utility.

Lipocalin-2, secreted by leukocytes and epithelial cells, is important for iron transport. Urinary levels were evaluated in 70 patients with lupus (with or without lupus nephritis) and controls, with normalization to urinary creatinine. Urinary levels were found to be predictive of active nephritis.[32]

Urinary MCP-1 has also been demonstrated to be predictive of disease activity. Increased levels were found to precede lupus flare by as much as 4 months, and urinary MCP-1 fell with successful treatment.[28] Also, polymorphism of the MCP-1 gene vary in predicting renal involvement in lupus (ie, A/A polymorphism indicates a lower likelihood of involvement compated with a A/G or G/G polymorphism).[33] In a study of 123 SLE patients and 53 controls, urinary MCP-1 was elevated in active lupus nephritis, whereas other markers (eg, IL-6, IL-10, and IL-8 [CXCL-8]) were not useful.[34] In separate studies, urinary message of MCP-1 and transforming growth factor β (TGF-β) correlated with active disease severity but not with the level of fibrosis. In a small group of pediatric patients, migration inhibition factor/creatinine ratio was elevated in the five active lupus nephritis patients versus the five inactive patients.

Zhang and colleagues[35] confirmed that infiltrating leukocytes in the kidney generated hepcidin, and they found that urinary hepcidin increased during active nephritis and decreased with disease resolution. Urinary hepcidin 20 was especially useful as a flare predictor, whereas urinary hepcidin 25 decreased during flares and increased during treatment. Urinary adiponectin (a cytokine produced by the adipodcytes with an anti-inflammatory effect) increased 2 months before flares, remained elevated during nephritic activity, and decreased 4 months postflare.

Various adhesion molecules have also been studied, including vascular cell adhesion molecule-1(VCAM-1), P-selectin, CXCL-16, and tumor necrosis factor receptor-1 (TNFR-1).[36] VCAM-1, which is found mostly in the kidney, recruits monocytes, dendritic cells, and endothelial cells to inflamed areas.[36,37] Urinary excretion of VCAM-1, P-selectin, CXCL-16, and TNFR-1 increased in lupus patients compared with the other groups. In separate studies, FOXP3 (forkhead family transcription factor 3, which is important for regulation of T cells) urinary messenger RNA levels correlated with proliferative lupus nephritis in a small cohort.

Chan and colleagues[38] analyzed T cells, B cells, and natural killer cells in the urine of 12 patients with active lupus nephritis, 17 patients in remission, and 12 lupus patients without renal involvement. CD3+ (T cells) and CD20+ (B cells) correlated best with lupus disease activity while the CD56+ cells did not recognize disease activity with any accuracy.

Chemokines

Avihingsanon and colleagues[39] studied urinary messenger RNA of various chemokines to differentiate the different classes of lupus nephritis. For diagnosing class IV nephritis, the messenger RNA of interferon-producing protein 10 (IP-10) was most useful, followed by vascular endothelial growth factor, and then CXCR3 (chemokine [C-X-C-motif] receptor 3).

Tumor necrosis factor–like weak inducer of apoptosis (TWEAK) regulates other chemokines, such as IP-10, RANTES, and MCP-1. Binding of TWEAK to the Fn14 receptor leads to activation of these chemokines. Schwartz and colleagues[40] evaluated this regulator in lupus nephritis in patients from the Ohio State SLE Study and the Albert Einstein College Lupus Cohort. TWEAK increased in active lupus nephritis patients compared with patients with only extrarenal lupus and with patients with inactive disease, and TWEAK levels appeared to increase with nephritic flares, but not extrarenal flares.

Osteoprotegerin

Osteoprotegerin (tumor necrosis factor family) causes bone reabsorption and is found in many other organs. Urinary levels of osteoprotegerin correlate well with the presence of renal lupus but not with the severity of disease.[41–102]

SUMMARY

Biomarkers provide the potential to noninvasively evaluate and help manage patients with lupus nephritis. Many candidates have been identified, but they require validation in larger cohorts. In the writers' opinion, it is likely that combinations of biomarker profiles, rather than individual markers, will emerge to help better predict the severity of inflammation, the extent of fibrosis, the degree of drug responsiveness, and other variables. This approach has the potential to limit use of the renal biopsy. Additionally, it should improve therapeutic efficacy and limit toxicity. We predict algorithms based on genotype and biomarkers combined with clinical presentation will emerge to help guide physicians in management. Ideally, the complexity of autoimmunity, inflammatory, and fibrogenic responses, along with predictions of pharmacologic utility, will better dictate what approaches are warranted in individual clinical presentations. Assays that show the most potential include serum erythrocyte bound complement C4d, IL-17, IL-23, IFN score/chemokine score ratio, and anti-C1q antibodies. Such urinary biomarkers as fractional excretion of ET-1, MCP-1, VCAM-1, and TWEAK may also be useful but require validations.

REFERENCES

1. Illei GG, Tackey E, Lapteva L, et al. Biomarkers in systemic lupus erythematosus. II. Markers of disease activity. Arthritis Rheum 2004;50(7):2048–65.
2. Illei GG, Tackey E, Lapteva L, et al. Biomarkers in systemic lupus erythematosus. I. General overview of biomarkers and their applicability. Arthritis Rheum 2004;50(6):1709–20.
3. Orbach H, Zandman-Goddard G, Amital H, et al. Novel biomarkers in autoimmune diseases: prolactin, ferritin, vitamin D, and TPA levels in autoimmune diseases. Ann N Y Acad Sci 2007;1109:385–400.
4. Almehed K, d'Elia HF, Bokarewa M, et al. Role of resistin as a marker of inflammation in systemic lupus erythematosus. Arthritis Res Ther 2008;10(1):R15.
5. Kyogoku C, Langefeld CD, Ortmann WA, et al. Genetic association of the R620W polymorphism of protein tyrosine phosphatase PTPN22 with human SLE. Am J Hum Genet 2004;75(3):504–7.
6. Liu CC, Ahearn JM. The search for lupus biomarkers. Best Pract Res Clin Rheumatol 2009;23(4):507–23.
7. Landolt-Marticorena C, Bonventi G, Lubovich A, et al. Lack of association between the interferon-alpha signature and longitudinal changes in disease activity in systemic lupus erythematosus. Ann Rheum Dis 2009;68(9):1440–6.
8. Manzi S, Navratil JS, Ruffing MJ, et al. Measurement of erythrocyte C4d and complement receptor 1 in systemic lupus erythematosus. Arthritis Rheum 2004;50(11):3596–604.
9. Navratil JS, Manzi S, Kao AH, et al. Platelet C4d is highly specific for systemic lupus erythematosus. Arthritis Rheum 2006;54(2):670–4.
10. Colburn KK, Green LM. Serum antiguanosine antibodies as a marker for SLE disease activity and pathogen potential. Clin Chim Acta 2006;370(1–2):9–16.
11. Liu CC, Manzi S, Kao AH, et al. Reticulocytes bearing C4d as biomarkers of disease activity for systemic lupus erythematosus. Arthritis Rheum 2005;52(10):3087–99.
12. Jacobi AM, Odendahl M, Reiter K, et al. Correlation between circulating CD27high plasma cells and disease activity in patients with systemic lupus erythematosus. Arthritis Rheum 2003;48(5):1332–42.
13. Baechler EC, Batliwalla FM, Karypis G, et al. Interferon-inducible gene expression signature in peripheral blood cells of patients with severe lupus. Proc Natl Acad Sci U S A 2003;100(5):2610–5.
14. Stohl W, Metyas S, Tan SM, et al. B lymphocyte stimulator overexpression in patients with systemic lupus erythematosus: longitudinal observations. Arthritis Rheum 2003;48(12):3475–86.
15. Chun HY, Chung JW, Kim HA, et al. Cytokine IL-6 and IL-10 as biomarkers in systemic lupus erythematosus. J Clin Immunol 2007;27(5):461–6.
16. Sabry A, Sheashaa H, El-Husseini A, et al. Proinflammatory cytokines (TNF-alpha and IL-6) in Egyptian patients with SLE: its correlation with disease activity. Cytokines 2006;35(3–4):148–53.

17. Robak E, Robak T, Wozniacka A, et al. Proinflammatory interferon-gamma–inducing monokines (interleukin-12, interleukin-18, interleukin-15)–serum profile in patients with systemic lupus erythematosus. Eur Cytokine Netw 2002;13(3): 364–8.

18. Lit LC, Wong CK, Tam LS, et al. Raised plasma concentration and ex vivo production of inflammatory chemokines in patients with systemic lupus erythematosus. Ann Rheum Dis 2006;65(2):209–15.

19. El-Shafey EM, El-Nagar GF, El-Bendary AS, et al. Serum soluble interleukin-2 receptor alpha in systemic lupus erythematosus. Iran J Kidney Dis 2008;2(2):80–5.

20. Fu Q, Chen X, Cui H, et al. Association of elevated transcript levels of interferon-inducible chemokines with disease activity and organ damage in systemic lupus erythematosus patients. Arthritis Res Ther 2008;10(5):R112.

21. Schiffer L, Kümpers P, Davalos-Misslitz AM, et al. B-cell-attracting chemokine CXCL13 as a marker of disease activity and renal involvement in systemic lupus erythematosus (SLE). Nephrol Dial Transplant 2009;24(12):3708–12.

22. Kong KO, Tan AW, Thong BY, et al. Enhanced expression of interferon-inducible protein-10 correlates with disease activity and clinical manifestations in systemic lupus erythematosus. Clin Exp Immunol 2009;156(1):134–40.

23. Cervera R, Viñas O, Ramos-Casals M, et al. Anti-chromatin antibodies in systemic lupus erythematosus: a useful marker for lupus nephropathy. Ann Rheum Dis 2003;62(5):431–4.

24. Simón JA, Cabiedes J, Ortiz E, et al. Anti-nucleosome antibodies in patients with systemic lupus erythematosus of recent onset. Potential utility as a diagnostic tool and disease activity marker. Rheumatology (Oxford) 2004;43(2):220–4.

25. Marto N, Bertolaccini ML, Calabuig E, et al. Anti-C1q antibodies in nephritis: correlation between titres and renal disease activity and positive predictive value in systemic lupus erythematosus. Ann Rheum Dis 2005;64(3):444–8.

26. Trendelenburg M, Lopez-Trascasa M, Potlukova E, et al. High prevalence of anti-C1q antibodies in biopsy-proven active lupus nephritis. Nephrol Dial Transplant 2006;21(11):3115–21.

27. Moroni G, Trendelenburg M, Del Papa N, et al. Anti-C1q antibodies may help in diagnosing a renal flare in lupus nephritis. Am J Kidney Dis 2001;37(3):490–8.

28. Rovin BH, Song H, Birmingham DJ, et al. Urine chemokines as biomarkers of human systemic lupus erythematosus activity. J Am Soc Nephrol 2005;16(2): 467–73.

29. Hamidou MA, Audrain MA, Masseau A, et al. Anti-topoisomerase I antibodies in systemic lupus erythematosus as a marker of severe nephritis. Clin Rheumatol 2006;25(4):542–3.

30. Mak A, Cheung BM, Mok CC, et al. Adrenomedullin—a potential disease activity marker and suppressor of nephritis activity in systemic lupus erythematosus. Rheumatology (Oxford) 2006;45(10):1266–72.

31. Dhaun N, Lilitkarntakul P, Macintyre IM, et al. Urinary endothelin-1 in chronic kidney disease and as a marker of disease activity in lupus nephritis. Am J Physiol Renal Physiol 2009;296(6):F1477–83.

32. Pitashny M, Schwartz N, Qing X, et al. Urinary lipocalin-2 is associated with renal disease activity in human lupus nephritis. Arthritis Rheum 2007;56(6):1894–903.

33. Tucci M, Barnes EV, Sobel ES, et al. Strong association of a functional polymorphism in the monocyte chemoattractant protein 1 promoter gene with lupus nephritis. Arthritis Rheum 2004;50(6):1842–9.

34. Li Y, Tucci M, Narain S, et al. Urinary biomarkers in lupus nephritis. Autoimmun Rev 2006;5(6):383–8.

35. Zhang X, Jin M, Wu H, et al. Biomarkers of lupus nephritis determined by serial urine proteomics. Kidney Int 2008;74(6):799–807.
36. Wu T, Xie C, Wang HW, et al. Elevated urinary VCAM-1, P-selectin, soluble TNF receptor-1, and CXC chemokine ligand 16 in multiple murine lupus strains and human lupus nephritis. J Immunol 2007;179(10):7166–75.
37. Wang G, Lai FM, Tam LS, et al. Urinary FOXP3 mRNA in patients with lupus nephritis—relation with disease activity and treatment response. Rheumatology (Oxford) 2009;48(7):755–60.
38. Chan RW, Lai FM, Li EK, et al. Urinary mononuclear cell and disease activity of systemic lupus erythematosus. Lupus 2006;15(5):262–7.
39. Avihingsanon Y, Phumesin P, Benjachat T, et al. Measurement of urinary chemokine and growth factor messenger RNAs: a noninvasive monitoring in lupus nephritis. Kidney Int 2006;69(4):747–53.
40. Schwartz N, Michaelson JS, Putterman C. Lipocalin-2, TWEAK, and other cytokines as urinary biomarkers for lupus nephritis. Ann N Y Acad Sci 2007;1109:265–74.
41. Kiani AN, Johnson K, Chen C, et al. Urine osteoprotegerin and monocyte chemoattractant protein-1 in lupus nephritis. J Rheumatol 2009;36(10):2224–30.
42. Becker-Merok A, Kalaaji M, Haugbro K, et al. Alpha-actinin-binding antibodies in relation to systemic lupus erythematosus and lupus nephritis. Arthritis Res Ther 2006;8(6):R162.
43. Cheng F, Guo Z, Xu H, et al. Decreased plasma IL22 levels, but not increased IL17 and IL23 levels, correlate with disease activity in patients with systemic lupus erythematosus. Ann Rheum Dis 2009;68(4):604–6.
44. Coremans I, Spronk P, Bootsma H, et al. Changes in antibodies to C1q predict renal relapses in systemic lupus erythematous. Am J Kidney Dis 1995;26(4):595–601.
45. Renaudineau Y, Croquefer S, Jousse S, et al. Association of alpha-actinin-binding anti-double-stranded DNA antibodies with lupus nephritis. Arthritis Rheum 2006;54(8):2523–32.
46. Rovin BH, Song H, Hebert LA, et al. Plasma, urine, and renal expression of adiponectin in human systemic lupus erythematosus. Kidney Int 2005;68(4):1825–33.
47. Otukesh H, Chalian M, Hoseini R, et al. Urine macrophage migration inhibitory factor in pediatric systemic lupus erythematosus. Clin Rheumatol 2007;26(12):2105–7.
48. Mizuno M, Blanchin S, Gasque P, et al. High levels of complement C3a receptor in the glomeruli in lupus nephritis. Am J Kidney Dis 2007;49(5):598–606.
49. Tumlin JA. Lupus nephritis: histology, diagnosis, and treatment. Bull NYU Hosp Jt Dis 2008;66(3):188–94.
50. Enghard P, Riemekasten G. Immunology and the diagnosis of lupus nephritis. Lupus 2009;18(4):287–90.
51. Liang MH, Simard JF, Costenbader K, et al. Methodologic issues in the validation of putative biomarkers and surrogate endpoints in treatment evaluation for systemic lupus erythematosus. Endocr Metab Immune Disord Drug Targets 2009;9(1):108–12.
52. Yang DH, Chang DM, Lai JH, et al. Usefulness of erythrocyte-bound C4d as a biomarker to predict disease activity in patients with systemic lupus erythematosus. Rheumatology (Oxford) 2009;48(9):1083–7.
53. Moroni G, Radice A, Giammarresi G, et al. Are laboratory tests useful for monitoring the activity of lupus nephritis? A 6-year prospective study in a cohort of 228 patients with lupus nephritis. Ann Rheum Dis 2009;68(2):234–7.

54. Ehrenstein MR, Alves JD. Antibodies and other biomarkers—pathological consequences (2). Lupus 2008;17(3):256–8.
55. Giles I, Putterman C. Autoantibodies and other biomarkers—pathological consequences (1). Lupus 2008;17(3):241–6.
56. Suh CH, Kim HA. Cytokines and their receptors as biomarkers of systemic lupus erythematosus. Expert Rev Mol Diagn 2008;8(2):189–98.
57. Waldman M, Madaio MP. Pathogenic autoantibodies in lupus nephritis. Lupus 2005;14(1):19–24.
58. Kallenberg CG, Stegeman CA, Bootsma H, et al. Quantitation of autoantibodies in systemic autoimmune diseases: clinically useful? Lupus 2006;15(7):397–402.
59. Rhodes B, Vyse TJ. The genetics of SLE: an update in the light of genome-wide association studies. Rheumatology (Oxford) 2008;47(11):1603–11.
60. Rovin BH. The chemokine network in systemic lupus erythematous nephritis. Front Biosci 2008;13:904–22.
61. Ferri GM, Gigante A, Ferri F, et al. Urine chemokines: biomarkers of human lupus nephritis? Eur Rev Med Pharmacol Sci 2007;11(3):171–8.
62. Varghese SA, Powell TB, Budisavljevic MN, et al. Urine biomarkers predict the cause of glomerular disease. J Am Soc Nephrol 2007;18(3):913–22.
63. Schwartz N, Su L, Burkly LC, et al. Urinary TWEAK and the activity of lupus nephritis. J Autoimmun 2006;27(4):242–50.
64. Bauer JW, Baechler EC, Petri M, et al. Elevated serum levels of interferon-regulated chemokines are biomarkers for active human systemic lupus erythematosus. PLoS Med 2006;3(12):e491.
65. Mosley K, Tam FW, Edwards RJ, et al. Urinary proteomic profiles distinguish between active and inactive lupus nephritis. Rheumatology (Oxford) 2006;45(12):1497–504.
66. Zhang B, Zhang X, Tang FL, et al. Clinical significance of increased CD4+CD25-Foxp3+ T cells in patients with new-onset systemic lupus erythematosus. Ann Rheum Dis 2008;67(7):1037–40.
67. O'Hara RM Jr, Benoit SE, Groves CJ, et al. Cell-surface and cytokine biomarkers in autoimmune and inflammatory diseases. Drug Discov Today 2006;11(7–8):342–7.
68. Oates JC, Varghese S, Bland AM, et al. Prediction of urinary protein markers in lupus nephritis. Kidney Int 2005;68(6):2588–92.
69. Vojdani A. Antibodies as predictors of complex autoimmune diseases. Int J Immunopathol Pharmacol 2008;21(2):267–78.
70. Renaudineau Y, Deocharan B, Jousse S, et al. Anti-alpha-actinin antibodies: a new marker of lupus nephritis. Autoimmun Rev 2007;6(7):464–8.
71. Paiva CN, Arras RH, Magalhães ES, et al. Migration inhibitory factor (MIF) released by macrophages upon recognition of immune complexes is critical to inflammation in Arthus reaction. J Leukoc Biol 2009;85(5):855–61.
72. Bonelli M, Savitskaya A, Steiner CW, et al. Phenotypic and functional analysis of CD4+ CD25- Foxp3+ T cells in patients with systemic lupus erythematosus. J Immunol 2009;182(3):1689–95.
73. Liu CC, Manzi S, Ahearn JM. Biomarkers for systemic lupus erythematosus: a review and perspective. Curr Opin Rheumatol 2005;17(5):543–9.
74. Manzi S, Ahearn JM, Salmon J. New insights into complement: a mediator of injury and marker of disease activity in systemic lupus erythematosus. Lupus 2004;13(5):298–303.
75. Cheema GS, Roschke V, Hilbert DM, et al. Elevated serum B lymphocyte stimulator levels in patients with systemic immune-based rheumatic diseases. Arthritis Rheum 2001;44(6):1313–9.

76. Chan RW, Lai FM, Li EK, et al. Expression of chemokine and fibrosing factor messenger RNA in the urinary sediment of patients with lupus nephritis. Arthritis Rheum 2004;50(9):2882–90.
77. Rönnblom L, Eloranta ML, Alm GV. The type I interferon system in systemic lupus erythematosus. Arthritis Rheum 2006;54(2):408–20.
78. Kalaaji M, Sturfelt G, Mjelle JE, et al. Critical comparative analyses of anti-alpha-actinin and glomerulus-bound antibodies in human and murine lupus nephritis. Arthritis Rheum 2006;54(3):914–26.
79. Feng X, Wu H, Grossman JM, et al. Association of increased interferon-inducible gene expression with disease activity and lupus nephritis in patients with systemic lupus erythematosus. Arthritis Rheum 2006;54(9):2951–62.
80. Spronk PE, Bootsma H, Huitema MG, et al. Levels of soluble VCAM-1, soluble ICAM-1, and soluble E-selectin during disease exacerbations in patients with systemic lupus erythematosus (SLE); a long term prospective study. Clin Exp Immunol 1994;97(3):439–44.
81. Pallis M, Robson DK, Haskard DO, et al. Distribution of cell adhesion molecules in skeletal muscle from patients with systemic lupus erythematosus. Ann Rheum Dis 1993;52(9):667–71.
82. Wellicome SM, Kapahi P, Mason JC, et al. Detection of a circulating form of vascular cell adhesion molecule-1: raised levels in rheumatoid arthritis and systemic lupus erythematosus. Clin Exp Immunol 1993;92(3):412–8.
83. Capper ER, Maskill JK, Gordon C, et al. Interleukin (IL)-10, IL-1ra and IL-12 profiles in active and quiescent systemic lupus erythematosus: could longitudinal studies reveal patient subgroups of differing pathology? Clin Exp Immunol 2004;138(2):348–56.
84. Oelzner P, Deliyska B, Fünfstück R, et al. Anti-C1q antibodies and antiendothelial cell antibodies in systemic lupus erythematosus—relationship with disease activity and renal involvement. Clin Rheumatol 2003;22(4–5):271–8.
85. Wada T, Yokoyama H, Su SB, et al. Monitoring urinary levels of monocyte chemotactic and activating factor reflects disease activity of lupus nephritis. Kidney Int 1996;49(3):761–7.
86. Karassa FB, Trikalinos TA, Ioannidis JP, et al. The Fc gamma RIIIA-F158 allele is a risk factor for the development of lupus nephritis: a meta-analysis. Fc gamma RIIIA-SLE meta-analysis investigators. Kidney Int 2003;63(4):1475–82.
87. Petri M, Buyon J, Kim M. Classification and definition of major flares in SLE clinical trials. Lupus 1999;8(8):685–91.
88. Eriksson C, Eneslätt K, Ivanoff J, et al. Abnormal expression of chemokine receptors on T-cells from patients with systemic lupus erythematosus. Lupus 2003;12(10):766–74.
89. Siegert CE, Daha MR, Tseng CM, et al. Predictive value of IgG autoantibodies against C1q for nephritis in systemic lupus erythematosus. Ann Rheum Dis 1993;52(12):851–6.
90. Brunner HI, Mueller M, Rutherford C, et al. Urinary neutrophil gelatinase-associated lipocalin as a biomarker of nephritis in childhood-onset systemic lupus erythematosus. Arthritis Rheum 2006;54(8):2577–84.
91. Das L, Brunner HI. Biomarkers for renal disease in childhood. Curr Rheumatol Rep 2009;11(3):218–25.
92. Suzuki M, Wiers K, Brooks EB, et al. Initial validation of a novel protein biomarker panel for active pediatric lupus nephritis. Pediatr Res 2009;65(5):530–6.
93. Keenan RT, Swearingen CJ, Yazici Y. Erythrocyte sedimentation rate and C-reactive protein levels are poorly correlated with clinical measures of disease

activity in rheumatoid arthritis, systemic lupus erythematosus and osteoarthritis patients. Clin Exp Rheumatol 2008;26(5):814–9.

94. Yao GH, Liu ZH, Zhang X, et al. Circulating thrombomodulin and vascular cell adhesion molecule-1 and renal vascular lesion in patients with lupus nephritis. Lupus 2008;17(8):720–6.

95. Zandman-Goddard G, Shoenfeld Y. Hyperferritinemia in autoimmunity. Isr Med Assoc J 2008;10(1):83–4.

96. Suzuki M, Wiers KM, Klein-Gitelman MS, et al. Neutrophil gelatinase-associated lipocalin as a biomarker of disease activity in pediatric lupus nephritis. Pediatr Nephrol 2008;23(3):403–12.

97. Rubinstein T, Pitashny M, Putterman C. The novel role of neutrophil gelatinase-B associated lipocalin (NGAL)/Lipocalin-2 as a biomarker for lupus nephritis. Autoimmun Rev 2008;7(3):229–34.

98. Cojocaru IM, Cojocaru M, Tănăsescu R, et al. Detection of autoantibodies to ribosome P in lupus patients with neurological involvement. Rom J Intern Med 2008;46(3):239–42.

99. Suzuki M, Ross GF, Wiers K, et al. Identification of a urinary proteomic signature for lupus nephritis in children. Pediatr Nephrol 2007;22(12):2047–57.

100. Amezcua-Guerra LM, Marquez-Velasco R, Bojali R. Erosive arthritis in systemic lupus erythematous is associated with high serum C-reactive protein and anti-cyclic citrullinated peptid antibodies. Inflamm Res 2008:75:555–7.

101. Efthimiou P, Blanco M. Pathogenesis of neuropsychiatric systemic lupus erythematous and potential biomarkers. Mod Rheumatol 2009;19(5):457–68.

102. Sun XY, Shi J, Han L, et al. Anti-histones antibodies in systemic lupus erythematous: prevelance and frequency in neuropsychiatric lupus. J Clin Lab Anal 2008;22(4):271–7.

Endothelial Function and its Implications for Cardiovascular and Renal Disease in Systemic Lupus Erythematosus

Robert Clancy, PhD[a,b],*, Ellen M. Ginzler, MD, MPH[c]

KEYWORDS

- Atherosclerosis • SLE nephritis • Adiponectin
- Membrane endothelial protein C receptor

Systemic lupus erythematosus (SLE) is a disease state posing several challenges to clinicians, including heterogeneity of presentation, undulating course, and an extraordinary risk for vascular injury,[1,2] including premature atherosclerosis and endothelial injury related to renal disease. Central to this concept is a focus on the endothelium, because it provides the physiologic boundary that limits extravasation and diapedesis of inflammatory cells. This article provides a clinical overview and outlines the putative pathogenic events that occur in SLE autoimmune-associated vasculopathy for atherosclerosis and renal disease.

Regarding premature cardiovascular disease, more than 3 decades ago investigators noted that most deaths in patients who had SLE with longer disease duration were attributed to atherosclerosis.[1] The rate of myocardial infarction in women aged 35 to 44 years is 50 times greater than expected.[2] Patients who have SLE have an increased atherosclerotic risk despite adjustment for traditional Framingham risk factors.[2,3] Risk factors among these patients are somewhat controversial but may include longer duration of disease and lower likelihood of treatment with prednisone, cyclophosphamide, or hydroxychloroquine.[4] Thus, inflammation related to underlying disease is likely to be contributory.

McMahon and coworkers[5] recently showed that plasma from patients who have SLE with premature atherosclerosis is enriched in proinflammatory high-density

[a] NYU Langone School of Medicine, New York, NY, USA
[b] 560 First Avenue, Tisch Hospital Tch4-407, New York, NY 10016, USA
[c] SUNY Downstate Medical Center, Brooklyn, New York, NY, USA
* Corresponding author. 560 First Avenue, Tisch Hospital Tch4-407, New York, NY 10016.
E-mail address: Bobdclancy@aol.com (R. Clancy).

Rheum Dis Clin N Am 36 (2010) 145–160
doi:10.1016/j.rdc.2009.12.011   **rheumatic.theclinics.com**
0889-857X/10/$ – see front matter © 2010 Elsevier Inc. All rights reserved.

lipoprotein (HDL). However, the inflammation may be clinically subtle because detectable cardiovascular events have been unexpectedly reported in patients who have SLE with extended periods of quiescence,[6] and subclinical atherosclerosis has not correlated with disease activity index scores.[4]

Functional impairment of the endothelium is reflected by the pattern of proinjury mediators, such as circulating endothelial cells (CECs), apoptotic circulating endothelial cells, and soluble E-selectin (sE-selectin). For example, generation of nitric oxide (NO) by the endothelium promotes relaxation of the contractile elements of the smooth muscle of the arterial blood vessels. In atherogenic disease, endothelial protection may be subverted because of a loss of boundary function through detachment of endothelial cells into the circulation or a change in the endothelial cell phenotype. Increased levels of CECs have been observed in patients who have active disease,[7] and apoptotic CECs have been reported in patients who have SLE with diminished flow-mediated dilatation.[8] sE-selectin, likely shed from an abnormally activated endothelium, was recently associated with atherosclerosis through an abnormal coronary artery calcium detected with electron beam CT.[9]

Blood vessel homeostasis involves a complex interplay between inflammatory signals, coagulation signals, and other mediators. T-cell recruitment of monocytes into artery walls may be a critical step in the effective handling of cholesterol. Cholesterol in the bloodstream is scavenged by a low-density lipoprotein molecule and deposited in the arterial wall, where monocytes, which have been recruited by activated T cells, are a part of normal homeostasis (**Fig. 1**). The monocyte should optimally serve as a temporary depot for fats, differentiating into an efficient cholesterol-metabolizing macrophage until the excess lipid can be picked up by HDL.

Phases of atherosclerosis development

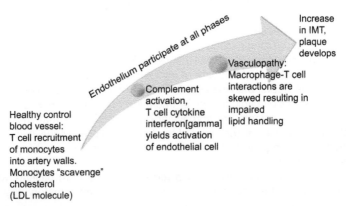

Endothelium participate at all phases

Healthy control blood vessel: T cell recruitment of monocytes into artery walls. Monocytes "scavenge" cholesterol (LDL molecule)

Complement activation, T cell cytokine interferon[gamma] yields activation of endothelial cell

Vasculopathy: Macrophage-T cell interactions are skewed resulting in impaired lipid handling

Increase in IMT, plaque develops

Fig. 1. Macrophage–T-cell interactions in atherosclerosis. Blood vessel homeostasis involves a complex interplay between inflammatory signals, coagulation signals, and other mediators. T-cell recruitment of monocytes into artery walls may be a critical step in the effective handling of cholesterol. Cholesterol in the bloodstream is scavenged by a low-density lipoprotein molecule and deposited in the arterial wall, where monocytes, which have been recruited by activated T cells, are a part of normal homeostasis. Complement activation, T-cell cytokine interferon-γ, or T-cell–stimulated immune complexes activate endothelial cells to express surface metalloproteinases, and concomitantly an impaired lipid handling occurs with a sequential narrowing of an artery. Once this system becomes overwhelmed, cholesterol plaques develop, which induce inflammatory and fibrotic reactions.

The scenario is dramatically altered when complement is activated. Complement activation, T-cell cytokine interferon -γ (IFN-γ), or T cell–stimulated immune complexes promote the activation of endothelial cells to express surface metalloproteinases; an impaired lipid handling with sequential arterial narrowing occurs concomitantly. Once this system becomes overwhelmed, cholesterol plaques develop, which induce both inflammatory and fibrotic reactions.

Lupus nephritis (LN) predominantly affects African American and Hispanic women of reproductive age. A higher incidence of progression to end-stage renal disease (ESRD) in these ethnic subsets has been shown, compared with other predominantly Caucasian populations.[10] Although the overall 10-year survival has improved to more than 90% in patients who have SLE,[11] the incidence of LN progressing to ESRD has remained constant.[10]

A literature review has shown a difference in response to treatment modalities for LN based on ethnic/racial differences. For patients who have proliferative forms of LN, renal survival is worse with progression to ESRD in African American and Hispanic patients despite treatment with intravenous cyclophosphamide (IVC), even after controlling for hypertension, initial renal functional impairment, and quantity of corticosteroid therapy.[12,13] Socioeconomic features (income, educational level, access to health care) may contribute to the poorer prognosis in these populations. In one study, however, the relative risk for progression to ESRD remained higher in the Hispanic population.[13] Several recent studies have found that African American and Hispanic populations had a better response to mycophenolate mofetil than to IVC.[14,15]

No new medications have been FDA approved specifically for treating SLE or LN in more than 50 years. Most drugs used in the treatment regimen are commercially available and prescribed off-label, or available only as part of an investigational protocol. Recent clinical trials for newer agents in the treatment of LN may not have achieved predetermined end points because of either an actual absence of efficacy or shortcomings in the design of the study protocol. Furthermore, pharmacogenomics may have a role in determining the efficacy and safety of a medication. Therefore, the effect a medication may have in improving the renal survival and overall outcome in select subgroups of patients or even individual patients is important to know before subjecting them to aggressive immunosuppression and its potential side effects.

Nephritis, a life-threatening manifestation of SLE, is strongly influenced by blood vessels partly because the vasculature plays a central role in supporting homeostasis. The contribution of the vascular endothelium to the pathogenesis of renal injury has not been emphasized in LN. Despite potential biologic insights and treatment strategies to be gained by studying the endothelium in LN, historic World Health Organization (WHO) classification, National Institutes of Health (NIH) chronicity (CI) and activity (AI) indices,[16] and recent International Society of Nephrology/Renal Pathology Society (ISN/RPS) 2003 pathologic classifications of LN[17] do not specifically address the state of the microvasculature in their definitions. However, recent murine data based on microarray analysis suggest that endothelial activation is a feature shared by progressive glomerulosclerosis compared with nonprogressive glomerulosclerosis.[18]

For one scenario of putative pathogenic events, exposure of healthy endothelial cells to potential stimuli such as circulating IFN-α, tumor necrosis factor α (TNF-α), or immune complexes present in patients who have active SLE results in the expression of NO synthase 2 (NOS2) and generation of NO and adhesion molecules. As shown in **Fig. 2**, this activated endothelium has now lost its function to serve as a physiologic brake, which normally prevents the infiltration of inflammatory cells that produce IL-18, a potent chemoattractant for plasmacytoid dendritic cells.[19]

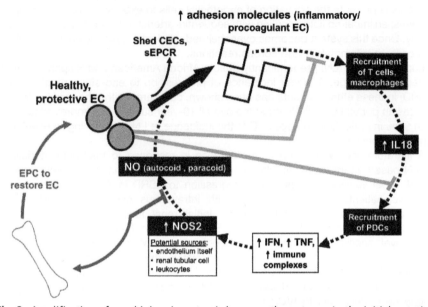

Fig. 2. Amplification of renal injury in systemic lupus erythematosus. In the initial putative pathogenic events, the exposure of healthy endothelial cells to potential stimuli such as circulating interferon (IFN)-α, tumor necrosis factor α, or immune complexes present in patients who have active SLE, results in the expression of nitric oxide synthase 2 and the generation of nitric oxide and adhesion molecules. This activated endothelium has now lost its ability to serve as a physiologic brake, which normally prevents the infiltration of inflammatory cells that produce interleukin (IL)-18, a potent chemoattractant for plasmacytoid dendritic cells (pDCs).[19] Endothelial cells may also be activated by IL-18. pDCs release IFNs which have a paracrine effect on other cell types to express nitric oxide synthase 2. In addition to the local inflammatory consequences of activation, endothelial cells are shed into the circulation, and membrane endothelial protein C receptor (EPCR) is lost, so that EPCR is now circulating as a soluble form (sEPCR), which produces a procoagulant effect. Prothrombin fragment F1+2 (a marker of thrombin generation) is generated, a consequence of thrombin, which is indirectly responsible for release of sEPCR. The increased release of sEPCR coupled with higher thrombin generation suggests that less membrane-bound EPCR will be available in these individuals for efficient protein C activation.

Endothelial cells may also be activated by IL-18.[20] Plasmacytoid dendritic cells release IFNs, which have a paracrine effect on other cell types to express NOS2. In addition to the local inflammatory consequences of activation, endothelial cells are shed into the circulation and membrane endothelial protein C receptor (EPCR) is lost so that EPCR circulates as a soluble form (sEPCR), with a procoagulant effect. Prothrombin F1+2 (a marker of thrombin generation) are generated, a consequence of thrombin that is indirectly responsible for release of sEPCR. The increased release of sEPCR coupled with higher thrombin generation suggests that less membrane-bound EPCR will be available in these individuals for efficient protein C activation.

Although prior studies on premature atherosclerosis and vascular injury in nephritis have highlighted the potential association of markers directly reflecting injury, absent is a focus on protective (anti-injury) molecules such as the adipocyte-derived protein, adiponectin, and membrane EPCR (mEPCR).

This article describes how adiponectin and mEPCR serve as a pathway that focuses on anti-injury. In addition, the authors propose that mEPCR and adiponectin may herald a thwarted attempt at protection in patients at risk for progression of atherosclerotic and renal disease. Moreover, the identification of these molecules as biomarkers may represent an incremental advance that offers insight into pathogenesis and therapy.

PROFILE OF ADIPONECTIN IN HEALTH AND DISEASE

Adiponectin (also known as 30-kd adipocyte complement-related protein [Acrp30]) is a secreted protein that is constitutively produced by adipocytes. Adiponectin, a trimer in serum, is a 30-kd protein consisting of four domains, including signal peptide at the N-terminus, a variable domain, a collagenous domain, and a C-terminal globular domain homologous to C1q. The protein is well characterized regarding its capacity to improve insulin sensitivity. During the early 1990s the best-characterized biologic property was enhancing glycogen accumulation and fatty acid oxidation in C2C12 myotubes. The in vivo action to regulate serum levels of fatty acids and glucose was linked to adiponectin's effect on the liver to suppress glucose output while acting on muscle to increase glucose uptake and fatty acid oxidation.

However, adiponectin's actions are not restricted to controlling glucose and lipid metabolism. Properties involving anti-inflammatory and anti-atherosclerotic functions have also been reported. Adiponectin accumulates in the subendothelium of injured human arteries, where it inhibits monocyte adhesion to endothelial cells and ultimately inhibits the migration and proliferation of vascular smooth muscle, which contribute to the atherosclerotic process[21] through a mechanism that partly involves the down-regulation of adhesion molecules through attenuating the nuclear factor κB pathway.[22,23]

Adiponectin also has been found in blood vessel walls after experimental endothelial injury,[24] and is strongly expressed around infarcted but not normal myocardium,[25] supporting a role in vascular and endothelial remodeling. Specifically, adiponectin was recruited to the affected area of an arterial injury site in balloon-injured rat carotid arteries. Adiponectin knockout (KO) mice were used to further study the relationship between adiponectin and the properties of the vasculature. The mice displayed an impaired endothelium-dependent vasodilation. A series of experiments were performed that suggested that adiponectin serves a role as a proangiogenic regulator. Angiogenic repair of ischemic hind limbs was impaired in adiponectin KO mice compared with wild-type. These data suggested that the exogenous supplementation of adiponectin could be a beneficial treatment for obesity-related vascular disorders.

MEMBRANE ENDOTHELIAL PROTEIN C RECEPTOR: PROTECTION OF THE ENDOTHELIUM

EPCR, which has been cloned in mice and human tissues,[26] is constitutively expressed by endothelial cells, particularly in large blood vessels and monocyte/macrophages. EPCR is a 46-kd type 1 transmembrane glycoprotein with structural features consistent with an antigen-presenting groove analogous to major histocompatibility complex (MHC) class 1 and the CD1 family of proteins. Its structure consists of a large extracellular domain (221 amino acids), a transmembrane domain (25 amino acids), and a short highly conserved cytoplasmic sequence (3 amino acids).

The 5' flanking region of the murine EPCR gene was recently examined and shown to contain elements that reflect involvement in cell growth and development and a thrombin response element. Endotoxin and thrombin elevate rodent EPCR mRNA levels and increase receptor shedding in vivo.[27] A phospholipid is tightly bound in the position of the antigen-presenting groove, suggesting that EPCR recycles to membrane endosomes and participates in antigen presentation.

A well-characterized biologic property of membrane EPCR is its role as an accessory factor to thrombin–thrombomodulin complexes causing a dramatic augmentation of the formation of activated protein C (APC).[28,29] For example, previous studies showed that APC generation was dependent on EPCR and that blocking protein C–EPCR interaction decreased APC formation approximately 10-fold.[30] In baboons, EPCR blocking antibodies were found to decrease protein C activation and increase susceptibility to bacterial sepsis.

These studies have advanced the notion that high levels of mEPCR are a beneficial property and that lower levels of are deleterious, which was supported by several studies focusing on genetic manipulation of EPCR in mice. Overexpression of EPCR under the control of an endothelium-specific Tie2 promoter was shown to dramatically alter patterns of EPCR expression,[31] although the mice did not exhibit any gross hemorrhagic abnormalities. They did, however, exhibit an eightfold increase in APC generation in response to infusion of thrombin, and were partially resistant to a lethal dose of bacterial lipopolysaccharide. These findings confirm and extend the results of previous studies, which used blocking antibodies.

Cleavage of EPCR from the cell surface by matrix metalloproteinases has been shown.[32] This action is initiated when endothelial cells are treated with lipopolysaccharide, inflammatory cytokines, and thrombin. A single nucleotide polymorphism (SNP) in exon 4 of the EPCR gene at 20q11, which converts serine 219 to glycine (219 Gly) in a region of the molecule close to the plasma membrane, is associated with increased basal and stimulated shedding of EPCR from endothelial cells.[33] The absence of membrane EPCR resulted in an attenuation of the thrombin–thrombomodulin complex–dependent protein C activation. Because sEPCR also binds to protein C and APC,[26] functionally it results in a loss of a brake to thrombosis and inflammation.

In a murine model using heterozygotes of EPCR knockout mice, administration of endotoxin-induced disseminated intravascular coagulation, which was aggravated in heterozygous protein C–deficient mice compared with wild-type. It is tempting to speculate that low levels of membrane EPCR secondary to high shedding of EPCR may also have deleterious consequences to coagulation and inflammation. However, studies in humans, which initially focused on deep vein thrombosis, have not shown uniform results of the risk for venous thrombosis for the genotype in separate cohorts.[33,34]

mEPCR may also have direct effects on endothelial cell phenotype. For example, the shedding of EPCR is associated with the activation of protease-activated receptors (PARs), a novel family of G-protein–coupled receptors that are constitutively expressed on endothelial cells and are involved in the early recruitment of leukocytes.[35]

ENDOTHELIAL DYSFUNCTION AND PROGRESSION OF ATHEROSCLEROSIS AND RENAL DISEASE

The usefulness of biomarkers, which identify patients who have endothelial dysfunction and progression of atherosclerosis and renal disease, has fallen short of the mark. This section reviews the biomarker discovery initiative in the context of inflammation hypothesis and Schwartzman phenomenon. Recent studies are then reviewed that offer a new direction for risk stratification. New mechanistic insights into the patho-physiology underlying accelerated atherogenesis and renal disease are then highlighted.

Many have speculated that inflammation, the central feature of SLE pathogenesis and clinical flares, is linked to the increased atherosclerotic risk among these patients, in addition to higher rates of traditional risk factors. However, the absence of an asso-ciation between carotid plaque and overt disease activity in this study and others contradicts the inflammation hypothesis. One simple explanation is that the SELENA-SLEDAI (SLE Disease Activity Index) instrument may underestimate disease activity. However, this instrument does capture current inflammation in the cutaneous, renal, serosal, hematologic, neurologic, and serologic systems. In fact, these clinical settings of activity are where the traditional markers of endothelial (luminal) injury have been identified.

However, the scope of the vasculopathy may include normal-appearing blood vessels. For example, in a skin biopsy obtained from nonlesional, non–sun exposed skin of the buttocks, immunohistochemistry found levels of adhesion molecules (VCAM1, ICAM1 and E selectin) to be significantly elevated in patients versus normal controls. Because these phenotypic changes occurred in normal-appearing tissue, the widespread endothelial activation was portrayed in the context of the Schwartz-man phenomenon. However, expression of the anti-injury molecules (eg, adiponectin, mEPCR) was not evaluated.

As the authors reported at the 2009 American College of Rheumatology meeting, in a cohort of 131 patients and 73 race/ethnicity-matched healthy controls, carotid pla-que was observed in more than twice the proportion of patients who had lupus compared with age-and sex-matched controls (43% vs 17%, P = .0002).[36] Excess prevalence of plaque was seen beginning in the fifth decade of life. On multivariate analysis, age, SLE disease duration, sE-selectin, and adiponectin were the only inde-pendent predictors of plaque.[36] Among patients who had lupus who showed plaque, elevations in these biomarkers were persistent over more than one visit in those who had multiple measurements. Elevation of sE-selectin was anticipated, because this biomarker reflects activation of the endothelium and has been previously associated with atherosclerosis and cardiovascular risk in both SLE and non-SLE cohorts.[9,37,38] The association with elevated adiponectin was unexpected because adiponectin is generally considered to be vasoprotective. In fact, the authors' hypothesis was that adiponectin would be decreased.

This finding led the authors to speculate that perhaps elevated adiponectin repre-sents a continued but unsuccessful attempt at vascular repair. **Table 1** reports percentage of plaque for different groups defined according to adiponectin and E-selectin levels. Given the study design, these percentages can be directly inter-preted as predictive values or, more accurately, predicted probabilities of plaque. For example, the probability of plaque is predicted to be 75% if an individual has high levels of both adiponectin and E-selectin, whereas the probability of plaque is 19% for individuals who have low levels of both biomarkers (see **Table 1**). The two biomarkers must be considered simultaneously when evaluating predictive values because each was found to be independently associated with plaque. Therefore, the predicted probability of plaque for adiponectin depends on whether the E-selectin level is high or low, and vice versa.

sE-selectin and adiponectin have been reported in patients who have active disease.[39–41] The elevation of sE-selectin in patients who have plaque despite clinical quiescence, and the stability of that elevation over time, likely indicate that a low level of inflammation or atherogenic injury independent of inflammation contributes to

Table 1
Patients who have biomarkers in group sE-selectin + adiponectin, high, associated with the development of atherosclerosis

Group	Plasma Biomarker Level	Plaque (%)
Patients, total	High + Low	43
sE-selectin	High	52
Adiponectin	High	55
sE-selectin + adiponectin	High	75
sE-selectin	Low	33
Adiponectin	Low	32
sE-selectin + adiponectin	Low	19[a]

[a] sE-selectin + Adiponectin High versus sE-selectin + Adiponectin Low (P = .002).

atherosclerosis in lupus.[42] Further precedent in SLE for endothelial activation in the absence of an inflammatory infiltrate has been reported in the kidney[43] and skin,[44] in which increased expression of adhesion molecules, including E-selectin, were observed in the microvasculature of nonlesional areas. Molecules including E-selectin were observed in the microvasculature of nonlesional areas.

Adiponectin has pleiotropic biologic activities, including improving insulin sensitivity.[45,46] Beyond these metabolic actions, considerable preclinical evidence also shows that adiponectin exerts direct anti-atherosclerotic and cardioprotective effects.[47] Epidemiologic studies evaluating the association of adiponectin with cardiovascular events have reported somewhat conflicting results and have been limited largely to men, especially older men.[48–52]

Based on a recent biomarker study from Vanderbilt, performed in a retrospective cross-sectional analysis of 65 patients who had SLE and 69 controls, no association was found between adiponectin levels and coronary calcium scores.[53–55] Although a definitive explanation for the disparate findings between this study and the one presented herein await larger longitudinal cohorts, several differences are noteworthy. The Vanderbilt cohort comprised a greater percentage of Caucasians, the adiponectin levels were higher in controls than most reported series, subset analysis of patients who had low SLEDAI scores was not performed, and assessment was limited to one sampling.

In the New York cohort, evaluation across visits in 60% of patients also showed a significant difference between sustained high levels in patients who had plaque compared with those who did not. This finding is relevant because cross-sectional evaluation of a biomarker for a condition that represents accrued insult has limitations. In both cohorts, the adiponectin levels were significantly higher overall in the patients who had SLE compared with healthy controls, yet these patients are at risk for premature atherosclerosis. This finding alone distinguishes SLE from most reports of men in which lower levels of adiponectin are associated with both atherosclerosis and risk for progression.[56]

The authors hypothesize that, for unknown reasons, the endothelial dysfunction characteristic of SLE (reflected by elevated sE-selectin in both studies) drives a higher adiponectin level, which nevertheless is not effective in protection. Therefore, increased adiponectin concentration could represent a compensatory mechanism to existing vascular damage. In fact, children who had diabetes (another high-risk group for premature atherosclerosis) were recently reported to have a higher concentration of adiponectin than healthy matched controls.[57]

Other biomarkers that were recently linked to endothelial damage per se or inflammatory luminal injury include CECs and sEPCR.[7,58] Neither tracked with plaque, suggesting that inflammation may not be the sole explanation.

Limitations of this study include the challenge of precisely quantifying the activity, severity, and disease treatment over the lifetime of patients who have SLE. Atherosclerosis develops over years. Because this study was limited to 1 year, evaluation is not necessarily reflective of the total burden of undulating activity that might lead to plaque. Reliable indices of the cumulative burden of inflammatory disease activity in SLE do not exist. The SLE Damage Index is the closest approximation, but it assesses damage accrued since diagnosis, some of which may not be directly related to the disease process per se, such as avascular necrosis or premature ovarian failure.[59] Although cardiovascular event rates in patients who have SLE are markedly higher than in matched healthy controls, the rates are too low to permit correlation with biomarkers, and therefore carotid ultrasound studies are used as proxies of actual events.

Skin biomarkers are present despite clinical quiescence. Diverse studies in patients who have SLE have confirmed the permissive role of vascular adhesion molecules in the pathogenesis of vasculitis and glomerulonephritis.[60–62] Widespread activation of the endothelium was suggested by the observation that even in nonlesional, non–sun-exposed skin (buttock) from patients who had active SLE, endothelial expression of adhesion molecules and inducible NOS (iNOS, NOS2) is up-regulated.[62,63] These findings support the notion that, in patients who have SLE, the vascular endothelium in general is primed for injury by activated leukocytes, although no overt injury is present. When another factor is superimposed on widespread priming, vascular lesions develop, contributing to specific organ injury. For example, deposition of immune complexes in renal tissue initiates a sequence that ultimately involves macrophages, which are recruited to the primed endothelium where they secrete inflammatory cytokines such as IFN-γ.[64]

mEPCR regulates the conversion of protein C to APC through presenting it to the thrombin–thrombomodulin complex.[58,65] mEPCR is shed in a pathologic state to a soluble form, sEPCR, increased levels of which have been reported in two lupus cohorts.[58,65] Patients who had LN had significantly higher levels of sEPCR than those who did not have nephritis.[58] mEPCR expression in the glomerular and interstitial microvasculature was reported to be increased in rodents with experimentally induced sepsis.[66] In this model, sepsis was associated with a depletion of APC, the consequence of which may be a compensatory increase in mEPCR as shown in the diseased renal parenchyma. Similarly, increased mEPCR was also seen in renal biopsies from patients who had acute kidney injury.[66]

In a recent retrospective study with chart review, the authors' group analyzed mEPCR (anti-injury molecule) using immunohistochemistry in 59 biopsies from 49 patients who had LN.[43] The focus was to score the expression of biomarker using a standard index that is widely used by pathologists during an evaluation of normal appearing cortical peritubular capillaries (PTCs). mEPCR was expressed in the medulla, arterial endothelium, and PTCs in all biopsies with LN but not in the cortical PTCs of normal kidney. Positive mEPCR staining in more than 25% of PTCs was observed in 16 of 59 biopsies and associated with poor response to therapy. At 6-months follow-up, 11 (84.6%) of 13 patients who had positive staining for mEPCR in greater than 25% of PTCs did not experience response to therapy, compared with 8 of 28 (28.6%) who had mEPCR staining in less than 25% PTCs ($P = .0018$).

Renal response was defined according to the FDA-sponsored trial led by Dr Ginzler that compared mycophenolate mofetil with IVC.[67] At 1 year, 10 (83.3%) of 12 patients who had positive mEPCR staining in greater than 25% of PTCs did not experience response to therapy (with two progressing to end-stage renal disease) compared with 8 of 24 (33.3%) with positive staining in less than 25% of PTCs (P = .0116). Although tubular-interstitial damage (TID) was always accompanied by mEPCR, this endothelial marker was extensively expressed in the absence of TID, suggesting that poor response could not be attributed solely to increased TID. mEPCR expression was independent of ISN/RPS class, activity, and chronicity indices.

The relationship between mEPCR expression and renal disease progression is intriguing, because mEPCR is generally considered a protective molecule based on its role in both inflammation and coagulation. mEPCR binds protein C, presenting it to the thrombin–thrombomodulin complex, thus regulating its conversion to APC.[29] Conditions that reduce surface expression of mEPCR on endothelial cells attenuate the efficiency of protein C activation.[68] The decrease in mEPCR is caused by a metalloproteinase-dependent cleavage that splits the molecule into a soluble form, sEPCR.[69]

Given the prediction that shed mEPCR impairs the integrity of the endothelium and places the net balance of this protective protein in biologic arrears, a decrease in mEPCR expression was the predicted result in patients who had progressive renal injury. Thus, finding increased mEPCR expression in the endothelium of PTCs, compared with controls, was unexpected.

The seemingly paradoxic finding of increased mEPCR in LN is provocative but not without precedent. Gupta and colleagues reported that mEPCR expression in the glomerular and interstitial microvasculature was increased in rodents with experimentally induced sepsis.[66] In this model, sepsis was associated with a depletion of APC, the consequence of which may be a compensatory increase in mEPCR as shown in the diseased renal parenchyma. Similarly, increased mEPCR was also seen in renal biopsies from patients who had acute kidney injury.[66]

One explanation for these findings is that increased mEPCR may represent a thwarted attempt at endothelial defense. An alternative hypothesis is that in LN, circulating or deposited immune complexes activate the classical complement pathway, generating C4b-binding protein, which in turn complexes with protein S, impairing its ability to generate APC.[70] Against this explanation is the absence of a correlation between mEPCR expression and local deposits of immune complexes or complement. However, circulating immune complexes, mimicking the effects of sepsis, may still possibly activate the endothelium of the microvasculature. Finally, as in sepsis, LN may induce a low protein C state.

Biomarker studies have corroborated the involvement of the endothelium in murine and human LN. In a murine study, severe LN was associated with high vascular cell adhesion molecule 1 levels in urine and increased expression in the tubules and vascular endothelium in LN.[71] In humans, urine levels of adiponectin were significantly elevated before and during renal flares.[39] In addition, adiponectin was expressed on endothelial surfaces in the renal microvasculature in patients who had LN.[39] Urine levels of the monocyte chemoattractant protein-1, produced by endothelial cells, have been shown to increase significantly during renal flares with decreases paralleling response.[72,73] Increased NO production, generated partly by vascular endothelial cells, has been associated with renal damage and poor response to therapy.[74]

Several shortcomings are acknowledged regarding interpretation of the overall data. This study was largely retrospective and the number of patients with biopsy tissue and data for clinical evaluation was limited. In addition, compliance with oral medication was difficult to address and patient numbers were too small to gain insight into the potential benefit of a specific therapy. The use of various treatments, each with

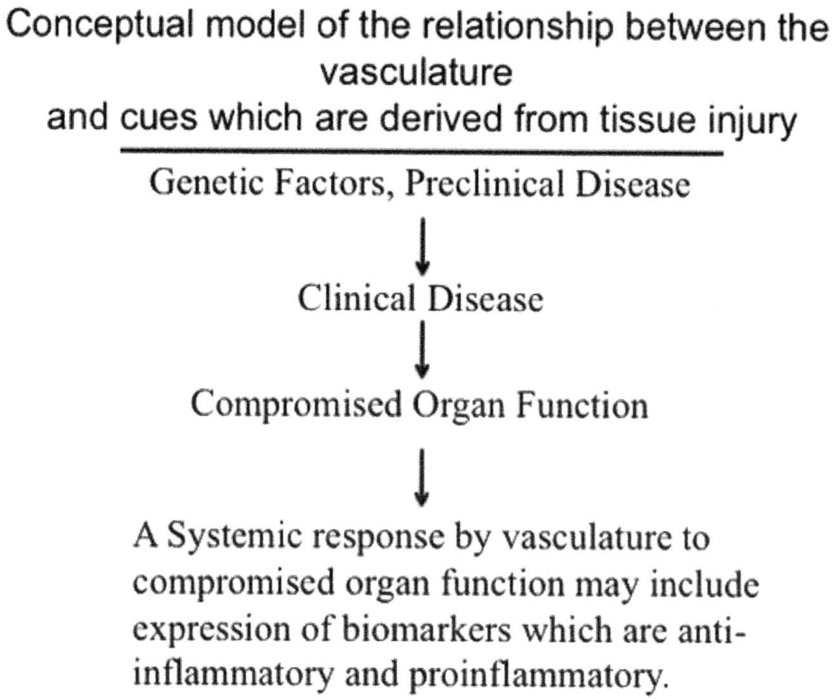

Conceptual model of the relationship between the vasculature and cues which are derived from tissue injury

Genetic Factors, Preclinical Disease

↓

Clinical Disease

↓

Compromised Organ Function

↓

A Systemic response by vasculature to compromised organ function may include expression of biomarkers which are anti-inflammatory and proinflammatory.

Fig. 3. Conceptual model of the relationship between the vasculature and cues that are derived from tissue injury. Genetic and environmental influence provoke an autoimmune response. At the efferent end, tissue injury will be sensed by organ systems throughout the body.

a different response rate and time of response, further dictates caution in interpreting these findings.

In summary, positive mEPCR staining greater than 25% in cortical PTCs is associated with a poor renal response to standard therapy. Although these results suggest a contribution of the endothelium of the renal parenchyma to the pathophysiology of more progressive lupus nephritis, further studies are needed to distinguish whether the endothelium plays an active or reactive role. Larger prospective studies are needed to affirm the significance of mEPCR expression as a novel biomarker of unanticipated renal progression and to address the usefulness of longitudinally measuring sEPCR in the serum and urine.

SUMMARY

Prior conceptual framework portrayed widespread endothelial activation in the context of the Schwartzman phenomenon. The focus was solely restricted to analysis of proinflammatory molecules. Findings suggested that the anti-injury molecules (eg, adiponectin, mEPCR) might be down-regulated. In fact, the authors' early hypothesis was that adiponectin might be lower in patients who have plaque, and mEPCR is lower in progressive nephritis. The fact that the opposite was observed challenges the initial conceptualizations.

Although further mechanistic studies are pending, the sustained expression of these anti-injury biomarkers might be a property to be exploited in a replication cohort. The hypothesis that the presentation, course, and prognosis of LN could be predicted by mEPCR expression in the renal microvasculature would be a strong potential biomarker. Most importantly, this would be observed at the clinically relevant time (renal biopsy) when a treatment decision must be made (**Fig. 3**).

Regarding adiponectin, how do we proceed in the future? Firstly, identification of biomarkers associated with atherogenic injury that might be present, independent of recognized lupus activity, should advance understanding of the pathology and guide prophylaxis for at-risk subgroups. Experts must acknowledge the limitation of relevance in biomarker studies that are restricted to a cross-sectional evaluation of a biomarker. Clearly under these circumstances, there are limitations to fit the condition that represents accrued insult. In studies described earlier, injury pathways clearly may vary according to site of the pathologic process (eg, for atherosclerosis, arterial blood vessels or for nephritis, peri tubular capillaries) and the adaptive responses of the target cell. Successful strategies to inhibit the excessive and damaging production of injury molecules in tissues in response to phlogistic cytokines must simultaneously spare the physiologic protective anti-injury molecules such as mEPCR and adiponectin, which exert action to preserve function at the vascular endothelium.

REFERENCES

1. Urowitz MB, Bookman AA, Koehler BE, et al. The bimodal mortality pattern of systemic lupus erythematosus. Am J Med 1976;60(2):221–5.
2. Manzi S, Meilahn EN, Rairie JE, et al. Age-specific incidence rates of myocardial infarction and angina in women with systemic lupus erythematosus: comparison with the Framingham Study. Am J Epidemiol 1997;145(5):408–15.
3. Esdaile JM, Abrahamowicz M, Grodzicky T, et al. Traditional Framingham risk factors fail to fully account for accelerated atherosclerosis in systemic lupus erythematosus. Arthritis Rheum 2001;44(10):2331–7.
4. Roman MJ, Shanker BA, Davis A, et al. Prevalence and correlates of accelerated atherosclerosis in systemic lupus erythematosus. N Engl J Med 2003;349(25): 2399–406.
5. McMahon M, Grossman J, FitzGerald J, et al. Proinflammatory high-density lipoprotein as a biomarker for atherosclerosis in patients with systemic lupus erythematosus and rheumatoid arthritis. Arthritis Rheum 2006;54(8):2541–9.
6. Doherty NE, Siegel RJ. Cardiovascular manifestations of systemic lupus erythematosus. Am Heart J 1985;110(6):1257–65.
7. Clancy R, Marder G, Martin V, et al. Circulating activated endothelial cells in systemic lupus erythematosus: further evidence for diffuse vasculopathy. Arthritis Rheum 2001;44(5):1203–8.
8. Rajagopalan S, Somers EC, Brook RD, et al. Endothelial cell apoptosis in systemic lupus erythematosus: a common pathway for abnormal vascular function and thrombosis propensity. Blood 2004;103(10):3677–83.
9. Rho YH, Chung CP, Oeser A, et al. Novel cardiovascular risk factors in premature coronary atherosclerosis associated with systemic lupus erythematosus. J Rheumatol 2008;35(9):1789–94.
10. Ward MM. Changes in the incidence of endstage renal disease due to lupus nephritis in the United States, 1996–2004. J Rheumatol 2009;36(1):63–7.
11. Isenberg D, Lesavre P. Lupus nephritis: assessing the evidence, considering the future. Lupus 2007;16(3):210–1.

12. Dooley MA, Hogan S, Jennette C, et al. Cyclophosphamide therapy for lupus nephritis: poor renal survival in black Americans. Glomerular Disease Collaborative Network. Kidney Int 1997;51(4):1188–95.

13. Barr RG, Seliger S, Appel GB, et al. Prognosis in proliferative lupus nephritis: the role of socio-economic status and race/ethnicity. Nephrol Dial Transplant 2003; 18(10):2039–46.

14. Isenberg D, Appel GB, Contreras G, et al. Influence of race/ethnicity on response to lupus nephritis treatment: the ALMS Study. Rheumatology (Oxford) 2010;49(1): 128–40.

15. Rivera TL, Belmont HM, Malani S, et al. Current therapies for lupus nephritis in an ethnically heterogeneous cohort. J Rheumatol 2009;36(2):298–305.

16. Austin HA 3rd, Muenz LR, Joyce KM, et al. Prognostic factors in lupus nephritis. Contribution of renal histologic data. Am J Med 1983;75(3):382–91.

17. Weening JJ, D'Agati VD, Schwartz MM, et al. The classification of glomerulonephritis in systemic lupus erythematosus revisited. J Am Soc Nephrol 2004; 15(2):241–50.

18. Berthier C, Bethunaickan R, Bottinger E, et al. Proliferative SLE nephritis and progressive non-inflammatory glomerulosclerosis share key gene expression profiles. Arthritis Rheum 2008;58(Suppl 9):902–3.

19. Kaser A, Kaser S, Kaneider NC, et al. Interleukin-18 attracts plasmacytoid dendritic cells (DC2s) and promotes Th1 induction by DC2s through IL-18 receptor expression. Blood 2004;103(2):648–55.

20. Yamagami H, Kitagawa K, Hoshi T, et al. Associations of serum IL-18 levels with carotid intima-media thickness. Arterioscler Thromb Vasc Biol 2005;25(7): 1458–62.

21. Kumada M, Kihara S, Sumitsuji S, et al. Association of hypoadiponectinemia with coronary artery disease in men. Arterioscler Thromb Vasc Biol 2003;23(1):85–9.

22. Ouchi N, Kihara S, Arita Y, et al. Adiponectin, an adipocyte-derived plasma protein, inhibits endothelial NF-kappaB signaling through a cAMP-dependent pathway. Circulation 2000;102(11):1296–301.

23. Ouchi N, Kihara S, Arita Y, et al. Novel modulator for endothelial adhesion molecules: adipocyte-derived plasma protein adiponectin. Circulation 1999;100(25): 2473–6.

24. Okamoto Y, Arita Y, Nishida M, et al. An adipocyte-derived plasma protein, adiponectin, adheres to injured vascular walls. Horm Metab Res 2000;32(2):47–50.

25. Ishikawa Y, Akasaka Y, Ishii T, et al. Changes in the distribution pattern of gelatin-binding protein of 28 kDa (adiponectin) in myocardial remodelling after ischaemic injury. Histopathology 2003;42(1):43–52.

26. Fukudome K, Kurosawa S, Stearns-Kurosawa DJ, et al. The endothelial cell protein C receptor. Cell surface expression and direct ligand binding by the soluble receptor. J Biol Chem 1996;271(29):17491–8.

27. Gu JM, Katsuura Y, Ferrell GL, et al. Endotoxin and thrombin elevate rodent endothelial cell protein C receptor mRNA levels and increase receptor shedding in vivo. Blood 2000;95(5):1687–93.

28. Fukudome K, Esmon CT. Molecular cloning and expression of murine and bovine endothelial cell protein C/activated protein C receptor (EPCR). The structural and functional conservation in human, bovine, and murine EPCR. J Biol Chem 1995; 270(10):5571–7.

29. Stearns-Kurosawa DJ, Kurosawa S, Mollica JS, et al. The endothelial cell protein C receptor augments protein C activation by the thrombin-thrombomodulin complex. Proc Natl Acad Sci U S A 1996;93(19):10212–6.

30. Taylor FB Jr, Peer GT, Lockhart MS, et al. Endothelial cell protein C receptor plays an important role in protein C activation in vivo. Blood 2001;97(6):1685–8.

31. Li W, Zheng X, Gu J, et al. Overexpressing endothelial cell protein C receptor alters the hemostatic balance and protects mice from endotoxin. J Thromb Haemost 2005;3(7):1351–9.

32. Xu J, Qu D, Esmon NL, et al. Metalloproteolytic release of endothelial cell protein C receptor. J Biol Chem 2000;275(8):6038–44.

33. Saposnik B, Reny JL, Gaussem P, et al. A haplotype of the EPCR gene is associated with increased plasma levels of sEPCR and is a candidate risk factor for thrombosis. Blood 2004;103(4):1311–8.

34. Medina P, Navarro S, Estelles A, et al. Contribution of polymorphisms in the endothelial protein C receptor gene to soluble endothelial protein C receptor and circulating activated protein C levels, and thrombotic risk. Thromb Haemost 2004;91(5):905–11.

35. Erlich JH, Boyle EM, Labriola J, et al. Inhibition of the tissue factor-thrombin pathway limits infarct size after myocardial ischemia-reperfusion injury by reducing inflammation. Am J Pathol 2000;157(6):1849–62.

36. Reynolds HR, Buyon J, Kim M, et al. Association of plasma soluble E-selectin and adiponectin with carotid plaque in patients with systemic lupus erythematosus. Atherosclerosis 2009. [Epub ahead of print].

37. Hwang SJ, Ballantyne CM, Sharrett AR, et al. Circulating adhesion molecules VCAM-1, ICAM-1, and E-selectin in carotid atherosclerosis and incident coronary heart disease cases: the Atherosclerosis Risk In Communities (ARIC) study. Circulation 1997;96(12):4219–25.

38. Rohde LE, Lee RT, Rivero J, et al. Circulating cell adhesion molecules are correlated with ultrasound-based assessment of carotid atherosclerosis. Arterioscler Thromb Vasc Biol 1998;18(11):1765–70.

39. Rovin BH, Song H, Hebert LA, et al. Plasma, urine, and renal expression of adiponectin in human systemic lupus erythematosus. Kidney Int 2005;68(4):1825–33.

40. Egerer K, Feist E, Rohr U, et al. Increased serum soluble CD14, ICAM-1 and E-selectin correlate with disease activity and prognosis in systemic lupus erythematosus. Lupus 2000;9(8):614–21.

41. Panes J, Perry M, Granger DN. Leukocyte-endothelial cell adhesion: avenues for therapeutic intervention. Br J Pharmacol 1999;126(3):537–50.

42. Roldan V, Marin F, Lip GY, et al. Soluble E-selectin in cardiovascular disease and its risk factors. A review of the literature. Thromb Haemost 2003;90(6):1007–20.

43. Izmirly PM, Barisoni L, Buyon JP, et al. Expression of endothelial protein C receptor in cortical peritubular capillaries associates with a poor clinical response in lupus nephritis. Rheumatology (Oxford) 2009;48(5):513–9.

44. Belmont HM, Buyon J, Giorno R, et al. Up-regulation of endothelial cell adhesion molecules characterizes disease activity in systemic lupus erythematosus. The Shwartzman phenomenon revisited. Arthritis Rheum 1994;37(3):376–83.

45. Okamoto Y, Kihara S, Ouchi N, et al. Adiponectin reduces atherosclerosis in apolipoprotein E-deficient mice. Circulation 2002;106(22):2767–70.

46. Shibata R, Ouchi N, Kihara S, et al. Adiponectin stimulates angiogenesis in response to tissue ischemia through stimulation of amp-activated protein kinase signaling. J Biol Chem 2004;279(27):28670–4.

47. Hopkins TA, Ouchi N, Shibata R, et al. Adiponectin actions in the cardiovascular system. Cardiovasc Res 2007;74(1):11–8.

48. Pischon T, Girman CJ, Hotamisligil GS, et al. Plasma adiponectin levels and risk of myocardial infarction in men. JAMA 2004;291(14):1730-7.
49. Frystyk J, Berne C, Berglund L, et al. Serum adiponectin is a predictor of coronary heart disease: a population-based 10-year follow-up study in elderly men. J Clin Endocrinol Metab 2007;92(2):571-6.
50. Sattar N, Wannamethee G, Sarwar N, et al. Adiponectin and coronary heart disease: a prospective study and meta-analysis. Circulation 2006;114(7):623-9.
51. Kanaya AM, Wassel Fyr C, Vittinghoff E, et al. Serum adiponectin and coronary heart disease risk in older Black and White Americans. J Clin Endocrinol Metab 2006;91(12):5044-50.
52. Kizer JR, Barzilay JI, Kuller LH, et al. Adiponectin and risk of coronary heart disease in older men and women. J Clin Endocrinol Metab 2008;93(9):3357-64.
53. Chung CP, Long AG, Solus JF, et al. Adipocytokines in systemic lupus erythematosus: relationship to inflammation, insulin resistance and coronary atherosclerosis. Lupus 2009;18(9):799-806.
54. Asanuma Y, Oeser A, Shintani AK, et al. Premature coronary-artery atherosclerosis in systemic lupus erythematosus. N Engl J Med 2003;349(25):2407-15.
55. Chung CP, Oeser A, Raggi P, et al. Increased coronary-artery atherosclerosis in rheumatoid arthritis: relationship to disease duration and cardiovascular risk factors. Arthritis Rheum 2005;52(10):3045-53.
56. Maahs DM, Ogden LG, Kinney GL, et al. Low plasma adiponectin levels predict progression of coronary artery calcification. Circulation 2005;111(6):747-53.
57. Heilman K, Zilmer M, Zilmer K, et al. Elevated plasma adiponectin and decreased plasma homocysteine and asymmetric dimethylarginine in children with type 1 diabetes. Scand J Clin Lab Invest 2009;69(1):85-91.
58. Sesin CA, Yin X, Esmon CT, et al. Shedding of endothelial protein C receptor contributes to vasculopathy and renal injury in lupus: In vivo and in vitro evidence. Kidney Int 2005;68(1):110-20.
59. Gladman D, Ginzler E, Goldsmith C, et al. The development and initial validation of the Systemic Lupus International Collaborating Clinics/American College of Rheumatology damage index for systemic lupus erythematosus. Arthritis Rheum 1996;39(3):363-9.
60. Robertson CR, McCallum RM. Changing concepts in pathophysiology of the vasculitides. Curr Opin Rheumatol 1994;6(1):3-10.
61. van Vollenhoven RF. Adhesion molecules, sex steroids, and the pathogenesis of vasculitis syndromes. Curr Opin Rheumatol 1995;7(1):4-10.
62. Belmont HM, Levartovsky D, Goel A, et al. Increased nitric oxide production accompanied by the up-regulation of inducible nitric oxide synthase in vascular endothelium from patients with systemic lupus erythematosus. Arthritis Rheum 1997;40(10):1810-6.
63. Weinberg JB, Granger DL, Pisetsky DS, et al. The role of nitric oxide in the pathogenesis of spontaneous murine autoimmune disease: increased nitric oxide production and nitric oxide synthase expression in MRL-lpr/lpr mice, and reduction of spontaneous glomerulonephritis and arthritis by orally administered NG-monomethyl-L-arginine. J Exp Med 1994;179(2):651-60.
64. Masutani K, Akahoshi M, Tsuruya K, et al. Predominance of Th1 immune response in diffuse proliferative lupus nephritis. Arthritis Rheum 2001;44(9):2097-106.
65. Kurosawa S, Stearns-Kurosawa DJ, Carson CW, et al. Plasma levels of endothelial cell protein C receptor are elevated in patients with sepsis and systemic lupus

erythematosus: lack of correlation with thrombomodulin suggests involvement of different pathological processes. Blood 1998;91(2):725–7.

66. Gupta A, Berg DT, Gerlitz B, et al. Role of protein C in renal dysfunction after polymicrobial sepsis. J Am Soc Nephrol 2007;18(3):860–7.

67. Ginzler EM, Dooley MA, Aranow C, et al. Mycophenolate mofetil or intravenous cyclophosphamide for lupus nephritis. N Engl J Med 2005;353(21):2219–28.

68. Ye X, Fukudome K, Tsuneyoshi N, et al. The endothelial cell protein C receptor (EPCR) functions as a primary receptor for protein C activation on endothelial cells in arteries, veins, and capillaries. Biochem Biophys Res Commun 1999; 259(3):671–7.

69. Qu D, Wang Y, Esmon NL, et al. Regulated endothelial protein C receptor shedding is mediated by tumor necrosis factor-alpha converting enzyme/ADAM17. J Thromb Haemost 2007;5(2):395–402.

70. Rezende SM, Simmonds RE, Lane DA. Coagulation, inflammation, and apoptosis: different roles for protein S and the protein S-C4b binding protein complex. Blood 2004;103(4):1192–201.

71. Wu T, Xie C, Bhaskarabhatla M, et al. Excreted urinary mediators in an animal model of experimental immune nephritis with potential pathogenic significance. Arthritis Rheum 2007;56(3):949–59.

72. Sica A, Wang JM, Colotta F, et al. Monocyte chemotactic and activating factor gene expression induced in endothelial cells by IL-1 and tumor necrosis factor. J Immunol 1990;144(8):3034–8.

73. Rovin BH, Song H, Birmingham DJ, et al. Urine chemokines as biomarkers of human systemic lupus erythematosus activity. J Am Soc Nephrol 2005;16(2): 467–73.

74. Oates JC, Shaftman SR, Self SE, et al. Association of serum nitrate and nitrite levels with longitudinal assessments of disease activity and damage in systemic lupus erythematosus and lupus nephritis. Arthritis Rheum 2008;58(1):263–72.

Cell-Bound Complement Biomarkers for Systemic Lupus Erythematosus: From Benchtop to Bedside

Chau-Ching Liu, MD, PhD[a], Susan Manzi, MD, MPH[a,b],
Amy H. Kao, MD, MPH[a], Jeannine S. Navratil, MS[a],
Joseph M. Ahearn, MD[a,*]

KEYWORDS

- Systemic lupus erythematosus
- Cell-bound complement activation products • Biomarkers

Systemic lupus erythematosus (SLE) is arguably the most clinically and serologically diverse autoimmune disease.[1,2] Currently available information suggests that intricate interactions between environmental factors, hormonal factors, and disease susceptibility genes may predispose an individual to develop aberrant immune responses leading to SLE. Such aberrant responses, characterized by polyclonal activation of autoreactive lymphocytes, autoantibody production, immune complex formation, and complement activation, lead to acute and chronic inflammation in various tissue and organ systems. Owing to its complex etiopathogenesis, heterogeneous presentation, and unpredictable course, SLE remains one of the greatest challenges to both investigators and physicians. Currently, the diagnosis of SLE primarily is based on the presence or absence of American College of Rheumatology (ACR) criteria.[3,4] Disease activity in SLE patients often is assessed using indices such as the Systemic Lupus Erythematosus Disease Activity Index (SLEDAI),[5] the Systemic Lupus Activity Measurement (SLAM),[6,7] and the British Isles Lupus Assessment Group (BILAG) index.[8] The lack of easy-to-measure, reliable, and specific biomarkers for SLE not only hampers precise assessment of disease activity and accurate evaluation of response to treatment, but also impedes the development of novel therapeutics

Investigations in the authors' laboratory were supported by grants from the National Institutes of Health (RO1HL074335, RO1AI077591, RO1 AR-46588, K23 AR-051044, and K24 AR-02213), the Department of Defense (W81XWH-06-2-0038), the Alliance for Lupus Research, and the Lupus Research Institute.

[a] Lupus Center of Excellence, University of Pittsburgh School of Health Sciences, Department of Medicine, University of Pittsburgh School of Medicine, Pittsburgh, PA 15260, USA
[b] Graduate School of Public Health, University of Pittsburgh, Pittsburgh, PA, USA
* Corresponding author.
E-mail address: joa8@pitt.edu (J.M. Ahearn).

Rheum Dis Clin N Am 36 (2010) 161–172
doi:10.1016/j.rdc.2009.12.003
0889-857X/10/$ – see front matter © 2010 Elsevier Inc. All rights reserved.

targeting key pathogenic factors. Therefore, there is an urgent need for reliable, specific biomarkers in not only lupus patient care, but also in research.

COMPLEMENT AND SLE: THE HISTORICAL BOND

The complement system has been linked more intimately to SLE than to any other human disease.[9–11] The involvement of complement proteins in the etiopathogenesis of SLE has been recognized and investigated for decades. In the current era of biomarkers and targeted therapeutic approaches, investigators' interest in the complement system has been reinvigorated.

The Complement System

The complement system comprises a group of plasma and membrane-bound proteins that form three distinct—classical, alternative, and lectin—pathways designed to protect the host against invasion of foreign pathogens. The classical pathway is activated by antibodies or antigen–antibody complexes (immune complexes).[12–14] Distinct from the antibody-dependent classical pathway, the alternative pathway is initiated when spontaneously generated complement components bind to surfaces of invading organisms or self-tissues, whereas the lectin pathway is triggered when mannose-binding lectins attach to polysaccharides uniquely expressed on the surface of microorganisms. Overall, the cascading reaction of complement activation generates proteolytic fragments that are capable of attracting inflammatory cells, inducing production and release of inflammatory mediators, and tagging invading organisms to be promptly phagocytosed by neutrophils and monocytes. Consequently, activation of the complement system may lead to not only physiologic immune responses but also to pathologic immune–inflammatory tissue damage. An unfortunate example of the latter is the myriad disease manifestations in SLE.

C3 is the most abundant protein in the complement system and also the indispensable molecule involved in all three activation pathways of the complement system.[12–14] C4 is the second most abundant component and is essential for the classical and lectin pathways. C3 and C4 are synthesized predominantly in the liver and undergo posttranslational modification to become 3-chain proteins linked by disulfide bonds. Both C3 and C4 contain an internal thioester site that is located within the C3d and C4d region in the α chain of each respective parental molecule.[15,16] During activation of the classical pathway, proteolytic cleavage of C4 by C1s generates a small peptide C4a and a major fragment C4b. C4b contains the activated, highly reactive thioester that can readily interact with hydroxyl or amino groups on the receptive surface (eg, pathogens, host cells, or immune complexes) to form covalent ester or amide linkages. Target-bound C4b then cleaves C2, resulting in the formation of C4bC2a complexes that function as the C3 convertase. Like C4, C3 is proteolytically cleaved during activation of the complement system, yielding a small peptide C3a and a large fragment C3b. Similar to C4b, C3b is capable of binding covalently to acceptor molecules on target surfaces via ester or amide linkages. C4b and C3b may be cleaved further by Factor I, yielding ultimately C4d and C3d.

Once C3b binds covalently to target cells, it recruits C5 and cleaves the latter into C5a and C5b. Binding of C5b to target cells initiates the formation of the C5b-9 membrane attack complexes (MAC). Perhaps in a dose-dependent manner, MAC inserted into the membrane can either activate (at sublytic levels) or cause lysis of target cells. In contrast to their larger, enzymatically active counterparts, the smaller fragments C4a, C3a, and C5a (collectively referred to as anaphylatoxins) are potent chemotactic factors that are capable of recruiting leukocytes into inflamed tissues.

Moreover, by binding to specific receptors expressed on most infiltrating leukocytes and endothelial cells, these anaphylatoxins can cause activation and release of numerous inflammatory mediators from host cells, thereby aggravating and perpetuating inflammatory tissue damage.

Soluble Complement Proteins as Lupus Biomarkers

Because antibody/immune complex-triggered activation of the complement system is thought to play an important role in the pathogenesis of SLE, one might expect complement proteins to be consumed to an extent proportional to the disease activity. Thus, measures of complement C3 and C4 have historically been viewed as gold standard laboratory tests for SLE. Many physicians consider decreases in serum C3 and C4 levels as indications of increased inflammation and SLE disease activity. There are several drawbacks to this approach, however. First, there is a wide range of variation in serum C3 and C4 levels among healthy individuals, and this range overlaps with the range observed in SLE patients. Second, standard laboratory tests measure the concentration of parental C3 and C4 molecules rather than products of activation. Third, acute-phase response during inflammation may lead to an increase in C4 and C3 synthesis, which can balance the activation and increased consumption of these proteins. Fourth, partial deficiencies of C4, which are commonly present in both the general population and SLE patients, may result in lower than normal serum C4 levels because of decreased synthesis rather than increased complement activation or active SLE. As a result of these confounding factors, there have been conflicting conclusions regarding the value of serial measurement of serum C4 in monitoring disease activity in SLE patients.[17–23] Some studies have found serum C4 and C3 levels valuable in this regard, while others have found C4 and C3 levels to remain normal during SLE flares. These conflicting results suggest that current standard tests, based on serum levels of the native form of complement proteins, are inadequate to accurately and promptly detect SLE disease flares. During the past several years, other investigators have explored the potential for measurement of soluble complement activation products such as C3a, C5a, and C4d to serve as biomarkers in SLE.[24–29] Despite some intriguing observations, serum levels of complement activation products have not replaced measurement of native C3 and C4 as gold standards.

CELL-BOUND COMPLEMENT BIOMARKERS: COMPLEMENT MEASURES AND LUPUS REVISITED

Given the less-than-satisfactory performance of soluble complement components as lupus biomarkers, there is strong incentive for developing alternative complement-based biomarkers.

Rationale for Cell-Bound Complement Biomarkers

Complement proteins are abundant in the circulation and in tissues. Besides floating freely as soluble proteins, both the parental molecules and their activation derivatives can readily interact with cells circulating in the blood (eg, erythrocytes and lymphocytes) or tissues (eg, endothelial cells). Conceivably, complement activation products generated during SLE flares may attach to various circulating and tissue cells and alter physiologic functions of those cells. The rationale for exploring cell-bound complement biomarkers is as follows. First, most soluble complement activation products are easily subjected to hydrolysis in circulation or in tissue fluids and thus are short-lived. Second, activation products derived from C3 and C4 contain thioester bonds capable of covalently attaching to circulating cells and may decorate the surfaces for the lifespan of those cells.[16] Third, many hematopoietic cells express receptors for proteolytic fragments generated upon complement activation. Fourth, products of C4 activation are known to be present on surfaces of erythrocytes of healthy individuals.[30,31] Therefore, cell-bound complement components have the potential to be long-lived and may perform more reliably than soluble complement proteins as biomarkers for SLE.

Experimental Studies of Cell-Bound Complement Activation Products

Recent studies in the authors' laboratory have been focused on discovery and validation of cell-bound complement activation products (CB-CAP) as potential lupus biomarkers. Using flow cytometry assays, a unique CB-CAP phenotype of circulating blood cells that is highly specific for SLE has been identified (**Fig. 1**).[32–35]

Considering the physiologic abundance and localization of erythrocytes, the authors have hypothesized that erythrocytes, circulating throughout the body and hence having easy assess to products derived from systemic as well as local activation of the complement system, may serve as biologic beacons of the inflammatory condition in vivo (and hence the disease activity) in patients with SLE or other

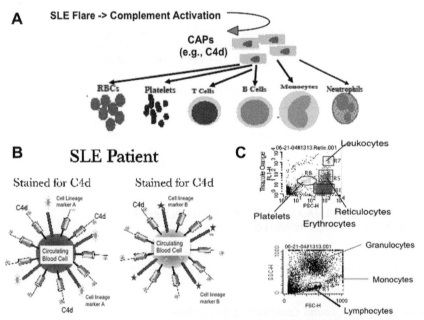

Fig. 1. Schematic summary of the rationale and methodology of the CB-CAP biomarkers. (*A*) Rationale: During SLE flares, considerable amounts of complement activation products may be generated. These CAPs may bind stably to various circulating cells in proportion to the extent of complement activation. (*B*) Schematic illustration of the multicolor staining of circulating cells for cell type-specific surface markers and surface-bound CAPs (eg, C4d). (*C*) Representative dot plots demonstrate the identification of erythrocytes, reticulocytes, platelets, lymphocytes, monocytes, and granulocytes. These cell types also can be differentiated using cell lineage-specific mAbs added to the cell suspension (eg, anti-CD3, anti-CD19, and others).

inflammatory diseases. To verify this hypothesis, the first CB-CAP study was a cross-sectional investigation examining erythrocyte-bound C4d (E-C4d) levels in patients with SLE (n = 100), patients with other inflammatory and immune-mediated diseases (n = 133), and healthy controls (n = 84).[32] In light of the previous reported association of low erythrocyte-complement receptor 1 (E-CR1) levels in SLE, E-CR1 was determined simultaneously. This study demonstrated unambiguously for the first time that patients with SLE have significantly higher levels of E-C4d (specific mean fluorescence intensity [SMFI] = 24.6 plus or minus 28.5) as compared with patients with other diseases (SMFI = 9.3 plus or minus 6.5; $P<.001$) and healthy individuals (SMFI = 6.7 plus or minus 5.3; $P<.001$).

A subsequent study took advantage of the knowledge that erythrocytes develop from hematopoietic stem cells in the bone marrow and emerge as reticulocytes, which then maintain distinct phenotypic features for 1 to 2 days before fully maturing into erythrocytes. Reticulocytes, if released into the peripheral circulation during an active disease state, may immediately be exposed to and bind C4-derived fragments generated from activation of the complement system. Therefore, it was hypothesized that the levels of C4d bound on reticulocytes (R-C4d) may effectively and precisely reflect the current disease activity in a given SLE patient at a specific point in time. The results of a cross-sectional study involving 156 patients with SLE, 140 patients with other autoimmune and inflammatory diseases, and 159 healthy controls showed that:

  R-C4d levels of patients with SLE (SM[median]FI = 5.5 plus or minus 9.0; range: 0.0 to 66.8) were significantly higher than those of patients with other diseases (SMFI = 1.8 plus or minus 2.0; range: 0.0 to 17.6) or healthy controls (SMFI = 1.4 plus or minus 0.7; range; 0.0 to 4.7)
  R-C4d levels fluctuated over time in patients with SLE and correlated with clinical disease activity as measured by the SLEDAI and SLAM indices.[33]

Additional studies explored the possibility that CAP also may bind to nonerythroid lineages of circulating cells such as platelets and lymphocytes. A cross-sectional comparison of platelet-bound C4d (P-C4d) in patients with SLE (n = 105), patients with other inflammatory and immune-mediated diseases (n = 115), and healthy controls (n = 100) showed that abnormal levels of C4d were present on platelets in 18% of SLE patients, 1.7% of patients with other diseases, and 0% of healthy controls.[34] More recently, the authors tested their hypothesis by flow cytometric analysis of C4d on T and B lymphocytes (referred to as T-C4d and B-C4d, respectively) from patients with SLE (n = 224), patients with other diseases (n = 179), and healthy controls (n = 114). Remarkably, both T-C4d and B-C4d levels were significantly and specifically elevated in SLE patients (SM[median]FI = 12.1 plus or minus 20.5 [T-C4d] and 49.0 plus or minus 73.2 [B-C4d]), as compared with healthy controls (SMFI = 1.7 plus or minus 1.0 [T-C4d] and 8.8 plus or minus 8.5 [B-C4d]; both $P<.001$) and patients with other diseases (SMFI = 2.5 plus or minus 3.0 [T-C4d] and 14.7 plus or minus 26.8 [B-C4d]; both $P<.001$).[35]

Collectively, these studies strongly suggest a CB-CAP phenotype that is highly specific for patients with SLE. Moreover, we have noticed that high levels of C4d are not necessarily concurrently present on erythrocytes, reticulocyte, platelets, and lymphocytes of a given SLE patient at a particular time (Liu and colleagues, unpublished data). These findings suggest that binding of CAP to circulating blood cells does not merely reflect complement activation occurring during SLE disease flares, but may also reflect specific cellular and molecular mechanisms in lupus pathogenesis.

CLINICAL APPLICATIONS OF CB-CAP AS LUPUS BIOMARKERS

Despite extensive research and numerous trials of potential new therapeutics, SLE remains one of the greatest challenges for physicians. This is a critical situation for several reasons. First, SLE is commonly misdiagnosed, even by experienced rheumatologists. As no single test is sufficiently sensitive and specific to be diagnostic, the diagnosis requires interpretation of complex ACR criteria, many of which are subject to interpretation and may require years to evolve. Second, the course of SLE in a given patient is characterized by unpredictable flares and remissions. Again, the monitoring of SLE disease activity relies on sophisticated indices such as the SLEDAI and BILAG index, since there is no laboratory test with reliable capacity to identify or predict a disease flare. Third, lack of biomarkers has impeded efforts to evaluate the response to treatment. Consequently, it is of importance to develop accurate and easy-to-use biomarkers to improve daily management of SLE patients and facilitate the development of new SLE therapeutics. CB-CAPs appear to have the potential to serve as clinically practical biomarkers for SLE (**Table 1**).

CB-CAP as Diagnostic Biomarkers for SLE

The diagnostic utility of CB-CAP has been demonstrated for E-C4d, P-C4d, T-C4d, and B-C4d. In the inaugural CB-CAP study, an abnormally high level of E-C4d in combination with an abnormally low level of E-CR1 was shown to be 72% sensitive and 79% specific in differentiating SLE from other inflammatory or immune-mediated diseases, and 81% sensitive and 91% specific in differentiating SLE from healthy conditions, with an overall negative predictive value of 92%.[32] Similarly, T-C4d and B-C4d levels, as diagnostic tools, were 56% sensitive/80% specific and 60% sensitive/82% specific in differentiating SLE from other diseases and healthy controls, respectively.[35] Remarkably, despite being present in only a subset of SLE patients evaluated in a cross-sectional study, an abnormal P-C4d test has high diagnostic specificity, being 100% specific for a diagnosis of SLE compared with healthy controls and 98% specific for SLE compared with patients with other diseases.[34]

Until recently, the single most useful laboratory test for confirming a diagnosis of SLE was determination of anti-double stranded DNA (dsDNA) antibodies. This test is highly specific for SLE, detected in less than 5% of patients with other diseases. The mean sensitivity of anti-dsDNA testing for SLE among published studies is only 57%, however.[36] In contrast, the commonly used antinuclear antibody (ANA) test is

Table 1
Potential clinical applications of CB-CAP as lupus biomarkers

Cell Type	CB-CAP	Clinical Application	References
Erythrocyte	E-C4d, E-C3d	Diagnosis; monitoring	32,38
Reticulocyte	R-C4d (R-C3d)	Monitoring	33
Platelet	P-C4d (P-C3d)	Diagnosis; stratification	34
T lymphocyte	T-C4d, T-C3d	Diagnosis; others (under investigation)	35
B lymphocyte	B-C4d, B-C3d	Diagnosis; others (under investigation)	35
Monocyte	M-C4d	Under investigation	
Granulocyte	G-C4d	Under investigation	
Circulating endothelial cell	CEC-C4d	Under investigation	

sensitive (>95%) but highly nonspecific for a diagnosis of SLE, with a positive predictive value as low as 11% in some studies.[37] Therefore, the reported diagnostic specificity and sensitivity of E-C4d, P-C4d, T-C4d, and B-C4d tests indicate that a single CB-CAP assay is in general more sensitive than the anti-dsDNA test and more specific than the ANA test. It remains to be investigated if combinations of CB-CAP assays of different cell types will provide greater diagnostic utility than individual CB-CAP assays of a particular cell type.

CB-CAP as Biomarkers for SLE Disease Activity

Initial studies demonstrated that E-C4d levels in the same SLE patient examined on different days varied considerably, suggesting that changes in E-C4d levels in SLE patients might reflect fluctuations in disease activity.[32] The utility of E-C4d as a biomarker for monitoring SLE disease activity was subsequently investigated through a longitudinal study.[38] This study was conducted with 157 patients with SLE, 290 patients with other diseases, and 256 healthy individuals who were followed prospectively over a 5-year period (2001 to 2005), encompassing 1005 patient visits (SLE patients), 660 patient visits (patients with other diseases), and 395 subject visits (healthy individuals). The disease activity in SLE patients was measured using the SLAM and the Safety of Estrogen in Lupus Erythematosus: National Assessment version of the SLEDAI index (SELENA-SLEDAI). Consistent with the initial cross-sectional study, the results showed that SLE patients had higher levels of E-C4d and E-C3d than did the healthy controls and patients with other diseases. The variances of E-C4d and E-C3d were high, not only within the same SLE patient, but also between different SLE patients, suggesting again the possibility that levels of these biomarkers may track with changes in disease activity over time. This possibility was verified by a regression formulation in which each patient's evolving clinical status was regressed on each of the biomarkers, using both univariate and multivariate analyses. Although the univariate analysis demonstrated that E-C4d and E-C3d, as well as the gold standards anti-dsDNA and serum C3 levels, were significantly associated with disease activity in SLE patients, the multivariate analysis showed that E-C4d and E-C3d remained significant predictors of SLE disease activity measured by SELENA-SLEDAI (E-C4d) or SLAM (E-C4d and E-C3d), even after adjusting for serum C3, C4, and anti-dsDNA antibody. These observations suggest that erythrocyte-bound CAP can serve as informative measures of SLE disease activity as compared with anti-dsDNA and serum complement levels and should be considered for monitoring disease activity in patients with SLE.

To devise a laboratory test that can differentiate ongoing active disease from cumulative past disease activity in an SLE patient, the authors have embarked on a series of studies focused on analyzing C4d levels on reticulocytes. The rationale underlying these studies is that the level of CAP bound to reticulocytes (eg, R-C4d), which are short-lived (0 to 2 days) intermediates transiting into mature erythrocytes, should reflect precisely and promptly the extent of complement activation (and disease activity) at the time of blood sample procurement. During longitudinal follow-up of 156 patients with SLE, it was noted that the R-C4d levels in a significant fraction of SLE patients varied considerably over time,[33] suggesting that fluctuations in R-C4d levels coincide with changes in disease activity. Indeed, initial studies showed that, within the SLE patient population, the level of R-C4d appeared proportionate to the clinical disease activity in a given SLE patient (ie, patients with higher R-C4d levels have higher disease activity as measured using the SLAM and SELENA-SLEDAI).[33] In cross-sectional comparison, patients with R-C4d levels in the highest quartile, compared with those in the lowest quartile, had significantly higher SELENA-SLEDAI

(P<.001) and SLAM (P = .02) scores. Moreover, longitudinal observations showed that the R-C4d levels appeared to change promptly in relation to the clinical course in individual SLE patients. Taken together, these results suggest that R-C4d levels, compared with C4d levels on the 120 day-lived erythrocytes, may reflect more precisely ongoing disease activity in an SLE patient, supporting a potential role for CAP-bearing reticulocytes as instant messengers of SLE disease activity.

CB-CAP as Biomarkers for Identifying Clinical Subsets of SLE Patients

The various studies outlined previously indicate that the paradigm CB-CAP as a lupus biomarker is not limited to a particular lineage of circulating cells. Observations also suggest that CB-CAP associated with a particular cell type may provide clues to clinical stratification or subsetting of SLE patients. In view of the biologic role of platelets in hemostasis and coagulation, the authors postulated that the presence of abnormal levels of CAPs on platelets may serve as a useful biomarker for SLE patients who are at increased risk of cardiovascular and cerebrovascular events. Indeed, the authors' previous cross-sectional study of 100 SLE patients showed that P-C4d correlated with a history of neurologic event (seizure and psychosis; P=.006) and positive antiphospholipid antibody tests (P = .013), a clinical manifestation and a known risk factor for thrombotic complications of SLE, respectively.[34] Recently, a longitudinal study of 341 SLE patients who had at least three consecutive office visits identified 57 patients (17%) with abnormal P-C4d levels. Moreover, the P-C4d-positive SLE patients, compared with the P-C4d-negative patients, were found to be more likely to have a history of seizure disorder (16% vs 7%, P = .04) and positive antiphospholipid antibody tests (46% vs 26%, P = .003). Furthermore, P-C4d-positive patients had a significantly higher frequency of cardiovascular events associated with acute thrombosis than did P-C4d-negative patients (P = .03) (Kao and colleagues, unpublished data). The results of the cross-sectional and longitudinal studies together suggest that SLE patients with abnormal P-C4d levels may represent a subset of patients with increased thrombotic tendency and risk of cardiovascular and cerebrovascular complications.

Associations between the CB-CAP phenotypes of other circulating cells (eg, lymphocytes) and clinical manifestations of SLE warrant further investigation.

EXPLORATORY STUDIES OF CB-CAP AS BIOMARKERS OF DISEASE COURSE IN SLE
CAP-bearing Erythrocytes as Time Capsules of SLE Disease Activity

Studies of E-C4d as a specific biomarker for lupus diagnosis led to the hypothesis that E-C4d also may be useful to monitor lupus disease activity. This hypothesis was based on the following rationale. Because the life span of human erythrocytes is approximately 120 days, erythrocytes ranging from 1 day to 120 days old are circulating at any given time. The natural course of SLE consists of intermittent episodes of disease flares and remission, which are thought to correlate with the extent of complement-involved inflammatory reactions. Together, these physiologic facts suggest that a disease flare in an SLE patient may lead to an increased level of C4 binding to erythrocytes circulating at that time. Once the flare subsides and the patient enters remission, erythrocytes that emerge from the bone marrow may have a lower (remission) level of surface C4. Thus, detection of erythrocyte subpopulations expressing distinct levels of C4d at a specific time point should theoretically reveal, much like time capsules, SLE disease activity during the preceding 120 days (**Fig. 2**).

To explore this hypothesis, erythrocytes from patients with SLE were fractionated using density gradient centrifugation, a widely accepted technique for separating erythrocytes of different ages,[39,40] and the C4d levels of different fractions of erythrocytes were determined by flow cytometry. These studies demonstrated that in some SLE patients, the levels of C4d on older erythrocytes were distinctively higher than levels of C4d on younger erythrocytes (see **Fig. 2**), suggesting there may have been an event such as a disease flare, that had occurred at a distinct time point before the day of examination. To date, pilot studies have identified three patterns of E-C4d on age-fractionated erythrocytes:

1. High E-C4d levels on old erythrocytes
2. Constant E-C4d levels on all fractions regardless of the age of erythrocytes
3. Elevated E-C4d levels associated with young erythrocytes (Liu and colleagues, unpublished data).

It is conceivable that these different E-C4d patterns may reflect a previously active, a stable (or chronically active), and a recently activated disease status, respectively. These findings have provided support for the time capsule hypothesis that CAP-bearing erythrocytes can contribute informative clues to the course of disease activity in a given SLE patient.

PERSPECTIVE

The studies summarized have not only identified a unique CB-CAP phenotype that appears to be highly specific for SLE, but they also have demonstrated the potential

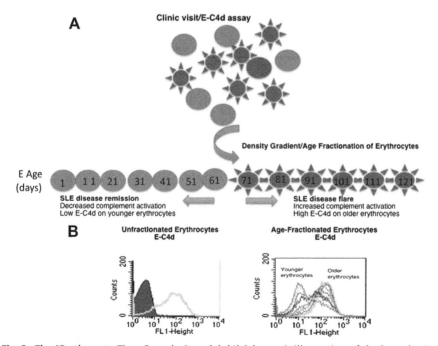

Fig. 2. The "Erythrocyte Time Capsules" model. (*A*) Schematic illustration of the hypothetical model. (*B*) Histograms of E-C4d levels on age-fractionated erythrocytes prepared from a representative SLE patient. The open histograms represent the C4d staining on the entire population (*left panel*) or density/age-fractionated erythrocytes (*right panel*). The purple closed peak depicts the background staining of erythrocytes using an istotype mouse immunoglobulin (Ig)G control.

for CB-CAPs to serve as diagnostic and monitoring biomarkers for SLE. Preliminary data have further suggested that complement activation products can bind to different combinations of circulating cell types in individual SLE patients. Therefore, it is plausible that a composite profile of CB-CAP biomarkers on different cell types may reflect a more complete picture of the underlying pathogenic process and correlate with specific clinical features/outcomes (eg, organ involvement) of individual patients, thereby serving as a novel class of personalized biomarkers for diagnosis and monitoring disease activity, assessment/prediction of clinical features, and stratification of SLE subtypes. Precise classification of SLE, in turn, may not only help customize therapeutic approaches suiting specific patients, but also assist in judicious trials of novel therapeutics.

ACKNOWLEDGMENTS

The authors thank their colleagues in the Lupus Center of Excellence and Division of Rheumatology and Clinical Immunology for providing clinical samples, helpful discussion, and skilled technical and administrative support.

REFERENCES

1. Sherer Y, Gorstein A, Fritzler MJ, et al. Autoantibody explosion in systemic lupus erythematosus: more than 100 different antibodies found in SLE patients. Semin Arthritis Rheum 2004;34(2):501–37.
2. Rahman A, Isenberg DA. Systemic lupus erythematosus. N Engl J Med 2008; 358(9):929–39.
3. Tan EM, Cohen AS, Fries JF. The 1982 revised criteria for the classification of systemic lupus erythematosus. Arthritis Rheum 1982;25:1271–7.
4. Hochberg MC. Updating the American College of Rheumatology revised criteria for the classification of systemic lupus erythematosus. Arthritis Rheum 1997;40: 1725.
5. Bombardier C, Gladman DD, Urowitz MB, et al. Derivation of the SLEDAI. A disease activity index for lupus patients. The Committee on Prognosis Studies in SLE. Arthritis Rheum 1992;35:630–40.
6. Liang MH, Socher SA, Larson MG, et al. Reliability and validity of six systems for the clinical assessment of disease activity in systemic lupus erythematosus. Arthritis Rheum 1989;32:1107–18.
7. Bae SC, Koh HK, Chang DK, et al. Reliability and validity of systemic lupus activity measure-revised (SLAM-R) for measuring clinical disease activity in systemic lupus erythematosus. Lupus 2001;10(6):405–9.
8. Hay EM, Bacon PA, Gordon C, et al. The BILAG index: a reliable and valid instrument for measuring clinical disease activity in systemic lupus erythematosus. QJM 1993;86(7):447–58.
9. Vaughan JH, Bayles TB, Favour CB. The response of serum gamma globulin level and complement titer to adrenocorticotropic hormone (ACTH) therapy in lupus erythematosus disseminatus. J Lab Clin Med 1951;37:698–702.
10. Schur PH, Sandson J. Immunological factors and clinical activity in systemic lupus erythematosus. N Engl J Med 1968;278:533–8.
11. Cook HT, Botto M. Mechanisms of disease: the complement system and the pathogenesis of systemic lupus erythematosus. Nat Clin Pract Rheumatol 2006;2(6):330–7.
12. Muller-Eberhard HJ. Molecular organization and function of the complement system. Annu rev Biochem 1988;57:321–47.

13. Liszewski MK, Farries TC, Lublin DM, et al. Control of the complement system. Adv Immunol 1996;61:201–83.
14. Walport MJ. Complement. First of two parts. N Engl J Med 2001;344:1058–66.
15. Law SK, Levine RP. Interaction between the third complement component and cell surface macromolecules. Proc Natl Acad Sci U S A 1977;74:2701.
16. Law SKA. The covalent binding reaction of C3 and C4. Ann N Y Acad Sci 1983; 421:246–58.
17. Lloyd W, Schur PH. Immune complexes, complement, and anti-DNA in exacerbations of systemic lupus erythematosus (SLE). Medicine 1981;60:208–17.
18. Valentijn RM, van Overhagen H, Hazevoet HM, et al. The value of complement and immune complex determinations in monitoring disease activity in patients with systemic lupus erythematosus. Arthritis Rheum 1985;28:904–13.
19. Ricker DM, Hebert LA, Rohde R, et al. Serum C3 levels are diagnostically more sensitive and specific for systemic lupus erythematosus activity than are serum C4 slevels. Am J Kidney Dis 1991;19:678–85.
20. Swaak AJ, Groenwold J, Bronsveld W. Predictive value of complement profiles and anti-dsDNA in systemic lupus erythematosus. Ann Rheum Dis 1986;45: 359–66.
21. Abrass CK, Nies KM, Louie JS, et al. Correlation and predictive accuracy of circulating immune complexes with disease activity in patients with systemic lupus erythematosus. Arthritis Rheum 1980;23:273–82.
22. Liu C-C, Ahearn JM, Manzi S. Complement as a source of biomarkers in systemic lupus erythematosus: past, present, and future. Curr Rheumatol Rep 2004;6:85–8.
23. Liu CC, Manzi S, Danchenko N, et al. New advances in measurement of complement activation: lessons of systemic lupus erythematosus. Curr Rheumatol Rep 2004;6(5):375–81.
24. Sturfelt G, Jonasson L, Sjoholm AG. Sequential studies of complement activation in systemic lupus erythematosus. Scand J Rheumatol 1985;14:184–96.
25. Hopkins P, Belmont HM, Buyon JP, et al. Increased levels of plasma anaphylatoxins in systemic lupus erythematosus predict flares of the disease and may elicit vascular injury in lupus cerebritis. Arthritis Rheum 1988;31:632–41.
26. Wild G, Watkins J, Ward AM, et al. C4a anaphylatoxin levels as an indicator of disease activity in systemic lupus erythematosus. Clin Exp Immunol 1990;80: 167–70.
27. Porcel JM, Ordi J, Castro-Salomo A, et al. The value of complement activation products in the assessment of systmeic lupus erythematosus flares. Clin Immunol Immunopathol 1995;74:283–8.
28. Manzi S, Rairie JE, Carpenter AB, et al. Sensitivity and specificity of plasma and urine complement split products as indicators of lupus disease activity. Arthritis Rheum 1996;39:1178–88.
29. Buyon JP, Tamerius J, Belmont HM, et al. Assessment of disease activity and impending flare in patients with systemic lupus erythematosus: comparison of the use of complement split products and conventional measurements of complement. Arthritis Rheum 1992;35:1028–37.
30. Tieley CA, Romans DG, Crookston MC. Localization of Chido and Rodgers determinants to the C4d fragment of human C4. Nature 1978;276:713–5.
31. Atkinson JP, Chan AC, Karp DR, et al. Origin of the fourth component of complement related Chido and Rodgers blood group antigens. Complement 1988;5:65–76.
32. Manzi S, Navratil JS, Ruffing MJ, et al. Measurement of erythrocyte C4d and complement receptor 1 in the diagnosis of systemic lupus erythematosus. Arthritis Rheum 2004;50:3596–604.

33. Liu CC, Manzi S, Kao AH, et al. Reticulocytes bearing C4d as biomarkers of disease activity for systemic lupus eryhematosus. Arthritis Rheum 2005;52: 3087–99.
34. Navratil JS, Manzi S, Kao AH, et al. Platelet C4d is highly specific for systemic lupus erythematosus. Arthritis Rheum 2006;54(2):670–4.
35. Liu CC, Kao AH, Hawkins DM, et al. Lymphocyte-bound complement activation products as biomarkers for diagnosis of systemic lupus erythematosus. Clin Transl Sci 2009;2(4):300–8.
36. Solomon DH, Kavanaugh AJ, Schur PH. American College of Rheumatology Ad Hoc Committee on Immunologic Testing G. Evidence-based guidelines for the use of immunologic tests: antinuclear antibody testing. Arthritis Rheum 2002; 47(4):434–44.
37. Slater CA, Davis RB, Shmerling RH. Antinuclear antibody testing. A study of clinical utility. Arch Intern Med 1996;156(13):1421–5.
38. Kao AH, Navratil JS, Ruffing MJ, et al. Erythrocyte C3d and C4d for monitoring disease activity in systemic lupus erythematosus. Arthritis Rheum, in press.
39. Rennie CM, Thompson S, Parker AC, et al. Human erythrocyte fractionation in Percoll density gradients. Clin Chim Acta 1979;98:119–25.
40. Piomelli S, Seaman C. Mechanism of red blood cell aging: relationship of cell density and cell age. Am J Hematol 1992;42:46–52.

Interferon-alpha: A Therapeutic Target in Systemic Lupus Erythematosus

Mary K. Crow, MD[a,b],*

KEYWORDS

- Systemic lupus erythematosus • Interferon-alpha
- Innate immune response

A role for type I interferon (IFN), predominantly IFN-α, in the pathogenesis of systemic lupus erythematosus (SLE) was first suggested based on the observation that serum from patients who had active SLE disease had augmented capacity to inhibit the death of virus-infected cells.[1] Those data, published in the late 1970s, found an association between IFN activity and the standard serologic indicators of disease activity: anti-DNA antibody titer and low complement levels. Recent re-examination of the IFN system using newer technology has heightened attention to this important immune system mediator.[2–6]

Along with clinical observations showing occasional induction of lupus-like autoantibodies and clinical disease in patients treated with recombinant IFN-α for hepatitis C infection or malignancy,[7] microarray gene expression analysis showing broad activation of IFN-inducible genes in blood cells of patients who have lupus has suggested that IFN-α may be a central player in systemic autoimmune disease.[2–4] As with any association between an immune system product and a clinical syndrome, it is important to address whether IFN-α plays a pathogenic role in the disease, is an innocent bystander, or is possibly playing a protective role. Increasing data relating IFN pathway activation to studies of genetic associations, clinical characterization of patients, murine models, and results from therapeutic interventions support an important, and possibly central, role for this cytokine family in SLE.[5,6] Together, the emerging data support the validity of IFN-α as a therapeutic target in patients who have SLE.

---

[a] Mary Kirkland Center for Lupus Research, Rheumatology Division, Hospital for Special Surgery, 535 East 70th Street, New York, NY 10021, USA
[b] Weill Cornell Medical College, New York, NY, USA
* Mary Kirkland Center for Lupus Research, Rheumatology Division, Hospital for Special Surgery, 535 East 70th Street, New York, NY 10021.
E-mail address: crowm@hss.edu

Rheum Dis Clin N Am 36 (2010) 173–186
doi:10.1016/j.rdc.2009.12.008
0889-857X/10/$ – see front matter
rheumatic.theclinics.com

TYPE I INTERFERON IN IMMUNE RESPONSES

The family of type I IFNs comprises the protein products of multiple related genes encoded on the short arm of human chromosome 9.[8] IFN-β may be the prototype member of the family, but IFN-α has the largest number of isoforms. Over time, 13 IFN-α genes have evolved, presumably selected to effectively combat infection by viruses. The type I IFNs are rapidly induced by infection with DNA and RNA viruses, either through intracellular nucleic acid receptors or after engagement of a Toll-like receptor (TLR) that recognizes nucleic acids, such as TLR3 for double-stranded RNA, TLR7 or -8 for single-stranded RNA, or TLR9 for demethylated CpG-rich DNA.[9] IFN-α can be synthesized by many cells, but plasmacytoid dendritic cells (pDCs) represent the cell type most capable of high-level IFN-α production.[10]

The broad expression of type I IFN receptor (IFNAR) on many cell types contributes to the diverse cellular responses induced by this cytokine family. Although T cells may be the conductors of the adaptive immune response orchestra, IFN-α is an innate immune system product that orchestrates the immune system's initial response to viral infection before T cell activation. Immune system functions implemented by IFN-α include differentiation of monocytes into dendritic-like cells capable of effective antigen presentation, induction of natural killer and natural killer T cells, promotion of IFN-γ production, support for B-cell differentiation into class-switched antibody-producing cells, and in some cases induction of apoptosis, resulting in release of cell debris, including potentially stimulatory self-antigens.[6,11]

The presenting clinical features of SLE can sometimes resemble those of some virus infections, and many of the immunologic alterations that are characteristic of SLE are similar to the immunologic effects of virus-induced IFN.

INSIGHTS FROM GENE EXPRESSION STUDIES IN PATIENTS WHO HAVE SYSTEMIC LUPUS ERYTHEMATOSUS

The advances in technology that permitted assessment of a broad spectrum of gene products in a population of cells emerged in the late 1990s and were used to show associations between the characteristic pattern of mRNA transcripts in monoclonal populations of cancer cells and disease prognosis.[12] Initially, experts believed that this experimental approach would not yield clinically relevant insights from microarray gene expression studies in complex diseases, including the systemic autoimmune diseases, because of the variability in representation of diverse cell types among individuals.

In fact, microarray studies of peripheral blood mononuclear cells (PBMC) from patients who had lupus were highly informative. Several laboratories analyzed large data sets and detected a pattern of gene expression rich in transcripts induced by IFNs.[2–4] Among the overexpressed mRNAs were some that are well-known as targets of type I IFN, such as MX1, the OAS family, and IFIT1. However the broad pattern of increased expression of IFN-regulated genes included many induced by both type I IFNs and type II IFN (IFN-γ).

To determine the relative roles of type I and type II IFN in the IFN signature, additional studies using more quantitative real-time polymerase chain reaction (PCR) focused more narrowly on genes preferentially regulated by either type I or type II IFN.[13] Those data clearly showed the predominant picture of increased levels of type I IFN–induced genes in lupus PBMCs. Moreover, the level of expression of those gene products across a population of patients who had lupus showed a high level of statistically significant correlation between each type I IFN-induced transcript and the others. This pattern strongly suggested that type I IFN present in vivo in many patients who had lupus was driving a broad gene expression program, similar to what has been seen in patients treated with either recombinant IFN-α or IFN-β for hepatitis C or multiple sclerosis.[14,15]

Some patients who had lupus also showed increased expression of genes preferentially regulated by IFN-γ, such as CXCL9 (monokine induced by gamma interferon [MIG]), but they were less frequent than those who showed activation of the type I IFN–induced genes.[13]

The type I IFN family includes not only multiple IFN-α isoforms but also products of related genes, including IFN-β. To determine which of these type I IFNs was most responsible for expression of the IFN-inducible genes, a functional assay of type I IFN activity in plasma or serum was developed and preferential inhibition of that activity in SLE plasmas by neutralizing antibodies to IFN-α was observed.[16] In contrast, only modest inhibition of type I IFN activity was seen when antibodies to IFN-β or IFN-θ were included in the cultures. The data led the authors to suggest that IFN-α represents the major type I IFN active in vivo in patients who have SLE, but that other isoforms probably contribute a small fraction of the type I IFN activity that alters immune system function in patients who have lupus.

The proportion of patients who have lupus who show the IFN signature varies among reports. In some studies of unselected adult patients, fewer than 50% show this gene expression pattern, whereas a study of pediatric patients who had lupus, most of whom were recently diagnosed and many who had not yet been treated aggressively, saw the IFN signature in nearly all patients.[3,13]

An association of IFN pathway activation with several clinical features of lupus, particularly a history of renal disease and anemia, has been shown in several cohorts, and a relative underrepresentation of IFN pathway activation has been seen in patients who have antiphospholipid antibodies.[2,13,14,17] Given the acknowledged diversity of disease manifestations in patients who have lupus, along with the fluctuating course of disease, it is not surprising that differences in prevalence of the IFN signature are seen in cross-sectional studies.

The demonstration of near-universal activation of the IFN pathway in pediatric patients who have lupus, with fewer adult patients showing this pattern, raises a question of whether the production or response to IFN-α is a function of age. In that regard, a study characterizing plasma type I IFN activity in patients who have SLE and healthy first-degree relatives based on age of the subjects showed similar patterns in women and men, but distinct levels of activity based on age.[18] The age at which plasma IFN activity was greatest corresponded to the peak reproductive years, with women between ages 12 and 22 years showing higher levels than those younger than 12 or older than 22. Women who had lupus and their first-degree relatives showed the lowest levels of type I IFN activity after 50 years of age. Men showed a similar pattern, but with a peak age range several years older (16–29 years). IFN levels were not significantly different between women and men in either the patients or relatives.

Together, these data suggest that age of the pediatric lupus cohort likely contributed to the higher prevalence of IFN signature. The molecular basis of this interesting age-related pattern of IFN pathway activation is not known.

ASSOCIATION OF INTERFERON-α WITH DISEASE ACTIVITY IN SYSTEMIC LUPUS ERYTHEMATOSUS

The first studies of IFN-α in SLE from the 1970s indicated that circulating levels of the cytokine were associated with serologic activity of the disease.[1] As microarray data from studies of PBMC in carefully characterized patients emerged from several laboratories in the early 2000s, measurements using standard tools such as systemic lupus erythematosus disease activity index and a quantitative real-time PCR measurement of IFN-inducible gene expression clearly showed a relationship to clinical disease activity.[2,13,14,17]

What has been less certain is the degree of fluctuation of IFN pathway activation over time in individual patients. The question remains whether the absence of IFN-inducible gene expression in PBMC or increased plasma type I IFN activity defines a distinct subset of lupus, reflects low disease activity, or indicates chronic disease that was earlier characterized by IFN pathway activation but is now burned-out, Arriving at an answer to this question has been difficult because of the inherent challenges of longitudinal clinical research studies and the technical difficulties and expense of quantifying IFN pathway activation. Validated disease activity measures are rarely applied to patients followed up in routine clinical care. Although several clinical investigator teams have established large cohorts of well-characterized patients and have followed up those patients over several years, appropriate biologic samples are rarely available and the clinical investigators who collect that data are rarely the same investigators who perform the laboratory analyses of IFN-inducible gene expression or plasma type I IFN activity.

Most commercially available enzyme-linked immunosorbent assay (ELISA) platforms for measuring IFN-α have not been useful for gaining insights into patterns of disease activity, most likely because of the limited range of IFN isoforms measured or possibly the presence of inhibitors or other plasma or serum components that obfuscate accurate measurement of the functionally active IFN.[19] The current available data do not definitively show whether and how IFN pathway activation relates to changes in immune function or disease activity, but the authors' group documents fluctuations in IFN-inducible gene expression in PBMC over time, in some cases, with close parallel to fluctuations in disease activity scores or response to therapy.[20] Additional longitudinal data will help determine whether IFN pathway activation can sometimes precede flares in disease activity and whether a causal link between those events can be established. Characterizing the changes in gene expression, serologic activity, or immune function that bridge a discrete increase in IFN pathway activation and a flare in disease activity could provide invaluable novel insights into lupus pathogenesis.

ADVANCES IN RESEARCH INTO MECHANISMS OF IFN PATHWAY ACTIVATION IN SYSTEMIC LUPUS ERYTHEMATOSUS
Genetic Contributions to Type I Interferon Production or Response

The major histocompatibility complex (MHC) provides the most significant contribution to the genetic variations that result in increased risk for developing SLE.[21,22] Alleles of MHC-encoded class II molecules are likely involved in the capacity to generate autoantigen-specific immune responses and production of autoantibodies. Recently developed candidate gene studies have identified several additional lupus-associated gene variants, and large-scale genome-wide association studies (GWAS) and their follow-up investigations, particularly two seminal collaborative studies published in 2008, have shown additional lupus-associated variants that identify up to 25 more genes, intronic regions, or gene loci.[23–25]

The single nucleotide polymorphisms (SNPs) identified in the published GWAS datasets represent common variants that are widespread in the population and confer a very modest increased risk for SLE. Additionally, several rare genetic variants associated with much greater risk for lupus-like disease have been found.[26]

Together, the increasing data on common variants conferring low risk and rare variants conferring higher risk for lupus indicate the most important molecular pathways involved in lupus pathogenesis.

When the list of lupus-associated gene variants is considered in the context of their known biologic function, the aggregate data collected strongly support the essential role of the immune system in disease pathogenesis.[27] Characterizing the precise functions that are altered by the nucleic acid variations enriched among patients who have lupus is the next major challenge, and will require the tools of genetics, molecular biology, and cell biology to provide a new understanding of lupus disease mechanisms and identify new therapeutic targets.

However, the data generated so far can be synthesized to propose several essential components of the disease, all of which reflect genetic factors that might augment likelihood of disease development. These include increased generation or impaired clearance of self-antigens, particularly nucleic acids, and capacity to activate autoantigen-specific immune response, including T- and B-cell activation and differentiation to plasma cells.[6,27] Most relevant to this review are a growing number of lupus-associated genetic variants, both common and rare, that impact type I IFN production or response.

A role for genetic variation in the increased production of type I IFN seen in many patients who have SLE was first supported by a family study in which plasma type I IFN activity was quantified in patients, their first-degree relatives, and unrelated individuals.[28] A significant increase in IFN level was documented in healthy first-degree relatives of patients compared with unrelated subjects. Moreover, high IFN levels tended to cluster in families. The conclusion that increased plasma type I IFN was a heritable trait led to subsequent efforts to relate lupus-associated genetic variants to activation of the IFN pathway and the publication of a series of papers by Timothy Niewold identifying contributions of specific gene variants to activation of that pathway.[29–32]

Abundant data have supported a complex set of SNPs in the interferon regulatory factor 5 (IRF5) gene that are associated with SLE.[33–35] Dissection of that association points to a role for particular autoantibody specificities, such as anti-Ro and anti-DNA, in the association with the IRF5 risk haplotype.[29] Moreover, that risk haplotype shows increased association with SLE and increased type I IFN activity in plasma of patients who have lupus who express those autoantibodies. Together those data link autoantibodies that target nucleic acids or nucleic acid-binding proteins, IRF5, and type I IFN production. With the knowledge that IRF5 is a signaling molecule downstream from several of the intracellular TLRs, the data support the concept that TLRs activated by DNA and RNA signal through IRF5 to induce type I IFN.

Additional lupus-associated gene variants that might modulate the TLR pathway and IFN production include IRF7 and TNFAIP3, encoding A20, an inhibitor of the TLR pathway.[27,36] An association between the lupus risk variants of PTPN22, a lymphocyte phosphatase, and secreted phosphoprotein 1 (SSP1; osteopontin) and plasma type I IFN activity have also been reported, although the exact mechanisms with which those variants impact IFN production have not been elucidated.[30,32] A relationship between polymorphisms in FCGRIIA, one of the first lupus-associated genes to be identified, and IFN production has not been investigated, although that might be a productive research direction considering the role that Fc receptor plays in internalizing immune complexes that induce IFN through TLRs.[9,37]

The response to type I IFN depends on sequential interaction of the cytokine with the two chains of IFNAR, the type I IFN receptor, and activation of a series of kinases, including members of the signal transducer and activator of transcription (STAT) and

Janus kinase (Jak) families. Although STAT1 has been most often implicated in signaling downstream of IFNAR, the STAT4 gene has been associated with SLE in several GWAS. A study of patients who had SLE with the risk allele of STAT4 showed normal or even decreased levels of plasma type I IFN activity but a significant association with increased IFN-inducible gene expression in the PBMC.[31] That is, for a given amount of type I IFN, patients who had the STAT4 risk allele seemed to have augmented transcription of genes regulated by type I IFN.

In some individuals the genetic makeup may favor autoantibody production over IFN pathway activation.[22] A study of serum from mothers of babies who had the neonatal lupus syndrome, in whom anti-Ro antibodies were universally present in high titer, showed that the antibodies were accompanied by high IFN activity only in those who had clinical features of SLE or Sjögren's syndrome.[38] These clinical data further support the concept that development of clinical lupus has several prerequisites. Some individuals have a genetic load for activation of the IFN pathway and others have increased capacity to form autoantibodies. The individuals who engage both arms of the immune system—the production of IFN through the innate immune response and the production of autoantibodies through the adaptive immune response—are most likely to develop clinical disease.[25]

The third important prerequisite, generation or impaired clearance of cell-derived self-antigens, may complete the requirements for disease pathogenesis. In that regard, although the lupus-associated genetic variants represent common variants that result in a modest increased risk for SLE, several recently described rare variants are associated with a greater risk for disease and seem to generate increased self-antigen. One of these genes, TREX1, encodes a DNAse, and another encodes an RNase.[26,39] Normal function of those gene products is required to dispose of endogenous nucleic acids that might otherwise stimulate an innate immune response. That concept is supported by studies in mice deficient in TREX1 that show increased production of type I IFN.[40]

The accumulated data implicate gene variants involved in the intracellular nucleic acid–response TLR pathways, and at least one gene that might contribute to signaling through the type I IFN receptor pathway, in susceptibility to SLE. A role for genetic variation in components of the TLR-independent cellular pathways in induction of type I IFN production is under investigation. In addition, rare variants are being identified that could result in generation of stimuli for immune responses that result in increased type I IFN. Additional research is required to determine whether analysis of lupus risk allelic variants or type I IFN activity, or the IFN signature will be practically useful for predicting increased susceptibility to lupus in individuals otherwise at risk (eg, sisters of patients who have lupus).

Molecular Pathways Mediating Production of Interferon-α

Numerous laboratories have supported an important capacity of nucleic acid–containing immune complexes to activate immune responses, particularly the innate immune response but also B-cell proliferation, through TLR pathways.[9,41–44] Investigators in the Ronnblom laboratory were the first to study the circulating factors in lupus serum or plasma that induced IFN-α production in vitro.[41] They showed that apoptotic or necrotic cell debris, when associated with SLE serum, could induce IFN. That response was inhibited by blockade of Fc receptors and chloroquine. At least one proposed mechanism of chloroquine's effects in vitro is its modification of the acidification of intracellular vesicles, which is likely to impact signaling downstream of TLRs engaged by nucleic acid ligands. A similar mechanism is likely to be operative in patients treated with hydroxychloroquine.

Studies from other groups have refined the mechanisms that account for immune complex stimulation of IFN production and have implicated TLR7, which is responsive to single-stranded RNA, and TLR9, which is responsive to hypomethylated CpG-rich DNA, in the induction of IFN by nucleic acid–containing immune complexes.[41–44] Although this mechanism is difficult to document in vivo in patients who have lupus, a striking association of IFN pathway activation with the presence of RNA-binding protein-specific autoantibodies (anti-RBP), such as anti-Ro, La, Sm, or ribonucleoprotein, has been observed.[14] The data from studies of the IRF5 lupus risk haplotype also support a functional link between anti-RBP and induction of IFN through the TLR7 pathway.[29]

Of course the induction of IFN by immune complexes cannot fully account for the increased production of type I IFN seen in SLE, because increased plasma IFN is observed in relatives who have lupus who do not express lupus autoantibodies, and some patients who have lupus with no measurable anti-RBP or anti-DNA antibodies do have an IFN signature.[28] However, the documented capacity of chloroquine to inhibit immune complex–mediated IFN production in vitro and the convincing data showing reduced frequency and severity of lupus flares in patients maintained on hydroxychloroquine support an important contribution of TLR signaling to clinical disease activity.[45–47] The author's current view is that induction of IFN-α by nucleic acid–containing immune complexes represents an important mechanism of augmenting type I IFN production that is influenced by genetic factors. However, it does not fully account for type I IFN produced early in the course of preclinical disease, before the development of autoantibodies. Additional studies addressing a role for environmental triggers, including virus infection, that act on a susceptible genetic substrate should provide more detailed understanding of lupus pathogenesis.

Interferon-α in Murine Lupus Models

In contrast to many aspects of lupus pathogenesis in which murine models have led the way in defining important disease mechanisms, the most significant milestones in elucidating the role of type I IFN in this disease pathway have derived from studies of patients. In fact, data from the standard murine lupus models pointed to a predominant role of IFN-γ rather than IFN-α in lupus pathology, based on knock-out and transgenic studies and documentation of increased IFN-γ levels in kidneys of mice with glomerulonephritis.[48] A role for IFN-γ in many patients who have lupus is also supported, but the data from the human system emphasize type I rather than type II IFN as the major player.

With attention focused on the type I IFN pathway in human lupus, new data from murine experiments are now supporting an important contribution of IFN-α to mouse lupus. This role has been shown through administering IFN-α to mice in the form of an adenoviral construct that leads to sustained increased levels of that cytokine.[49–51] The result is accelerated development of autoimmunity, renal disease, and death. A proposed effect of adenoviral IFN or type I IFN induced by poly (I-C), a surrogate double-stranded RNA ligand for TLR3, on recruitment of activated monocytes to kidneys may also suggest additional mechanisms of tissue fibrosis and damage that could be modified by targeting IFN-α.[51]

A murine model with very high fidelity to human lupus, or at least the aspects of human lupus associated with IFN-α, has been studied in detail by the laboratory of Westley Reeves.[52] Administering 2,6,10,14-tetramethylpentadecane (pristane) to healthy mice activates immature monocytes that produce type I IFN that is dependent on signaling through TLR7. Typical lupus autoantibodies are produced and the mice develop lupus nephritis. Although the precise mechanisms accounting for activation of the monocyte targets by pristane are not yet described, this model is arguably the ideal experimental system for gaining new understanding of a potential role for environmental triggers in initiating IFN pathway activation and disease in a manner highly similar to that observed in human patients.

INTERFERON-α AND ITS TARGETS AS LUPUS BIOMARKERS

The data supporting IFN-α as a central pathogenic mediator in lupus have contributed to interest in investigating IFN-α or expression of its gene targets as candidate biomarkers of severe or active disease or as predictors of disease flare, or for identifying patients likely to respond in clinical trials involving agents that might modify the IFN pathway. The rationale for these studies is strong, but the practical considerations involved in quantitatively assessing IFN protein, IFN activity, or IFN-inducible gene expression have been challenging. Moreover, the limited number of registries of patients who have lupus who have been longitudinally followed up with collection of disease activity data using validated instruments and with paired biologic samples stored has provided a hurdle to biomarker discovery in SLE that has not been fully overcome, despite excellent biomarker candidates for further study.

Based on the author's experience, real-time PCR quantification of a small panel of IFN-inducible genes in RNA isolated from PBMC lysates provides the most sensitive and specific measure of IFN pathway activation. Data being developed by MacDermott and colleagues[53] has shown fluctuations in IFN-inducible gene expression over up to 3 years of follow-up in patients who had lupus and were preselected to enrich for those who were likely to have IFN pathway activation based on the presence of anti-RBP autoantibodies.[53] Approximately half of the patients show a parallel pattern of fluctuations in disease activity with changes in IFN score, consistent with prior cross-sectional data.[14]

Another group of patients shows an intriguing pattern of IFN-inducible gene expression that peaks months before clinical disease flare.[53] Additional data are required to determine whether the relationship of these two events—IFN score and disease activity score—over time has functional significance or is an arbitrary concurrence of an immunologic response and a clinical presentation.

The authors used an assay of type I IFN functional activity in plasma or serum, based on induction of type I IFN-inducible gene expression in the WISH epithelial cell line that is highly responsive to IFN, to identify patients who had increased production of IFN.[16] This assay has been highly useful in relating levels of IFN activity to various lupus-associated gene alleles and for monitoring IFN production over time. However, this assay measures IFN present in the circulation but does not reflect the contribution of expression of IFN receptors or the efficiency of signaling and new gene transcription downstream of IFNAR in patient cells. Therefore, it does not fully reflect the many determinants of IFN pathway activation and may be less useful as a biomarker of disease activity than the IFN score, which measures expression of IFN-inducible genes in PBMC. Any conclusion regarding the optimal experimental approach to assessing IFN pathway activation will await a comprehensive comparison of IFN activity and PBMC IFN score in a well-characterized lupus cohort followed up regularly for at least 2 or 3 years, allowing sufficient examples of disease flare to assess the relationship of the candidate biomarkers to disease activity.

With the challenges of accurately measuring IFN pathway activation, some investigators have addressed the hypothesis that some of the chemokines that are induced by type I IFN and other stimuli might serve as a more reliable and useful biomarker of lupus disease activity or future flare.[54–56] Several chemokines are highly induced by type I IFN but many of those are also induced by IFN-γ, other cytokines, or microbial or endogenous stimuli of TLRs.

Despite issues regarding specificity of chemokines as biomarkers of disease activity, several studies suggest that measuring serum chemokines, or alternatively PBMC chemokine transcripts through PCR, might reflect IFN pathway activation, along with other inflammatory triggers, in a manner helpful in predicting generalized lupus flares or occurrence of lupus nephritis. Most promising is a recent study showing the capacity of a chemokine score to predict future flares of lupus nephritis.[56] Whether an assay is based on IFN activity, its specific gene targets, or a broader array of chemokine targets, additional studies based on collaborations among several centers and investigators are required to determine a practically useful biomarker that can aid in patient management.

PROMISE AND RISK OF THERAPIES THAT TARGET THE INTERFERON PATHWAY

With this strong case for type I IFN's important role as a heritable risk factor, a correlate of disease activity, and a global immune response modifier central to the pathogenesis of SLE (and some other systemic autoimmune diseases), many groups have concluded that this cytokine is an appropriate target for therapeutic modulation. Current efforts are directed at understanding the impact of currently available therapies on IFN pathway activation and development of new agents to inhibit the pathway, directly or indirectly.

Arguably the most effective approach to inhibiting production of IFN-α is administration of intravenous high-dose methylprednisolone. This treatment virtually ablates the IFN signature based on microarray or real-time PCR data from patient PBMC before and after pulse steroid treatment.[3] The presumed basis of this effect is death of the major producers of IFN-α, pDCs, by the high-dose steroids. Recent data suggest that additional mechanisms that modulate the capacity of interferon regulatory factors to regulate gene transcription might also contribute to reduced IFN pathway activation by high-dose steroids.[57] Although the mechanism through which other frequently used therapeutic agents, such as mycophenolate mofetil (MMF), might inhibit IFN production are only recently being studied, the author's preliminary data suggest that MMF treatment is associated with reduction of the IFN score derived from PBMC in patients who have lupus.[58] A recent study implicates a possible effect of MMF on autophagy and the TLR-independent innate immune system pathway, but additional investigation is required to pursue that suggestion.[59]

Hydroxychloroquine inhibits acidification of intracellular vesicles, and in vitro studies clearly document that chloroquine inhibits IFN production induced by nucleic acid–containing immune complexes. Additional mechanisms likely account for the positive impact of hydroxychloroquine therapy on reduction of lupus flares, but the strong rationale for its use based on the recent IFN pathway data suggests that additional approaches to inhibiting TLR activation might be even more productive in SLE. Among the approaches under investigation is inhibition of nucleic acid–mediated TLR activation by oligonucleotide inhibitors of TLR7, TLR8, or TLR9. This approach is attractive if the oligonucleotide inhibitors can be modified to assure adequate delivery to target cells.

The most active area of clinical development of therapeutics targeting the IFN pathway involves current clinical trials of monoclonal antibodies specific for numerous IFN-α isoforms. At least three of these monoclonal agents are in clinical development, each presumably slightly different from the others in the range of isoforms targeted. Very promising pharmacodynamic data from MedImmune have shown inhibition of the IFN signature in PBMC and skin biopsies from at least some patients who have lupus treated with Medi-545.[60] Currently, blocking the interaction of IFN-α with its receptor using monoclonal anti-IFN-α antibodies seems to be the most feasible and specific approach to controlling this important innate immune system pathway. Additional antibodies are available that block the IFN receptor. Because the receptor not only binds IFN-α but is also activated by the other type I IFNs, including IFN-β and IFN-θ, receptor blockade may produce a more complete blockade of downstream gene expression than the anti-IFN-α antibodies, for better or worse.

The essential role of type I IFN in host defense against virus infection is evident from the obvious effort expended by the collective human genome over evolutionary time to generate various similar but nonidentical type I IFN isoforms. Of those, IFN-α has the most variants.[8] The high impact of this system on generating effective and comprehensive immune responses triggered by virus infection is emphasized when considering the numerous approaches used by viruses to hijack the normal host response.[61] Virus-encoded proteins have been shown to block induction of type I IFN and response to that cytokine. In fact, study of the mechanisms used by viruses to paralyze the host IFN response has provided important insights into the essential components of that response. Blockade of any system that maintains the intactness of the host in the setting of a viral assault should be modulated with great care. Development of any therapeutic approaches will be accompanied by careful monitoring for viral infection. Considering the different options, blockade of IFNAR might be most risky, whereas TLR blockade or inhibition of selective type I IFNs (such as inhibition of IFN-α with monoclonal antibodies) would allow some other routes for production of IFN or response to other isoforms. Although the role of type I IFN in viral host defense has been extensively investigated, IFN-α is also active in modulating certain hematologic malignancies, such as hairy cell leukemia, and the role of the type I IFNs in regulating myeloid differentiation is not fully understood, suggesting continued need for caution as therapeutic trials move forward.

SUMMARY

The long history of elevated IFN-α in association with disease activity in patients who have SLE has assumed high significance in the past decade, with accumulating data strongly supporting broad activation of the type I IFN pathway in cells of patients who have lupus, and association of IFN pathway activation with significant clinical manifestations of SLE and increased disease activity based on validated measures. In addition, a convincing association of IFN pathway activation with the presence of autoantibodies specific for RNA-binding proteins has contributed to delineation of an important role for TLR activation by RNA-containing immune complexes in amplifying innate immune system activation and IFN pathway activation. Although the primary triggers of SLE and the IFN pathway remain undefined, rapid progress in lupus genetics is helping define lupus-associated genetic variants with a functional relationship to IFN production or response in patients. Together, the explosion of data and understanding related to the IFN pathway in SLE have readied the lupus community for translation of those insights to improved patient care. Patience will be needed to allow collection of clinical data and biologic specimens across multiple clinical centers required to support testing of IFN activity, IFN-inducible gene expression and chemokine gene products as candidate biomarkers. Meanwhile, promising clinical trials are moving forward to test the safety and efficacy of monoclonal antibody inhibitors of IFN-α. Other therapeutic approaches to target the IFN pathway may follow close behind.

REFERENCES

1. Hooks JJ, Moutsopoulos HM, Geis SA, et al. Immune interferon in the circulation of patients with autoimmune disease. N Engl J Med 1979;301(1):5–8.
2. Baechler EC, Batliwalla FM, Karypis G, et al. Interferon-inducible gene expression signature in peripheral blood cells of patients with severe lupus. Proc Natl Acad Sci U S A 2003;100(5):2610–5.
3. Bennett L, Palucka AK, Arce E, et al. Interferon and granulopoiesis signatures in systemic lupus erythematosus blood. J Exp Med 2003;197(6):711–23.
4. Crow MK, Kirou KA, Wohlgemuth J. Microarray analysis of interferon-regulated genes in SLE. Autoimmunity 2003;36(8):481–90.
5. Crow MK. Interferon-α. A new target for therapy in systemic lupus erythematosus? Arthritis Rheum 2003;48(9):2396–401.
6. Crow MK. Type I interferon in systemic lupus erythematosus. Curr Top Microbiol Immunol 2007;316:359–86.
7. Ronnblom LE, Alm GV, Oberg KE. Possible induction of systemic lupus erythematosus by interferon-alpha treatment in a patient with a malignant carcinoid tumour. J Intern Med 1990;227(3):207–10.
8. Woelk CH, Frost SD, Richman DD, et al. Evolution of the interferon alpha gene family in eutherian mammals. Gene 2007;397(1–2):38–50.
9. Lövgren T, Eloranta ML, Båve U, et al. Induction of interferon-alpha production in plasmacytoid dendritic cells by immune complexes containing nucleic acid releases by necrotic or late apoptotic cells and lupus IgG. Arthritis Rheum 2004;50(6):1861–72.
10. Rönnblom L, Alm GV. A pivotal role for the natural interferon alpha-producing cells (plasmacytoid dendritic cells) in the pathogenesis of lupus. J Exp Med 2001;194(12):F59–63.
11. Blanco P, Palucka AK, Gill M, et al. Induction of dendritic cell differentiation by IFN-alpha in systemic lupus erythematosus. Science 2001;294(5546):1540–3.
12. Alizadeh AA, Eisen MB, Davis RE, et al. Distinct types of diffuse large B-cell lymphoma identified by gene expression profiling. Nature 2000;403(6769):503–11.
13. Kirou KA, Lee C, George S, et al. Coordinate overexpression of interferon-alpha-induced genes in systemic lupus erythematosus. Arthritis Rheum 2004;50(12):3958–67.
14. Kirou KA, Lee C, George S, et al. Interferon-alpha pathway activation identifies a subgroup of systemic lupus erythematosus patients with distinct serologic features and active disease. Arthritis Rheum 2005;52(5):1491–503.
15. Singh MK, Scott TF, LaFramboise WA, et al. Gene expression changes in peripheral blood mononuclear cells from multiple sclerosis patients undergoing beta-interferon therapy. J Neurol Sci 2007;258(1–2):52–9.
16. Hua J, Kirou K, Lee C, et al. Functional assay of type I interferon in systemic lupus erythematosus plasma and association with anti-RNA binding protein autoantibodies. Arthritis Rheum 2006;54(6):1906–16.
17. Feng X, Wu H, Grossman JM, et al. Association of increased interferon-inducible gene expression with disease activity and lupus nephritis in patients with systemic lupus erythematosus. Arthritis Rheum 2006;54(9):2951–62.
18. Niewold TB, Adler JE, Glenn SB, et al. Age- and sex-related patterns of serum interferon-alpha activity in lupus families. Arthritis Rheum 2008;58(7):2113–9.
19. Jabs WJ, Hennig C, Zawatzky R, et al. Failure to detect antiviral activity in serum and plasma of healthy individuals displaying high activity in ELISA for IFN-alpha and IFN-beta. J Interferon Cytokine Res 1999;19(5):463–9.

20. Barillas-Arias L, MacDermott EJ, Duculan R, et al. Longitudinal prospective study of Type I Interferon pathway activation as a biomarker of disease activity in patients with systemic lupus erythematosus(SLE) - Interim analysis. Arthritis Rheum 2007;56(12):4245.
21. Harley IT, Kaufman KM, Langefeld CD, et al. Genetic susceptibility to SLE: new insights from fine mapping and genome-wide association studies. Nat Rev Genet 2009;10(5):285–90.
22. Ramos PS, Kelly JA, Gray-McGuire C, et al. Familial aggregation and linkage analysis of autoantibody traits in pedigrees multiplex for systemic lupus erythematosus. Genes Immun 2006;7(5):417–32.
23. International Consortium for Systemic Lupus Erythematosus Genetics (SLEGEN), Harley JB, Alarcón-Riquelme ME, et al. Genome-wide association scan in women with systemic lupus erythematosus identifies susceptibility variants in ITGAM, PXK, KIAA1542 and other loci. Nat Genet 2008;40(2):204–10.
24. Hom G, Graham RR, Modrek B, et al. Association of systemic lupus erythematosus with C8orf13-BLK and ITGAM-ITGAX. N Engl J Med 2008;358(9):900–9.
25. Crow MK. Developments in the clinical understanding of lupus. Arthritis Res Ther 2009;11(5):245.
26. Rice G, Newman WG, Dean J, et al. Heterozygous mutations in TREX1 cause familial chilblain lupus and dominant Aicardi-Goutieres syndrome. Am J Hum Genet 2007;80(4):811–5.
27. Crow MK. Collaboration, genetic associations, and lupus erythematosus. N Engl J Med 2008;358(9):956–61.
28. Niewold TB, Hua J, Lehman TJ, et al. High serum IFN-alpha activity is a heritable risk factor for systemic lupus erythematosus. Genes Immun 2007;8(6):492–502.
29. Niewold TB, Kelly JA, Flesch MH, et al. Association of the IRF5 risk haplotype with high serum interferon-alpha activity in systemic lupus erythematosus patients. Arthritis Rheum 2008;58(8):2481–7.
30. Kariuki SN, Crow MK, Niewold TB. The PTPN22 C1858T polymorphism is associated with skewing of cytokine profiles toward high IFN-alpha activity and low tumor necrosis factor-alpha levels in patients with lupus. Arthritis Rheum 2008;58(9):2818–23.
31. Kariuki SN, Kirou KA, MacDermott EJ, et al. Cutting edge: autoimmune disease risk variant of STAT4 confers increased sensitivity to IFN-alpha in lupus patients in vivo. J Immunol 2009;182(1):34–8.
32. Kariuki SN, Moore KA, Kirou KA, et al. Age- and gender-specific modulation of serum osteopontin and interferon-α by osteopontin genotype in systemic lupus erythematosus. Genes Immun 2009;10(5):487–94.
33. Graham RR, Kozyrev SV, Baechler EC, et al. A common haplotype of interferon regulatory factor 5 (IRF5) regulates splicing and expression and is associated with increased risk of systemic lupus erythematosus. Nat Genet 2006;38(5):550–5.
34. Graham RR, Kyogoku C, Sigurdsson S, et al. Three functional variants of IFN regulatory factor 5 (IRF5) define risk and protective haplotypes for human lupus. Proc Natl Acad Sci U S A 2007;104(16):6758–63.
35. Sigurdsson S, Goring HH, Kristjansdottir G, et al. Comprehensive evaluation of the genetic variants of interferon regulatory factor 5 (IRF5) reveals a novel 5 bp length polymorphism as strong risk factor for systemic lupus erythematosus. Hum Mol Genet 2008;17(6):872–81.

36. Musone SL, Taylor KE, Lu TT, et al. Multiple polymorphisms in the TNFAIP3 region are independently associated with systemic lupus erythematosus. Nat Genet 2008;40(9):1062–4.

37. Salmon JE, Millard S, Schachter LA, et al. Fc gamma RIIA alleles are heritable risk factors for lupus nephritis in African Americans. J Clin Invest 1996;97(5): 1348–54.

38. Niewold TB, Rivera TL, Buyon JP, et al. Serum type I interferon activity is dependent on maternal diagnosis in anti-SSA/Ro-positive mothers of children with neonatal lupus. Arthritis Rheum 2008;58(2):541–6.

39. Perrino FW, Harvey S, Shaban NM, et al. RNaseH2 mutants that cause Aicardi-Goutieres syndrome are active nucleases. J Mol Med 2009;87(1):25–30.

40. Stetson DB, Ko JS, Heidmann T, et al. Trex1 prevents cell-intrinsic initiation of autoimmunity. Cell 2008;134(4):569–71.

41. Vallin H, Perers A, Alm GV, et al. Anti-double-stranded DNA antibodies and immunostimulatory plasmid DNA in combination mimic the endogenous IFN-alpha inducer in systemic lupus erythematosus. J Immunol 1999;163(11):6306–13.

42. Vollmer J, Tluk S, Schmitz C, et al. Immune stimulation mediated by autoantigen binding sites within small nuclear RNAs involves Toll-like receptors 7 and 8. J Exp Med 2005;202(11):1575–85.

43. Barrat FJ, Meeker T, Gregorio J, et al. Nucleic acids of mammalian origin can act as endogenous ligands for Toll-like receptors and may promote systemic lupus erythematosus. J Exp Med 2005;202(8):1131–9.

44. Kelly KM, Zhuang H, Nacionales DC, et al. "Endogenous adjuvant" activity of the RNA components of lupus autoantigens Sm/RNP and Ro60. Arthritis Rheum 2006;54(5):1557–67.

45. The Canadian Hydroxychloroquine Study Group. A randomized study of the effect of withdrawing hydroxychloroquine sulfate in systemic lupus erythematosus. N Engl J Med 1991;324(3):150–4.

46. Tsakonas E, Joseph L, Esdaile JM, et al. A long-term study of hydroxychloroquine withdrawal on exacerbations in systemic lupus erythematosus. The Canadian Hydroxychloroquine Study Group. Lupus 1998;7(2):80–5.

47. Meinao IM, Sata EI, Andrade LE, et al. Controlled trial with chloroquine diphosphate in systemic lupus erythematosus. Lupus 1996;5(3):237–41.

48. Theofilopoulos AN, Baccala R, Beutler B, et al. Type I interferons (alpha/beta) in immunity and autoimmunity. Annu Rev Immunol 2005;23:307–36.

49. Mathian A, Weinberg A, Gallegos M, et al. IFN-alpha induces early lethal lupus in preautoimmune (New Zealand Black x New Zealand White) F1 but not in BALB/c mice. J Immunol 2005;174(5):2499–506.

50. Ramanujam M, Kahn P, Huang W, et al. Interferon-alpha treatment of female (NZW x BXSB)F(1) mice mimics some but not all features associated with the Yaa mutation. Arthritis Rheum 2009;60:1096–101.

51. Davidson A, Aranow C. Lupus nephritis: lessons from murine models. Nat Rev Rheumatol 2009. [Epub ahead of print].

52. Reeves WH, Lee PY, Weinstein JS, et al. Induction of autoimmunity by pristane and other naturally occurring hydrocarbons. Trends Immunol 2009;30(9):455–64.

53. MacDermott EJ, Cherian J, Santiago AG, et al. Type 1 interferon pathway activation predicts flares of disease activity in SLE. Arthritis Rheum 2008;58(12): 3974–5.

54. Bauer JW, Baechler EC, Petri M, et al. Elevated serum levels of interferon-regulated chemokines are biomarkers for active human systemic lupus erythematosus. PLoS Med 2006;3(12):e491.

55. Fu Q, Chen X, Cui H, et al. Association of elevated transcript levels of interferon-inducible chemokines with disease activity and organ damage in systemic lupus erythematosus patients. Arthritis Res Ther 2008;10(5):R112.

56. Bauer JW, Petri M, Batliwalla FM, et al. Interferon-regulated chemokines as biomarkers of systemic lupus erythematosus disease activity: a validation study. Arthritis Rheum 2009;60(10):3098–107.

57. Chinenov Y, Rogatsky I. Glucocorticoids and the innate immune system: crosstalk with the toll-like receptor signaling network. Mol Cell Endocrinol 2007;275(1–2): 30–42.

58. Gold S, Cherian J, Santiago A, et al. Type I interferon pathway activation parallels therapeutic response in patients with SLE. Arthritis Rheum 2009;60(10):S338–9.

59. Chaigne-Delalande B, Guidincelli G, Couzi L, et al. The immunosuppressor mycophenolic acid kills activated lymphocytes by inducing a nonclassical actin-dependent necrotic signal. J Immunol 2008;181(11):7630–8.

60. Yao Y, Richman L, Higgs BW, et al. Neutralization of interferon-alpha/beta-inducible genes and downstream effect in a phase I trial of an anti-interferon-alpha monoclonal antibody in systemic lupus erythematosus. Arthritis Rheum 2009; 60(6):1785–96.

61. Kumar H, Kawai T, Akira S. Pathogen recognition in the innate immune response. Biochem J 2009;420(1):1–16.

Glutamate Receptor Biology and its Clinical Significance in Neuropsychiatric Systemic Lupus Erythematosus

Cynthia Aranow, MD, Betty Diamond, MD*,
Meggan Mackay, MS, MD

KEYWORDS

- Neuropsychiatric SLE • Cognitive impairment
- Emotional impairment • NMDAR • Anti-NR2 antibody

In the past few decades, as patients with systemic lupus erythematosus (SLE) are experiencing increased longevity, there has been increasing awareness of the late sequelae of this disease.[1,2] It is clear that most patients with SLE develop some manifestation of neuropsychiatric systemic lupus erythematosus (NPSLE) and that the incidence of NPSLE is greater in those with longer duration of disease. It is also clear that many of the most common manifestations of NPSLE do not associate with other metrics of disease, such as flare or severity. Thus, there is a need for exploring new paradigms for pathophysiologic mechanisms to explain this paradoxic and increasingly vexing problem in NPSLE. This article discusses the effect of the classification scheme for NPSLE and new thoughts regarding the role of anti–N-methyl-D-aspartate receptor (NMDAR) antibodies in the pathogenesis of some of the diffuse central nervous system (CNS) manifestations of NPSLE.

NPSLE

Before 1999, characterization of CNS events in lupus was hampered by confusing terminology and differences among studies in attribution and methods of ascertainment. A consensus conference convened by the American College of Rheumatology (ACR) in 1999 to facilitate clinical and basic research of NPSLE resulted in the

All authors contributed equally.
Feinstein Institute for Medical Research, 350 Community Drive, Manhasset, NY 11030, USA
* Corresponding author.
E-mail address: bdiamond@nshs.edu (B. Diamond).

Rheum Dis Clin N Am 36 (2010) 187–201
doi:10.1016/j.rdc.2009.12.007   rheumatic.theclinics.com
0889-857X/10/$ – see front matter

elucidation of 19 different neuropsychiatric syndromes attributable to SLE (**Box 1**).[3] Case definitions, reporting standards, and diagnostic criteria were provided by the group. Identification of these 19 syndromes has allowed the rheumatology community to classify more precisely and universally individual clinical presentations, thereby paving the way for translational research investigating mechanisms of disease.

Effective use of the NPSLE classification scheme relies on correct attribution of the NP event. Approximately two-thirds of NP events occurring in patients with SLE are attributable to other causes; it is critically important that all other possible entities have been investigated and excluded for each syndrome.[4,5] Three conditions, in particular, must be excluded as they may mimic CNS disease resulting from active SLE. First, infections are a major confounding condition. Immunosuppressive therapies and inherent immune abnormalities in patients with SLE contribute to the increased infectious risk in SLE. In North America and Western Europe, most infections are bacterial, whereas in other parts of the world, fungal and mycobacterial infections are common. If unrecognized and untreated, these conditions can be fatal. Reports of progressive multifocal leukoencephalopathy (PML) in patients with SLE treated with rituximab or other immunosuppressive therapies highlight the need for increased vigilance in detecting infection in immunosuppressed patients with altered NP status.[6,7] Another condition, thrombotic thrombocytopenic purpura (TTP), presents with mental status changes and thrombocytopenia, microanigopathic hemolytic anemia, renal disease, and fever. Appropriate treatment is mandatory; untreated, TTP is always fatal. The pathologic lesion is platelet microthrombi, often a result of failure to

---

Box 1
ACR case definitions of neuropsychiatric syndromes in SLE

Acute confusional state

Cognitive dysfunction

Myasthenia gravis

Acute inflammatory demyelinating polyradiculoneuropathy (Guillain-Barré syndrome)

Demyelinating syndrome

Myelopathy

Anxiety disorder

Headache

Neuropathy, cranial

Aseptic meningitis

Mononeuropathy (single/multiplex)

Plexopathy

Autonomic disorder

Mood disorders

Polyneuropathy

Cerebrovascular disease

Movement disorder (chorea)

Psychosis

Seizures

cleave von Willebrand factor and ensuing platelet activation. Treatment of hypertension in patients with SLE is crucial. Posterior reversible encephalopathy syndrome (PRES) occurs in patients with hypertensive lupus, frequently in the setting of acute renal failure, recent cyclophosphamide treatment, TTP, or preeclampsia, and leads to increased cerebral vascular permeability and brain edema. Thus, 3 potentially fatal conditions (infection, TTP, and PRES) may be confused with SLE disease activity as they can all mimic an acute diffuse presentation of CNS NPSLE.

The 1999 classification scheme has been useful to the clinician considering diagnostic and therapeutic options in an individual patient, but is perhaps less useful in probing disease pathogenesis. Of the multiple symptoms encompassed by NPSLE, CNS symptoms occur much more frequently than peripheral nervous system symptoms.[4] Moreover, diffuse CNS symptoms, such as cognitive dysfunction, psychosis, acute confusional state, anxiety, and mood disorders, occur more commonly than focal CNS symptoms in most studies. The focal CNS symptoms, including stroke, demyelinating syndromes, movement disorders, and transverse myelitis, are most frequently secondary to vascular events caused by antiphospholipid antibodies.[8,9] The diffuse CNS symptoms have a less certain pathogenic mechanism. Cognitive impairment and mood disturbance are among the most frequently reported diffuse CNS syndromes. The cognitive impairment derives most often from memory impairment involving verbal memory and executive function and attention. These symptoms are insidious and usually develop slowly over time, independent of disease activity. Their presence is also independent of current or previous medication use and cannot be explained solely on the basis of coexisting antiphospholipid antibodies that are known to cause chronic cerebrovascular disease that may result in cognitive difficulty.

Multiple studies conducted in lupus cohorts worldwide have consistently reported that cognitive impairment occurs with a high frequency.[4,9–12] However, comparisons among studies are difficult. Variability in reported results is attributable to the different instruments used for cognitive assessment, differences in definition of impairment, and potential inherent differences in selected populations.[13] Traditionally, cognitive ability has been assessed in a one-on-one setting by a neuropsychologist who administers a battery of tests. Assessment of cognitive ability recommended by the ACR consensus panel includes 10 tests administered over 1 hour that evaluate 8 cognitive domains (intelligence, reasoning, attention, learning, recall, fluency, language, perception). However, despite these recommendations, there has been little uniformity in the selection of tests used. More recently, a computer-based neuropsychiatric assessment (ANAM) has been used to assess cognitive function.[14] This is, in general, less time consuming, less dependent on strong language skills, and less dependent on the establishment of a rapport between the tester and the subject. The ANAM has the additional advantage that the practice effect, improvement over time from repeated performances of the test, is less pronounced in longitudinal studies of cognitive function. However, the individual tests chosen by investigative groups remain variable. More significantly, the performance criteria to identify impairment vary among investigators. The lower frequency of cognitive impairment in some cohorts reflects a more stringent definition of impairment. Patients with memory deficits only are not identified as cognitively impaired in those cohorts, although they would be considered impaired by investigators reporting on other lupus cohorts.[4]

MECHANISTIC STUDIES OF NPSLE

The etiopathogenesis of cognitive impairment and mood disorder remain a mystery. Studies of serum antibodies and cytokines have failed to show a reproducible signal that predicts the development of diffuse NPSLE symptoms in the CNS or that correlates with the presence of these symptoms. For example, serum antiphospholipid antibodies have been shown to correlate with cognitive decline in some studies but not in others.[10,15–18] Numerous studies of serum antineuronal and antiribosomal p antibodies report inconclusive results.[18–20] Further complexity is introduced because these symptoms can wax and wane, or can be irreversible. Thus, it is not clear whether one mechanism or multiple mechanisms are responsible for these symptom complexes. Many, if not most, neuroimaging studies of NPSLE have sought to associate active NPSLE with reproducible neuroimaging abnormalities. Given that active NPSLE comprises a fairly large group of disparate syndromes, it is not surprising that this has proven to be extremely difficult, despite the use of numerous imaging modalities including computerized tomography (CT), magnetic resonance imaging (MRI), functional MRI (fMRI), magnetic resonance spectroscopy (MRS), diffusion tensor imaging (DTI), and positron emission tomography (PET) scans.[21–25] Differences in patient populations, instrumentation, technique, and metrics for interpretation all prevent comparisons among studies. Nonetheless, MRS identified regional increased choline/creatine ratios in gray and white matter in patients with cognitive dysfunction.[26,27] Functional MRI also distinguished differences in global and regional brain activation patterns between patients with SLE, healthy controls, and disease controls (rheumatoid arthritis [RA]) in response to specific memory tasks.[28,29]

Studies of cerebrospinal fluid (CSF) in patients with active NPSLE have proven to be more revealing and are furthering our understanding of the pathophysiology of NPSLE. Significantly elevated interleukin (IL)-6 levels are a consistent finding in patients with active CNS disease, particularly psychosis, and the concentration of this cytokine correlates with symptom severity.[30–32] Additionally, patients with active NP disease (defined as ≥ 2 of the following: psychosis, aseptic meningitis, transverse myelitis, seizures, pathologic brain MRI, severely abnormal NP tests, oligoclonal bands in CSF) have 20- and 200-fold increases in intrathecal levels of a proliferation-inducing ligand (APRIL) and B-cell activating factor (BAFF), respectively, compared with patients without NPSLE.[33] Immune complexes formed by autoantibodies in CSF from patients with active diffuse CNS symptoms (psychosis, acute confusional state, seizure disorders, mood and anxiety disorders) and added apoptotic debris has been shown to significantly induce production of IFNα by IFN-producing cells, although CSF alone does not do so.[34] Other inflammatory mediators identified in CSF of patients with active NPSLE include chemokines (MCP-1, RANTES, MIG, IP-10), IL-8, and MMP-9.[35,36] There are no studies of CSF abnormalities specific for insidious manifestations of NPSLE, such as cognitive impairment, as CSF is not routinely obtained from these individuals. Markers for cognitive impairment and mood disorder that can be reliably measured in an easy-to-use assay are clearly needed. The inability to identify such a marker for these manifestations of NP disease has hampered our understanding of its pathogenesis and has also made design of clinical trials in NPSLE extremely problematic. Clinical investigation of the course of NPSLE is also made difficult as there is no reliable assessment for measurement of improvement in symptoms or to determine whether progression of symptoms has been retarded.

ANTIBODIES AND THE BRAIN

In SLE, tissue injury is initiated by antibodies. This observation is true in the kidneys, skin, blood vessels, and in all organs for which there is an appreciation of pathogenesis and inflammatory pathways. For decades it has been known that the serum of many patients with SLE contains brain-reactive antibodies. The specific antigens that are recognized by these antibodies were not identified, nor was their functionality known. Additionally, no correlations were found between the presence of these antibodies in serum and aspects of NPSLE. Antiribosomal p antibody has been extensively studied with respect to NPSLE. Several clinical studies examining whether serum antiribosomal p correlates with psychosis have yielded conflicting results, and a recent meta-analysis of 14 published studies concluded that serum antiribosomal p measurements were not sensitive in diagnosing NPSLE and did not distinguish between NPSLE subsets.[18,37–40] Interest in the antibody diminished because it was also not clear how an antibody directed against an intracellular protein could mediate brain dysfunction. Recently, a team of investigators from Chile has showed that the antiribosomal p antibody cross-reacts with a membrane protein on neurons and that binding of the antibody to neurons can initiate an apoptotic cascade.[41] Thus, there is now a plausible mechanism for brain pathology resulting from antiribosomal p antibodies.

ANTIBODIES TO THE N-METHYL-D-ASPARTATE RECEPTOR AND FUNCTION OF THE NMDAR

Our own interest is in a subset of anti-DNA antibodies that cross-reacts with a consensus pentapeptide present in the NR2A and NR2B subunits of the NMDAR.

Many anti-DNA antibodies derived from patients with lupus and from some spontaneous mouse models of SLE are of the IgG isotype and display extensive somatic mutation in variable region sequences.[42] These are characteristics of the molecular signature of a T-cell–dependent, germinal center matured B-cell response. Generally, protein antigens induce a germinal center B-cell response; we therefore asked whether an anti-DNA antibody can bind to a peptide sequence. The anti-DNA antibody that we used in these studies, R4A, deposits in glomeruli, causes proteinuria, and therefore has features of a pathogenic lupus anti-DNA antibody. R4A binds a consensus pentapeptide sequence (D/E W D/E Y S/G) comprising L or D amino acids.[43] This sequence is contained within the NR2A and NR2B subunits of rodent and human NMDARs. The antibody binds each subunit on ELISA and Western blot, and can immunoprecipitate the subunits from a mouse brain lysate.[44]

NMDARs are receptors for the neurotransmitter glutamate, the major excitatory neurotransmitter in the brain and critically important for many brain functions. Most neurons in the brain contain high levels of glutamate stored inside synaptic vesicles that is released, in a carefully controlled fashion, to convey sensory information, respond to motor commands, and to form thoughts and memories that translate to cognitive and emotional abilities. Excessive exposure to glutamate results in increased excitotoxic cell death,[45] and disturbances of glutamate or NMDAR activity have been implicated in several neurologic syndromes including traumatic brain and cord injuries, stroke, Alzheimer disease, Huntington disease, Parkinson disease, seizures, multiple sclerosis, HIV-associated dementia, schizophrenia, and amyotrophic lateral sclerosis.[46]

NMDARs are present throughout the brain and subunits are differentially expressed regionally in the brain and temporally during development. They are composed of 2 NR1 subunits that have a binding site for glycine, a coagonist, and 2 of any 4 NR2 subunits (A–D).[47] Receptors containing NR2A and NR2B are most dense on neurons in the CA1 region of the hippocampus, and in the amygdala.[48–50] Pertinent to our concerns in SLE, hippocampal NMDARs subserve learning and memory and, in the amygdala, NMDARs are critical in the fear-conditioning response. These receptors function as voltage-gated calcium channels; following electrical stimulation to the nerve, glutamate and glycine bind an NR2 or NR1 subunit respectively and allow calcium to flux into the cell. Activation of the receptor requires that magnesium exits from the pore of the receptor, at which time calcium is free to enter.[51] The magnitude of the calcium influx is proportional to the time the pore remains in the open position. The change in intracellular calcium is crucial for cellular function. An excessive flux of calcium into neurons causes mitochondrial stress and activates caspase cascades, leading to neuronal death.[52–54] Proper regulation of NMDAR activation is, therefore, essential for cognitive performance and appropriate emotional responses. Consequences of alterations in NMDAR function can be severe; MK-801 is an NMDAR antagonist that effectively blocks excitotoxicity but can produce seizures and coma. Memantine is another NMDAR antagonist that successfully blocks the open channel with few of the sedating side effects.[55] Other NMDAR antagonists with different kinetics produce hallucinations (phencyclidine/PCP/angel dust) or excessive drowsiness (ketamine).[56] The observation that PCP produces hallucinations suggests the possibility that NMDAR abnormalities may contribute to schizophrenia.[57]

The murine monoclonal antibody R4A, which binds DNA and NMDAR, functions to enhance NMDAR activation. Studies of hippocampal slices from mice show that binding of cross-reactive, anti-DNA antibodies to NMDARs on neurons results in apoptotic neuronal death.[44] Further study has shown that the antibody modulates NMDAR activation, synergizing with the natural agonist glutamate to increase excitatory postsynaptic potentials. At higher concentrations, it synergizes with glutamate to cause mitochondrial stress and caspase activation. The death-inducing function is mediated through NMDAR binding as NMDAR antagonists block caspase activation. The antibody's effects are dependent only on antibody binding and do not require complement activation or antibody-dependent cell-mediated cytotoxicity as Fab′$_2$ fragments of antibody provoke cell death.[44]

Mechanistic studies of the interaction of R4A with NMDARs show that R4A preferentially binds the NMDAR when the pore is open; thus, the antibody can be presumed to augment the time of opening of the pore and enhances the calcium influx. R4A decreases the concentration of glutamate needed to trigger excitatory postsynaptic potentials and to induce apoptosis.

REGIONAL BRAIN EFFECTS OF ANTI-NMDAR ANTIBODIES: MURINE MODELS OF COGNITIVE AND BEHAVIORAL EFFECTS

To study the potential effects of anti-NMDAR antibody on cognition we immunized mice with a multimeric form of the DWEYS peptide. These mice develop anti-DNA/anti-NMDAR cross-reactive antibodies. Although these antibodies are present in the circulation, there is no evidence of brain pathology and no alteration of learning or memory, presumably because the endothelial cells in the brain microvasculature form a blood-brain barrier (BBB) that is impenetrable to antibody.[58] There are, however, conditions known to compromise the integrity of the BBB. Infection has long been recognized as a threat to barrier integrity. Bacterial lipolysaccharide (LPS) induces production of IL-1 and tumor necrosis factor, both of which alter permeability of the BBB. When mice immunized with the multimeric peptide are subsequently given LPS, antibody penetrates the BBB and preferentially targets the hippocampus. Anti-NMDAR antibodies bind hippocampal neurons with an ensuing death of hippocampal neurons that is immediate. As the BBB integrity is reconstituted quickly following LPS administration, there is no accumulation of damage following the initial event. Most notably, there is no inflammation in regions of neuronal loss, nor activation of resident inflammatory cells in the brain, and no influx of blood borne inflammatory cells. Mice with antibody-mediated neuronal loss perform poorly on several tests of memory function, but are unimpaired in tasks that measure other cognitive domains.[58]

Similar findings are observed when normal mice are given human lupus serum or CSF containing anti-DNA/anti-NMDAR antibody followed by administration of LPS. Human lupus anti-NMDAR antibody binds to hippocampal neurons in the mouse, causing apoptotic neuronal loss.[44] These mice also perform poorly in tests of memory function.

Another agent recognized to compromise the integrity of the BBB is epinephrine. When mice immunized with multimeric peptide and harboring high titers of anti-DNA/anti-NMDAR antibodies are given epinephrine systemically, the antibodies transit from the vasculature into the amygdala. The hippocampi of these mice are histologically normal and there are no cognitive deficits detected in testing of memory and learning functions.[59] However, these mice do have impaired performance in a fear-conditioning paradigm. In this paradigm, normal mice exposed to a neutral stimulus followed by a noxious stimulus learn to associate the noxious stimulus with the neutral one. Therefore, conditioned mice will freeze as soon as the neutral stimulus is delivered in anticipation of the noxious stimulus. Mice with antibody-mediated amygdala damage fail to freeze appropriately. Because there is no impairment of memory, the failure to freeze is a behavioral impairment. This study was highly informative for several reasons. It showed that anti-NMDAR antibodies could cause behavioral changes. It also showed that the same anti-NMDAR antibodies could result in two distinct manifestations of NPSLE. Finally, it showed that agents that breach the BBB do so with regional specificity. Thus antibody-related brain symptoms will depend on the nature of the agent that permits antibody penetration into brain, and the specific antibody.

These models show permanent loss of function in the hippocampus or the amygdala. However, it is clear that some cognitive or behavioral changes in patients are transient. We postulate that this reflects the observation that lower concentrations of antibodies are needed to affect synaptic plasticity than to cause apoptosis. Thus, low titers of antibody may lead to transient dysfunction and high titers lead to permanent impairment (**Fig. 1**).

ANTI-NMDAR ANTIBODIES AND SLE

Multiple studies performed on cohorts in Asia, Europe, and North America report that approximately 40% to 50% of patients have antibody reactivity to the DWEYS peptide. This reactivity is only observed in patients with anti-DNA antibody and,

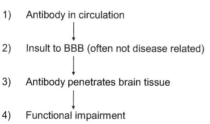

1)   Antibody in circulation

2)   Insult to BBB (often not disease related)

3)   Antibody penetrates brain tissue

4)   Functional impairment

•Nature of impairment depends on location of antibody penetration
•Transient impairment with low titers of antibody; permanent impairment with high antibody titers

Fig. 1. Proposed mechanism for anti-NMDAR antibody-mediated neurotoxicity.

when the peptide-reactive antibodies are purified, they display cross-reactivity to DNA.[60] Many studies have attempted to correlate the presence of these antibodies in serum with aspects of NPSLE. Two cross-sectional studies found correlations with cognitive impairment and depression,[27,61] and another study reported a weak association between decreased amygdala size and serum anti-NMDAR antibody,[62] but several other studies, including a prospective, longitudinal study, have found no correlations.[63–65] In general, there are no reproducible data to correlate serum titers of anti-NMDAR antibodies with any aspect of NPSLE.

More recently, some studies have explored CSF titers of these antibodies. Anti-NMDAR antibody present in CSF of patients with SLE cross-reacts with DNA, is neurotoxic, and is functionally indistinguishable from the serum antibody. In contrast to serum titers, the presence of these antibodies in the CSF correlates with acute, diffuse CNS manifestations of NPSLE that include seizure disorders, acute confusional state, psychosis, severe refractory headache, and cerebrovascular disease. Moreover, titers correlate with symptom severity.[66,67] A 6-month follow-up of CSF from patients studied at the time of an acute episode showed a decrease, but not a total absence, of CSF anti-NMDAR antibody.[68] Thus, antibody may be present in the CSF of patients without clinically apparent CNS disease. Further studies may determine whether antibody, anti-NMDAR antibody, or others can account for the insidious manifestations of disease and the changes in cognitive function and mood that occur in individuals who have never manifested acute clinical CNS disease.

The presence of anti-NMDAR antibody in serum or in CSF fails to correlate with peripheral nervous system manifestations of SLE. This reflects the absence of NMDARs on peripheral nerves. Compared with other autoantibodies studied; anti-DNA, antinuclear antibody, antiribosomal p, and anticardiolipin antibodies, anti-NMDAR antibodies have been shown to clearly distinguish between patients with central, diffuse CNS manifestations and those with peripheral nervous system involvement and those with no NP. It also underscores the need when studying NPSLE to consider central and peripheral manifestations separately, as the pathogenic agents and mechanisms are likely to be distinct.

How anti-NMDAR antibodies access the brain in human SLE remains unclear. Raised intrathecal levels imply two possible mechanisms: intrathecal production and increased permeability of the BBB. Grossly elevated intrathecal levels of all autoantibodies, including anti-NMDAR antibodies, occurs during a clear state of BBB disruption such as septic meningitis. Although intrathecal production may occur in some patients, it would seem an unlikely event in all patients.

ANTI-NMDAR ANTIBODIES AND BRAIN TISSUE

In addition to serum and CSF, anti-NMDAR antibody may be found in brain tissue. We have eluted anti-NMDAR antibody from postmortem brain tissue of a patient with SLE who died with severe cognitive deficits.[69] The eluted antibody displays neurotoxic effects when injected into a mouse brain. In several other brains, it has been possible to discern antibody bound to neurons and colocalizing with NMDARs.[69] It is clear that, under some circumstances, brain parenchyma is exposed to anti-NMDAR antibody.

ANTI-NMDAR ANTIBODIES AND FETAL BRAIN DEVELOPMENT

It has been reported in several small studies that the children of women with SLE have an increased frequency of learning disorders.[70–74] These disabilities are not related to birth weight or prematurity. Only one study has asked whether the offspring of male patients with SLE are similarly affected, and it found no evidence for this.[74] These observations suggest that the in utero environment might be a major contributor to abnormal fetal brain development. It is known that, after the first trimester of pregnancy, maternal antibody crosses the placenta and enters the fetal circulation. Because there is no BBB during fetal development, the fetal brain is exposed to circulating maternal antibody. We therefore studied whether anti-NMDAR antibody can impair normal brain development in pregnant mice.

To address the possibility that maternal anti-NMDAR antibody impaired normal brain development, female mice were immunized with multimeric peptide and high titers of anti-DNA anti-NMDAR antibodies were found. They were then mated with male mice. On day 15 of embryonic development (E15), fetal brains exposed to anti-NMDAR antibody display a thin cortical plate with an increase in the number of apoptotic neurons.[75] When mice exposed to anti-NMDAR antibody during gestation are born, they exhibit a delay in acquisition of neonatal reflexes. As adults, they display normal function of the hippocampus and amygdala, but are impaired in a few isolated tasks requiring intact cortical function.[75] Although these impairments cannot be called learning disabilities (learning disabilities refer specifically to difficulties with reading or mathematical skills), they are isolated impairments of cortical function and, in that respect, they are similar to learning disabilities. Thus, anti-NMDAR antibodies have the potential to affect fetal brain development in mice. To date there are no studies in humans, but intravenous administration of human monoclonal anti-DNA/anti-NMDAR antibodies to pregnant mice causes the same histologic insult to the brains of their offspring as that seen in the brains of immunized mice with polyclonal anti-NMDAR antibody. Administration of soluble DWEYS peptide during pregnancy in immunized mice blocks antibody-mediated damage, presumably by formation of peptide-antibody immune complexes and prevention of antibody binding to fetal tissue. This technique may be a useful therapeutic strategy if it becomes clear that the offspring of women with lupus can be damaged by this antibody during pregnancy.

NON-SLE ANTI-NMDAR ANTIBODIES

Anti-NMDAR antibodies and their toxic effects are not limited to SLE. Anti-NMDAR encephalitis is a recently described syndrome characterized by diffuse cerebral dysfunction with acute organic psychiatric disturbances progressing to seizures, dyskinesias, autonomic instability, abnormal cardiac conduction, decreased level of consciousness, and central hypoventilation.[76] This syndrome is highly associated with ovarian teratomas but can occur in the absence of tumor.[77] It has also been implicated in the pathogenesis of new-onset seizure disorder in young women.[78] All patients with anti-NMDAR–associated encephalitis or seizure disorder have the antibody in serum and CSF, and measurements of BBB integrity suggest intrathecal synthesis of the antibody. The target antigen for this anti-NMDAR antibody differs from that seen in patients with SLE. Whereas the lupus-associated anti-DNA/anti-NMDAR antibodies target the NR2A and NR2B subunits of the NMDAR, the nonlupus-associated anti-NMDAR antibodies bind the NR1 subunit and the two antibodies are not cross-reactive. In contrast, perhaps, to the apoptotic neuronal death induced by the lupus-associated antibody, the nonlupus-associated antibody produces a selective and reversible concentration-dependent decrease in the cell-surface density of NMDA receptors.[77] Generally, these patients do well with removal of the tumor (if present) or immunosuppressive therapy; clinical symptoms and abnormal MRI findings are reversed as the antibody titer declines. Other anti-NMDAR antibodies have been reported. An anti-NMDAR antibody directed against epitopes on the NR2A subunit was seen in 18% of a cohort of pediatric patients with epilepsy[79] suggesting the possibility of autoimmune epilepsy or that these antibodies can develop after neuronal damage.

SUMMARY

Studies to date show that cross-reactive anti-DNA/anti-NMDAR antibodies are present in serum, CSF, and brain tissue of a significant number of patients with SLE. Using a mouse model, it has been possible to show that these antibodies can cause cognitive or behavioral impairments. The nature of the brain dysfunction depends on the region of the brain exposed to antibody, which, in turn, is influenced by the agent breaching the BBB. These studies explain why serum titers of a pathologic antineuronal antibody will not correlate with CNS symptoms; antibodies must first gain access to brain tissue before causing neuronal dysfunction. In contrast, antibodies present within the CSF are closely related to disease manifestation.

The demonstration that anti-NMDAR antibody alters synaptic activity at concentrations below those needed to cause neuronal death explains how some episodes of CNS disease are characterized by transient symptomalogy and recovery, whereas others lead to a fixed impairment. Moreover, antibody synergizes with ligand, but does not bind a quiescent receptor, which suggests that regions of brain experiencing synaptic activity will be preferentially targeted.

Whether these antibodies can affect the offspring of mothers with lupus is a fascinating area that needs further study.

In summary, three important points need to be made. First, it is highly likely that there are multiple lupus autoantibodies that can bind targets in the brain and mediate aspects of CNS NPSLE. Of course, there will also be nonantibody-mediated mechanisms of brain injury. Second, to study CNS aspects of NPSLE further, noninvasive assessments of BBB integrity and reliable markers for changes in brain function are needed. Third, if brain dysfunction in patients with SLE is indeed mediated by anti-NMDAR antibody, it may be possible to develop the D-DWEYS peptide as a therapeutic to prevent neuronal damage from antibody. Similarly, it may be possible to use D-DWEYS to protect the fetal brain. Thus, this mechanism of tissue injury may be treatable, as there is no evidence that antibody triggers any inflammatory cascades in the adult or fetal brain.

Finally, the paradigm that has been developed suggests that it may be useful to reclassify NPSLE according to region of damage: vascular, CNS, or peripheral nerve. Antibodies or other toxic agents that differentially affect brain endothelial cells, brain cells (neurons, astrocytes, and microglia), or peripheral nerves, will result in distinct symptomatologies. This classification scheme (vascular, central, and peripheral) may facilitate mechanistic studies of NPSLE, and ultimately clinical trials.

REFERENCES

1. Ginzler EM, Dvorkina O. Newer therapeutic approaches for systemic lupus erythematosus. Rheum Dis Clin North Am 2005;31(2):315–28.
2. Scolding NJ, Joseph FG. The neuropathology and pathogenesis of systemic lupus erythematosus. Neuropathol Appl Neurobiol 2002;28(3):173–89.
3. The American College of Rheumatology nomenclature and case definitions for neuropsychiatric lupus syndromes. Arthritis Rheum 1999;42(4):599–608.
4. Hanly JG, McCurdy G, Fougere L, et al. Neuropsychiatric events in systemic lupus erythematosus: attribution and clinical significance. J Rheumatol 2004; 31(11):2156–62.

5. Hanly JG, Urowitz MB, Sanchez-Guerrero J, et al. Neuropsychiatric events at the time of diagnosis of systemic lupus erythematosus: an international inception cohort study. Arthritis Rheum 2007;56(1):265–73.

6. Molloy ES, Calabrese LH. Progressive multifocal leukoencephalopathy in patients with rheumatic diseases: are patients with systemic lupus erythematosus at particular risk? Autoimmun Rev 2008;8(2):144–6.

7. Carson KR, Evens AM, Richey EA, et al. Progressive multifocal leukoencephalopathy after rituximab therapy in HIV-negative patients: a report of 57 cases from the Research on Adverse Drug Events and Reports project. Blood 2009; 113(20):4834–40.

8. Love PE, Santoro SA. Antiphospholipid antibodies: anticardiolipin and the lupus anticoagulant in systemic lupus erythematosus (SLE) and in non-SLE disorders. Prevalence and clinical significance. Ann Intern Med 1990;112(9):682–98.

9. Sanna G, Bertolaccini ML, Cuadrado MJ, et al. Neuropsychiatric manifestations in systemic lupus erythematosus: prevalence and association with antiphospholipid antibodies. J Rheumatol 2003;30(5):985–92.

10. Brey RL, Holliday SL, Saklad AR, et al. Neuropsychiatric syndromes in lupus: prevalence using standardized definitions. Neurology 2002;58(8):1214–20.

11. Ainiala H, Loukkola J, Peltola J, et al. The prevalence of neuropsychiatric syndromes in systemic lupus erythematosus. Neurology 2001;57(3):496–500.

12. Sibbitt WL Jr, Brandt JR, Johnson CR, et al. The incidence and prevalence of neuropsychiatric syndromes in pediatric onset systemic lupus erythematosus. J Rheumatol 2002;29(7):1536–42.

13. Brey RL, Petri MA. Neuropsychiatric systemic lupus erythematosus: miles to go before we sleep. Neurology 2003;61(1):9–10.

14. Bleiberg J, Kane RL, Reeves DL, et al. Factor analysis of computerized and traditional tests used in mild brain injury research. Clin Neuropsychol 2000;14(3): 287–94.

15. Menon S, Jameson-Shortall E, Newman SP, et al. A longitudinal study of anticardiolipin antibody levels and cognitive functioning in systemic lupus erythematosus. Arthritis Rheum 1999;42(4):735–41.

16. McLaurin EY, Holliday SL, Williams P, et al. Predictors of cognitive dysfunction in patients with systemic lupus erythematosus. Neurology 2005;64(2):297–303.

17. Hanly JG, Hong C, Smith S, et al. A prospective analysis of cognitive function and anticardiolipin antibodies in systemic lupus erythematosus. Arthritis Rheum 1999;42(4):728–34.

18. Hanly JG, Urowitz MB, Siannis F, et al. Autoantibodies and neuropsychiatric events at the time of systemic lupus erythematosus diagnosis: results from an international inception cohort study. Arthritis Rheum 2008;58(3):843–53.

19. Trysberg E, Nylen K, Rosengren LE, et al. Neuronal and astrocytic damage in systemic lupus erythematosus patients with central nervous system involvement. Arthritis Rheum 2003;48(10):2881–7.

20. Waterloo K, Omdal R, Sjoholm H, et al. Neuropsychological dysfunction in systemic lupus erythematosus is not associated with changes in cerebral blood flow. J Neurol 2001;248(7):595–602.

21. Jarek MJ, West SG, Baker MR, et al. Magnetic resonance imaging in systemic lupus erythematosus patients without a history of neuropsychiatric lupus erythematosus. Arthritis Rheum 1994;37(11):1609–13.

22. Kao CH, Lan JL, ChangLai SP, et al. The role of FDG-PET, HMPAO-SPET and MRI in the detection of brain involvement in patients with systemic lupus erythematosus. Eur J Nucl Med 1999;26(2):129–34.

23. Lim MK, Suh CH, Kim HJ, et al. Systemic lupus erythematosus: brain MR imaging and single-voxel hydrogen 1 MR spectroscopy. Radiology 2000;217(1):43–9.

24. Kaell AT, Shetty M, Lee BC, et al. The diversity of neurologic events in systemic lupus erythematosus. Prospective clinical and computed tomographic classification of 82 events in 71 patients. Arch Neurol 1986;43(3):273–6.

25. Axford JS, Howe FA, Heron C, et al. Sensitivity of quantitative (1)H magnetic resonance spectroscopy of the brain in detecting early neuronal damage in systemic lupus erythematosus. Ann Rheum Dis 2001;60(2):106–11.

26. Kozora E, Arciniegas DB, Filley CM, et al. Cognition, MRS neurometabolites, and MRI volumetrics in non-neuropsychiatric systemic lupus erythematosus: preliminary data. Cogn Behav Neurol 2005;18(3):159–62.

27. Lapteva L, Nowak M, Yarboro CH, et al. Anti-*N*-methyl-D-aspartate receptor antibodies, cognitive dysfunction, and depression in systemic lupus erythematosus. Arthritis Rheum 2006;54(8):2505–14.

28. DiFrancesco MW, Holland SK, Ris MD, et al. Functional magnetic resonance imaging assessment of cognitive function in childhood-onset systemic lupus erythematosus: a pilot study. Arthritis Rheum 2007;56(12):4151–63.

29. Fitzgibbon BM, Fairhall SL, Kirk IJ, et al. Functional MRI in NPSLE patients reveals increased parietal and frontal brain activation during a working memory task compared with controls. Rheumatology (Oxford) 2008;47(1):50–3.

30. Fragoso-Loyo HE, Sanchez-Guerrero J. Effect of severe neuropsychiatric manifestations on short-term damage in systemic lupus erythematosus. J Rheumatol 2007;34(1):76–80.

31. Katsumata Y, Harigai M, Kawaguchi Y, et al. Diagnostic reliability of cerebral spinal fluid tests for acute confusional state (delirium) in patients with systemic lupus erythematosus: interleukin 6 (IL-6), IL-8, interferon-alpha, IgG index, and Q-albumin. J Rheumatol 2007;34(10):2010–7.

32. Hirohata S, Kanai Y, Mitsuo A, et al. Accuracy of cerebrospinal fluid IL-6 testing for diagnosis of lupus psychosis. A multicenter retrospective study. Clin Rheumatol 2009;28(11):1319–23.

33. George-Chandy A, Trysberg E, Eriksson K. Raised intrathecal levels of APRIL and BAFF in patients with systemic lupus erythematosus: relationship to neuropsychiatric symptoms. Arthritis Res Ther 2008;10(4):R97.

34. Santer DM, Yoshio T, Minota S, et al. Potent induction of IFN-alpha and chemokines by autoantibodies in the cerebrospinal fluid of patients with neuropsychiatric lupus. J Immunol 2009;182(2):1192–201.

35. Fragoso-Loyo H, Richaud-Patin Y, Orozco-Narvaez A, et al. Interleukin-6 and chemokines in the neuropsychiatric manifestations of systemic lupus erythematosus. Arthritis Rheum 2007;56(4):1242–50.

36. Trysberg E, Blennow K, Zachrisson O, et al. Intrathecal levels of matrix metalloproteinases in systemic lupus erythematosus with central nervous system engagement. Arthritis Res Ther 2004;6(6):R551–6.

37. Bonfa E, Golombek SJ, Kaufman LD, et al. Association between lupus psychosis and anti-ribosomal P protein antibodies. N Engl J Med 1987; 317(5):265–71.

38. Schneebaum AB, Singleton JD, West SG, et al. Association of psychiatric manifestations with antibodies to ribosomal P proteins in systemic lupus erythematosus. Am J Med 1991;90(1):54–62.

39. Karassa FB, Afeltra A, Ambrozic A, et al. Accuracy of anti-ribosomal P protein antibody testing for the diagnosis of neuropsychiatric systemic lupus erythematosus: an international meta-analysis. Arthritis Rheum 2006;54(1):312–24.

40. Isshi K, Hirohata S. Association of anti-ribosomal P protein antibodies with neuropsychiatric systemic lupus erythematosus. Arthritis Rheum 1996;39(9): 1483–90.

41. Matus S, Burgos PV, Bravo-Zehnder M, et al. Antiribosomal-P autoantibodies from psychiatric lupus target a novel neuronal surface protein causing calcium influx and apoptosis. J Exp Med 2007;204(13):3221–34.

42. Paul E, Manheimer-Lory A, Livneh A, et al. Pathogenic anti-DNA antibodies in SLE: idiotypic families and genetic origins. Int Rev Immunol 1990;5(3–4): 295–313.

43. Gaynor B, Putterman C, Valadon P, et al. Peptide inhibition of glomerular deposition of an anti-DNA antibody. Proc Natl Acad Sci U S A 1997;94(5):1955–60.

44. DeGiorgio LA, Konstantinov KN, Lee SC, et al. A subset of lupus anti-DNA antibodies cross-reacts with the NR2 glutamate receptor in systemic lupus erythematosus. Nat Med 2001;7(11):1189–93.

45. Olney JW, Ho OL. Brain damage in infant mice following oral intake of glutamate, aspartate or cysteine. Nature 1970;227(5258):609–11.

46. Chen HS, Lipton SA. The chemical biology of clinically tolerated NMDA receptor antagonists. J Neurochem 2006;97(6):1611–26.

47. Kutsuwada T, Kashiwabuchi N, Mori H, et al. Molecular diversity of the NMDA receptor channel. Nature 1992;358(6381):36–41.

48. Collingridge GL, Kehl SJ, McLennan H. Excitatory amino acids in synaptic transmission in the Schaffer collateral-commissural pathway of the rat hippocampus. J Physiol 1983;334:33–46.

49. Huntley GW, Vickers JC, Morrison JH. Cellular and synaptic localization of NMDA and non-NMDA receptor subunits in neocortex: organizational features related to cortical circuitry, function and disease. Trends Neurosci 1994;17(12):536–43.

50. Ozawa S, Kamiya H, Tsuzuki K. Glutamate receptors in the mammalian central nervous system. Prog Neurobiol 1998;54(5):581–618.

51. Coan EJ, Collingridge GL. Magnesium ions block an N-methyl-D-aspartate receptor-mediated component of synaptic transmission in rat hippocampus. Neurosci Lett 1985;53(1):21–6.

52. Choi DW, Rothman SM. The role of glutamate neurotoxicity in hypoxic-ischemic neuronal death. Annu Rev Neurosci 1990;13:171–82.

53. Laube B, Hirai H, Sturgess M, et al. Molecular determinants of agonist discrimination by NMDA receptor subunits: analysis of the glutamate binding site on the NR2B subunit. Neuron 1997;18(3):493–503.

54. Lipton SA, Rosenberg PA. Excitatory amino acids as a final common pathway for neurologic disorders. N Engl J Med 1994;330(9):613–22.

55. Erdo SL, Schafer M. Memantine is highly potent in protecting cortical cultures against excitotoxic cell death evoked by glutamate and N-methyl-D-aspartate. Eur J Pharmacol 1991;198(2–3):215–7.

56. Ellison G. The N-methyl-D-aspartate antagonists phencyclidine, ketamine and dizocilpine as both behavioral and anatomical models of the dementias. Brain Res Brain Res Rev 1995;20(2):250–67.

57. Gaspar PA, Bustamante ML, Silva H, et al. Molecular mechanisms underlying glutamatergic dysfunction in schizophrenia: therapeutic implications. J Neurochem 2009;111(4):891–900.

58. Kowal C, DeGiorgio LA, Nakaoka T, et al. Cognition and immunity; antibody impairs memory. Immunity 2004;21(2):179–88.

59. Huerta PT, Kowal C, DeGiorgio LA, et al. Immunity and behavior: antibodies alter emotion. Proc Natl Acad Sci U S A 2006;103(3):678–83.

60. Sharma A, Isenberg D, Diamond B. Studies of human polyclonal and monoclonal antibodies binding to lupus autoantigens and cross-reactive antigens. Rheumatology (Oxford) 2003;42(3):453–63.

61. Omdal R, Brokstad K, Waterloo K, et al. Neuropsychiatric disturbances in SLE are associated with antibodies against NMDA receptors. Eur J Neurol 2005;12(5): 392–8.

62. Emmer BJ, van der Grond J, Steup-Beekman GM, et al. Selective involvement of the amygdala in systemic lupus erythematosus. PLoS Med 2006;3(12):e499.

63. Hanly JG, Robichaud J, Fisk JD. Anti-NR2 glutamate receptor antibodies and cognitive function in systemic lupus erythematosus. J Rheumatol 2006;33(8): 1553–8.

64. Harrison MJ, Ravdin LD, Lockshin MD. Relationship between serum NR2a antibodies and cognitive dysfunction in systemic lupus erythematosus. Arthritis Rheum 2006;54(8):2515–22.

65. Steup-Beekman G, Steens S, van Buchem M, et al. Anti-NMDA receptor autoantibodies in patients with systemic lupus erythematosus and their first-degree relatives. Lupus 2007;16(5):329–34.

66. Arinuma Y, Yanagida T, Hirohata S. Association of cerebrospinal fluid anti-NR2 glutamate receptor antibodies with diffuse neuropsychiatric systemic lupus erythematosus. Arthritis Rheum 2008;58(4):1130–5.

67. Yoshio T, Onda K, Nara H, et al. Association of IgG anti-NR2 glutamate receptor antibodies in cerebrospinal fluid with neuropsychiatric systemic lupus erythematosus. Arthritis Rheum 2006;54(2):675–8.

68. Fragoso-Loyo H, Cabiedes J, Orozco-Narvaez A, et al. Serum and cerebrospinal fluid autoantibodies in patients with neuropsychiatric lupus erythematosus. Implications for diagnosis and pathogenesis. PLoS One 2008;3(10):e3347.

69. Kowal C, Degiorgio LA, Lee JY, et al. Human lupus autoantibodies against NMDA receptors mediate cognitive impairment. Proc Natl Acad Sci U S A 2006;103(52): 19854–9.

70. McAllister DL, Kaplan BJ, Edworthy SM, et al. The influence of systemic lupus erythematosus on fetal development: cognitive, behavioral, and health trends. J Int Neuropsychol Soc 1997;3(4):370–6.

71. Ross G, Sammaritano L, Nass R, et al. Effects of mothers' autoimmune disease during pregnancy on learning disabilities and hand preference in their children. Arch Pediatr Adolesc Med 2003;157(4):397–402.

72. Neri F, Chimini L, Bonomi F, et al. Neuropsychological development of children born to patients with systemic lupus erythematosus. Lupus 2004;13(10): 805–11.

73. Tincani A, Nuzzo M, Motta M, et al. Autoimmunity and pregnancy: autoantibodies and pregnancy in rheumatic diseases. Ann N Y Acad Sci 2006;1069:346–52.

74. Lahita RG. Systemic lupus erythematosus: learning disability in the male offspring of female patients and relationship to laterality. Psychoneuroendocrinology 1988; 13(5):385–96.

75. Lee JY, Huerta PT, Zhang J, et al. Neurotoxic autoantibodies mediate congenital cortical impairment of offspring in maternal lupus. Nat Med 2009;15(1):91–6.

76. Dalmau J, Tuzun E, Wu HY, et al. Paraneoplastic anti-N-methyl-D-aspartate receptor encephalitis associated with ovarian teratoma. Ann Neurol 2007;61(1): 25–36.

77. Dalmau J, Gleichman AJ, Hughes EG, et al. Anti-NMDA-receptor encephalitis: case series and analysis of the effects of antibodies. Lancet Neurol 2008;7(12): 1091–8.

78. Niehusmann P, Dalmau J, Rudlowski C, et al. Diagnostic value of *N*-methyl-D-aspartate receptor antibodies in women with new-onset epilepsy. Arch Neurol 2009;66(4):458–64.
79. Ganor Y, Goldberg-Stern H, Lerman-Sagie T, et al. Autoimmune epilepsy: distinct subpopulations of epilepsy patients harbor serum autoantibodies to either glutamate/AMPA receptor GluR3, glutamate/NMDA receptor subunit NR2A or double-stranded DNA. Epilepsy Res 2005;65(1–2):11–22.

Index

Note: Page numbers of article titles are in **boldface** type.

A

Actinin antibodies, in lupus nephritis, 136
Adhesion molecules, in lupus nephritis, 137, 151, 153
Adiponectin
    in lupus nephritis, 137
    in metabolic syndrome, 87
    pathogenic effects of, 149–154
Adrenomedullin, in lupus nephritis, 136
Alopecia, 37–38
Amenorrhea, 64, 100
Anemia, 62–63
Antibody(ies). *See also specific antibodies.*
    as biomarkers, 133
    in cutaneous lupus, 38–39
    in lupus nephritis, 133, 136
    in pediatric SLE, 60, 63–65
Anticardiolipin antibodies, in pediatric SLE, 63
Antigen presentation, B cells in, 113–114
Antimalarials, for pediatric SLE, 66–67
Antinuclear antibodies
    appearance of, 110
    in pediatric SLE, 64–65
Antiphospholipid antibody syndrome, 63–64
Apoptosis defects, loss of B-cell tolerance in, 110–111
Ascites, 62
Aspreva Lupus Management trial, 105
Atacicept, 123
Atherosclerosis, 64, **145–160**
Autoimmunity and Rituximab French registry, 118
Azathioprine
    as cyclophosphamide alternative, 105
    for pediatric SLE, 67

B

B cells, in SLE
    abnormal, 111, 113
    autoantibody-independent functions of, 114–115
    in autoimmunity initiation and propagation, 113–114
    in innate/adaptive immunity interface, 115–116
    loss of tolerance of, 110–112
    therapies targeting, 116–123

Rheum Dis Clin N Am 36 (2010) 203–212
doi:10.1016/S0889-857X(10)00009-8
0889-857X/10/$ – see front matter © 2010 Elsevier Inc. All rights reserved.

Moving?

Make sure your subscription moves with you!

To notify us of your new address, find your **Clinics Account Number** (located on your mailing label above your name), and contact customer service at:

Email: journalscustomerservice-usa@elsevier.com

800-654-2452 (subscribers in the U.S. & Canada)
314-447-8871 (subscribers outside of the U.S. & Canada)

Fax number: 314-447-8029

Elsevier Health Sciences Division
Subscription Customer Service
3251 Riverport Lane
Maryland Heights, MO 63043

*To ensure uninterrupted delivery of your subscription, please notify us at least 4 weeks in advance of move.

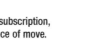

Printed and bound by CPI Group (UK) Ltd, Croydon, CR0 4YY

03/10/2024

01040452-0004